# Health Informatics

*(formerly Computers in Health Care)*

Kathryn J. Hannah    Marion J. Ball
Series Editors

# Health Informatics Series
*(formerly Computers in Health Care)*

*Series Editors*
Kathryn J. Hannah  Marion J. Ball

*(continued after index)*

Daniel F. Cowan
Editor

# Informatics for the Clinical Laboratory
## *A Practical Guide for the Pathologist*

With 42 Illustrations

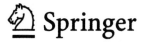
Springer

Daniel F. Cowan, M.D., C.M.
Professor of Pathology
and
Director, Laboratory Information Services
Department of Pathology
The University of Texas Medical Branch at Galveston
Galveston, TX 77555, USA

Series Editors:

Kathryn J. Hannah, Ph.D., R.N.
Adjunct Professor, Department
of Community Health Sciences
Faculty of Medicine
The University of Calgary
Calgary, Alberta, T2N 4N1, Canada

Marion J. Ball, Ed.D.
Vice President, Clinical Informatics Strategies
Healthlink, Inc.
Baltimore, MD, 21210, USA
and
Adjunct Professor
Johns Hopkins University School
of Nursing
Baltimore, MD 21205, USA

Library of Congress Cataloging-in-Publication Data
A catalog record for this book is available from the Library of Congress

ISBN 0-387-24449-2          Printed on acid-free paper.

Printed in the United States of America.

9 8 7 6 5 4 3 2 1

springeronline.com

# Series Preface

This series is directed to healthcare professionals who are leading the transformation of health care by using information and knowledge. Launched in 1988 as Computers in Health Care, the series offers a broad range of titles: some addressed to specific professions such as nursing, medicine, and health administration; others to special areas of practice such as trauma and radiology. Still other books in the series focus on interdisciplinary issues, such as the computer-based patient record, electronic health records, and networked healthcare systems.

Renamed Health Informatics in 1998 to reflect the rapid evolution in the discipline now known as health informatics, the series will continue to add titles that contribute to the evolution of the field. In the series, eminent experts, serving as editors or authors, offer their accounts of innovations in health informatics. Increasingly, these accounts go beyond hardware and software to address the role of information in influencing the transformation of healthcare delivery systems around the world. The series also increasingly focuses on "peopleware" and the organizational, behavioral, and societal changes that accompany the diffusion of information technology in health services environments.

These changes will shape health services in this new millennium. By making full and creative use of the technology to tame data and to transform information, health informatics will foster the development of the knowledge age in health care. As coeditors, we pledge to support our professional colleagues and the series readers as they share advances in the emerging and exciting field of health informatics.

*Kathryn J. Hannah*
*Marion J. Ball*

# Preface

This book developed out of a course in laboratory informatics for residents in training in pathology and for fellows in the clinical laboratory sciences given over a period of years. The topics covered and the approach taken were strongly influenced by real-life experience. Pathology residents and clinical laboratory scientists, like the general population, vary greatly in familiarity with information issues in the laboratory and the computer system and infrastructure that supports an information system. Some know essentially nothing at all, while others have considerable expertise in some aspect, such as microcomputer functions or even computer engineering. For all, the idea of the clinical diagnostic laboratories as primarily an information center is a new idea, and for many it is a not entirely comfortable idea.

Our objective in the instructional program and in this book is to level the knowledge of all concerned without boring those who might already have considerable knowledge. It is not possible to bring everyone to the level of expert in all areas. Our object here is literacy and familiarity with the major issues and tools, not expertise. It should be evident that for us the clinical laboratory includes both anatomic and clinical pathology as those areas are usually defined. We expect to substantially exceed the informatics requirements of the American Board of Pathology for general certification in anatomic and clinical pathology.

The contributors are all members of the faculty and staff of the Department of Pathology of the University of Texas Medical Branch, and all have years of experience in the areas in which they write. They are all workers in the fields and the vineyard, and none is a technician. The editor is a working surgical pathologist as well as Director of Laboratory Information Services.

The book is organized into three sections, the first group of chapters dealing with the concept, organization, and management of laboratory information services; the second with technical aspects of computer systems; and the third with applications. Each chapter more or less stands alone, so they do not have to be read in any particular order, although the complete computer novice, if any exist in this computer age, might do well to begin with Chapter 6. Each chapter is accompanied by a glossary and all chapter glossaries are compiled into a comprehensive glossary at the end of the book.

Throughout the book references are made to particular products supplied by various commercial vendors. This is not to be taken as an endorsement of those products or vendors, and most especially, failure to mention a product or vendor is not to be taken as a judgment. Citations of products or vendors are made to keep discussions from being hopelessly abstract and to suggest to beginners where they may start in evaluating and selecting products. The life expectancy of vendor companies and the rapid turnover of versions of products, often measured in months rather than years, are such that no recommendations or criticisms are offered or implied. We have used most or all of the applications software products mentioned.

It is difficult to know just who should be accorded thanks for the development of a book such as this, and the program that it represents. Many contribute to the development of knowledge, and often their contribution is not noticed at the time. I suspect we learn less from our friends than we do from our critics, of whom there are many and faithful ones. We would like to acknowledge the assistance of B.A. Rampy, D.O., Ph.D., for great help in the preparation of illustrations.

Finally, I would like to remember our friend and colleague, Dr. Gbo Yuoh, a fine teacher-pathologist and a gentle soul whose untimely death cut short a promising career.

*Daniel F. Cowan*

# Contents

# Contributors

*Beverly C. Campbell, B.S.*
Manager, Laboratory Information Services, Department of Pathology, The University of Texas Medical Branch at Galveston, Galveston, TX 77555, USA

*Gerald A. Campbell, M.D., Ph.D.*
Professor of Pathology, Department of Pathology, The University of Texas Medical Branch at Galveston, Galveston, TX 77555, USA

*Daniel F. Cowan, M.D., C.M.*
Professor of Pathology and Director, Laboratory Information Services, Department of Pathology, The University of Texas Medical Branch at Galveston, Galveston, TX 77555, USA

*R. Zane Gray, B.S.*
Automated Systems Manager, Department of Pathology, The University of Texas Medical Branch at Galveston, Galveston, TX 77555, USA

*Amin A. Mohammad, Ph.D.*
Assistant Professor and Associate Director, Division of Clinical Chemistry and Associate Director, Laboratory Information Services, Department of Pathology, The University of Texas Medical Branch at Galveston, Galveston, TX 77555, USA

*Anthony O. Okorodudu, Ph.D., M.B.A.*
Associate Professor and Director, Division of Clinical Chemistry, Department of Pathology, The University of Texas Medical Branch at Galveston, Galveston, TX 77555, USA

*John R. Petersen, Ph.D.*
Associate Professor and Associate Director, Division of Clinical Chemistry, Department of Pathology, The University of Texas Medical Branch at Galveston, Galveston, TX 77555, USA

*Sue Schneider, B.S.*
Database Manager, Laboratory Information Services, Department of Pathology, The University of Texas Medical Branch at Glaveston, Galveston, TX 77555, USA

*Michael B. Smith, M.D.*
Assistant Professor and Director, Division of Clinical Microbiology, and Associate Director, Laboratory Information Services, Department of Pathology, The University of Texas Medical Branch at Galveston, Galveston, TX 77555, USA

*Gbo Yuoh, M.D. (deceased)*
Assistant Professor, Department of Pathology, The University of Texas Medical Branch at Galveston, Galveston, TX  77555, USA

# 1
# Laboratory Informatics and the Laboratory Information System

DANIEL F. COWAN

The primary objective of clinical laboratorians is to provide the highest possible quality of service to patients and those who care for patients. High-quality service encompasses accurate and precise analysis, timely, clear, and concise reporting, and delivery of the service to a location in a format most valuable to the user of the service. Quality has also come to include elements of efficiency, effectiveness, analysis of diagnostic utility, and decision support.[1,2] Delivery of the service has come to mean that integration into a comprehensive electronic medical record (EMR) is to be expected.[3,4] Although it is widely accepted that about 70% of the information used in the management of patients comes from the clinical and anatomical pathology laboratories,[5] in one large medical center in which information flow is tracked, about 94% of requests to the EMR are for laboratory results.[4] In addition, a critical quality feature is the transformation of laboratory data into information.[2,5,6–8]

Drives for improved quality, integration, and efficiency have resulted in the incorporation of information technology and the personnel, policy, and procedural changes needed to exploit the technology into the clinical service laboratory.[9–11] This applies equally well to anatomic and clinical pathology. It seems clear enough that the managers of laboratory operations must understand information, the purpose of information, and the proper management of information in order to survive and prosper in an environment that demands an orientation to service and a full appreciation for the inter-relationship between processes and events. This is especially so when more information is being produced than can be assimilated, far beyond the limitations of memory-based learning, and the future is uncertain. The ability to respond and adapt to change requires recognition of changes in an early stage and understanding of the changes in qualitative and quantitative terms. This means that decision makers must have full and ready access to high-quality, accurate information.

The flow and management of information is made possible by the technology of computers and other information devices. Although the technology is fascinating, the important issues for the laboratorian are the purpose and management of information. The laboratorian must understand that the laboratory is a knowledge- and service-based enterprise. Information management is an essential task of leadership, and like other aspects of management, if it is not done well in the laboratory, either it will be taken away by a higher level of administration or by an institutional information services organization or it will be outsourced.

The pathology laboratory must be run as a business, and usually it is a component of a larger business: a hospital, medical center, or some other enterprise.[12] This perception should not be much of a surprise, but for the laboratorian whose orientation is technical, academic, or altruistic, it requires a drastic reorientation of thinking. Laboratory leadership is responsible not only for technical and scientific matters but also for the jobs of people employed by the laboratory. Skill in business matters may be the critical factor in the viability of the laboratory and hence in the livelihood of those who work in it. Business tends to be a very competitive affair. Some businesses succeed and some fail. The struggle of business is and will always be a struggle for advantage. Those who build and sustain competitive advantage will win; those who do not will lose. Competition is all about advantage.[13] Advantages over business competitors seldom are quantum jumps. They are much more likely to be the accumulation of small incremental gains realized over time resulting from careful management. Every human enterprise, even if not competitive in a direct way, must be run in a businesslike fashion; otherwise its resources, always limited, will not be used in a way that enhances the purposes of the organization. This principle applies as much to churches as to commercial establishments.

The purpose of information technology, or as it is sometimes called, information movement and management, is competitiveness. It allows an organization to build and sustain a competitive advantage. All other activities, such as increasing efficiency, developing a better product, and decision support, are contributors to that objective, not the objective itself.[13] After all, if the business fails, the laboratory closes or is sold and whatever high-minded or altruistic motives that might have driven it cannot be realized. The successful leader balances his or her attention between the present and the future; understands that today's success is temporary; while enjoying today's success is preparing for tomorrow's greater success; and cultivates the ability to see the world as it is, not as it ought to be.

The effective use of information services in any enterprise requires an understanding of the environment, structure, function, and politics of the organization, as well as the role of management and management decision making in it. Six types of information systems or subsystems are used in various organizational levels.

**Executive support systems (ESSs)** are used at the strategic decision level of an organization; they are designed to address unstructured decision making using advanced graphics and communication representing vast amounts of structured and processed information.

**Management information systems (MISs)** provide current and historical performance data to middle managers who use it in planning, controlling, and decision making.

**Decision support systems (DSSs)** are similar to MISs but tend to be more analytical; they deal with semistructured problems using data from both internal and external sources.

**Knowledge work systems (KWSs)** are used by knowledge workers (scientists, engineers, and so on) to help create and distribute new knowledge.

**Office automation systems (OASs)** are used to increase the productivity of data workers (secretaries, bookkeepers, and so on) but may also be used by knowledge workers.

**Transaction processing systems (TPSs)** are basic business systems used at the operations level of an organization to keep track of daily transactions in the course of business. TPS might include databases and spread sheets.

# Business of Pathology

Because it primarily involves the acquisition, creation, evaluation, and dissemination of information, the practice of pathology can be characterized as a complex information system designed to produce useful information for individual or groups of patients. An information system can be formally defined as interrelated components working together to collect, process, store, and disseminate information to support decision making, coordination, control analysis, and visualization within an organization.[14] This information function of the service department complements pathology's traditional role as a method for systematic study of disease as seen in a patient, living or dead. In addition to its basis in laboratory testing, pathology also includes collection, processing, and dispensing of blood and blood products and consultation in their appropriate use. Each step in these processes requires the accumulation, organization, validation, storage, and transmission of information. Therefore, it is apparent that the laboratorian is continually involved in information processing and communication tasks. Indeed, as actual analytical processes are done more and more by automated machines, the laboratorian is becoming *primarily* an information manager.[10] The choice is not whether to be an information manager; it is to be a competent or an incompetent one.

# *Information Product of the Laboratory*

The **business product** of the laboratory, aside from the exception of blood and blood products, is information.[2,9,15–17] As with any business enterprise, the product offered by the laboratory, information, must be delivered to the user in a timely manner, in a comprehensible precise form and format, and at a location satisfactory to the user. One hopes to make a profit by so doing, or if in a capitated or other cost-limiting system, do it in the way that uses the smallest possible amount of money.

As a practical matter, information generated in the laboratory can be classified as **product information**, information intended to be used outside the laboratory, such as patient results, and **process information**, information produced in the course of receiving, processing, and testing specimens, organizing of reports, and all the financial, scheduling and other operational matters necessary to run the laboratory. Thus, in the generation of information, the laboratory has both product goals and process goals. The product goals of the laboratory are service related, including promptness, clarity in communication, accuracy, and error reduction. The process goals of the laboratory are efficiency in the use of resources and documentation for management and for accreditation. The overall goal of laboratory information management is to obtain, create, manage, and use information to improve patient services and individual and laboratory performance in contributing to patient care, business management, and support processes.

## Pathologist as Information Manager

This approach to the specialty is novel for many pathologists, who may see themselves first as histologic diagnosticians, clinical consultants, or overseers of analytic processes, and many of whom have had no training or orientation in information management. Certainly the pathologist does all those things, but in so doing is primarily giving or receiving information. In one sense the business of the laboratory is constant and unchanging over the years. It consists of the timely delivery of reliable results, the responsive support of clinicians, effective cost management, and proper billing.[17] While the essence of the business may be relatively unchanging, the organizing concepts, ethics, tools, and financial basis of the laboratory's operations are not. In recent years the practice of pathology has been transformed under the pressures of technological innovation and changes in financing, and it is evolving in directions that cannot be easily foreseen. The rate of change is so great that it seems inevitable that the practice of pathology and laboratory medicine will become qualitatively different from what it is and has been. Automation and miniaturization of testing processes have turned the clinical laboratory into something like a light industrial mass production line. The use of robotics in laboratory operations, once a fanciful notion, is becoming more and more an integral component of work flow. Many clinical laboratories have expanded and taken on new sources of business, while others have participated in mergers with other laboratories to form large testing organizations. With increased size has come a disproportionate increase in operational complexity. Computerization has allowed the aggregation and manipulation of masses of data and speeded up and changed modes of communication. The combination of complexity and computerization tended to promote centralization of laboratories in the past, but it is now supporting distributed or on-site testing equally well, in a way not possible only a few years ago.[18]

Changes in financing have transformed the clinical laboratories from hospital profit centers to cost centers, on a par with housekeeping. Whatever weight the laboratory had in the past, now it is an expense to be trimmed and minimized. Quality care, as an abstract ideal, may be important to doctors, but to administrators with budgets to balance, payrolls to meet, and profit objectives to fulfill, the bottom line carries the day. Withdrawal of money from the laboratory and intense scrutiny of budgets adds almost intolerable pressures for efficiency. A well-run laboratory is supposed to do more with less. With the evolution from a craftlike cottage industry to an industrial mode of production has come an industrial approach to management. Greater attention to the articulation of the laboratory as part of a "healthcare system" is required. Each of these transformations in technology and finance have brought other changes. The director of the laboratory is responsible not only to the medical staff for the quality of the data provided by the laboratory but also to the hospital administration for the management of scarce resources, to third-party payers for charges, and finally to inspectors and accreditors, who increasingly talk about quality and appropriateness of services. Successful performance of all these tasks requires all laboratory leaders to have a good understanding of information processes and the tools that support them; in essence, it requires them to become information managers.[7] This does not mean that they must become computer gurus any more than they must be able to repair their own chemistry analyzers. Highly technical problems are better handled by highly trained technicians, for whom it is not necessary to develop a broader world view. The leaders of the laboratory, as information managers, must be prepared to anticipate and answer certain questions. What changes in health care will affect the laboratory? What technology investments will be needed to meet demands imposed by clinical changes? What advances in information technology will be important to the laboratory? How is the introduction of new technology best managed?[17]

## Information Management in the Laboratory Organization

Organizations tend to have an individual who functions to some degree as the chief information officer (CIO). Where that individual fits in a formal table of organization reflects the importance that top management places on information movement and management. In many successful corporations, the CIO is a senior vice president, reporting directly to the president or chief executive officer (CEO). The CIO manages the information enterprise, decides on which information processes and devices will be used, and sets information policies and procedures. More important, the CIO provides information about the organization's business directly to the top decision makers, unfiltered and uncolored by the biases and interests of intervening layers of the organization. After all, the information provided may include things that suggest changes in the organization that could cost someone position or prestige. In this kind of organization, the CIO and the information process are staff functions serving the organization through the topmost executive. The CIO leads the ultimate executive support system in the organization, assuring its optimal functioning in part by preventing unpopular information from being stifled at a lower level either because it includes threatening performance data or simply because of resistance to change. In some organizations, probably for historical reasons, the information function is left to the finance department, usually not a good idea because of the narrow focus that often characterizes financial officers. Indeed, such an arrangement expresses the idea, whether realized or not, that information services are to be treated as a cost center to be minimized rather than a critically important strategic asset to be maximally exploited. A strange notion to be sure, considering the millions or tens of millions of dollars spent to develop and run an information system.

Most laboratories are small organizations and neither need nor can afford a complex dedicated information structure. In laboratories with a supporting business staff, the effective CIO might be the laboratory business manager. This can be very functional, since the leader of the organization is likely to be a pathologist with a broad view, who can interpret the information provided by the laboratory manager and appreciate its implications. In a large group practice, one of the pathologists or a clinical laboratory scientist may take on the role of CIO as a major responsibility.

In some large pathology departments, the information flow and management function has been given division status, and it has been proposed that laboratory informatics be made into a separately recognized subspecialty within a department of pathology.[19,20] The benefits from such an arrangement are said to be enhanced productivity and efficiency in the development of alignment and impact applications, better management of the information product of pathology and the informaticians themselves; increased political power and influence for pathology; and increased awareness and sophistication on the part of department leaders about information processing.[19] Division status might be appropriate in large medical centers, perhaps university medical center pathology departments, in which such an organization might be associated with an informatics training program and research. In our view, laboratory informatics should be a special section within a large department, but there seems to be little need for subspecialty certification, since a basic understanding of information flow and management should be part of the intellectual furniture of every pathologist, clinical laboratory scientist, senior technologist, and manager. Having a certified specialist in the department, in addition to adding a layer of bureaucracy, might be taken as relieving others of their need to understand the basic nature of pathology as an information science and behave accordingly.

## What Is Information?

Information is defined in different ways. In one sense, information is merely the summarization of **data**, which are raw facts and figures that are processed in such a way as to provide a higher order of meaning, such as summaries and totals. Since information prepared at one level may be used as data at a higher level, the terms data and information are sometimes used interchangeably. Not so here.

We can think of a hierarchy of data, information, knowledge, and wisdom or judgment. This can be illustrated in the following way. The comedian George Carlin has a routine in which he gives baseball scores: 3–2, 1–0, 7–5, 10–1. The humor consists in the presentation of numbers (data) out of a familiar and interpretable context, in all seriousness, and with impeccable timing. The numbers may be right, but they don't mean anything. We can add more data—the names of the teams—to give a little more meaning to the numbers. Now we have information. Information alone is not enough; we must know more to see how it fits. In our hierarchy, that might be the season records of the teams to date and the status of the players. Call this knowledge. Finally, using the accumulation of information from current scores, season records, and the state of the players, we may make a judgment about which teams are likely to make it to the World Series.

Another way to look at information is the way data are defined and used. Data may be numbers collected in discretely defined fields, words collected as text, numbers in an organized matrix or spreadsheet, frames of bits or vectors that define images (pictures), streams of sound interpretable as voice, or video, a sequence of frames.

## Information Technology in the Laboratory

The laboratory is both a light industry and an office workplace. It is no longer feasible to administer a busy laboratory without the aid of electronic data processing. Data are plentiful; useful information tends to be scarce. Data are not necessarily information. Information is developed by the accumulation of data in a structured, organized way. The task is to define the kind and amount of information that must be collected and analyzed, the use to which it will be put and by whom, then organize to do it. That is, the task is to develop a laboratory information system, much of which will be built around electronic data processors, or computers. An **information system** may be defined as interrelated components working together to collect, process, store, and disseminate information to support decision making, coordination, control analysis, and visualization in an organization.[14] It cannot be overemphasized that the information system transcends the computer, and indeed, one must be ready on occasion, using manual procedures, to do without computer support. The computer and its programs support the information system; they are not the system itself.

## Evolving Role of the Computer

In earlier days of computerization, the task uses to which the technology was applied were narrow and deep and focused in an area such as finance. The orientation was vertical; that is, concerned with a relatively small number of tasks and controlled by a relatively expert "power user" who was comfortable with the technology. It served administrative functions but provided little support for professional decision making. In contrast, modern computerization is aimed mainly toward horizontal integration and decision support. The medical user approaches computerization as an intrinsically different sort of activity than the task orientation of the traditional power user. The orientation toward solution of problems rather than performance of tasks demands that, unlike the traditional power user, the laboratory user must be able to use a broad array of functions. One of the most obvious and familiar transitions, apart from the use of computers to automate general office functions, has been in literature searching. At one time the province of a research librarian, routine searching has shifted to the user of the information, who can conduct an on-line, exploratory evolving search using one of several search tools.

## Cost, Quality, and Efficiency Considerations

New information technology is brought into an enterprise on the expectation that it will improve quality and efficiency and in the long run save money. It will **add value.** Quality may be easily defined as the degree of excellence of a product or service, efficiency as the effective use of resources to obtain an objective. Cost considerations are more complex and abstract. As new devices and procedures are brought into the operation, costs increase, not only by the price of the purchase of the technology, but also because the change required to assimilate it means a period of learning and inefficiency in a system that previously may have been running well at its lower level. Increased resource utilization in the laboratory may be justified internally in that at its new level of sophistication, productivity may increase at a rate faster than increase in costs. Efficiency may make a disproportionate gain. New work may be brought in or new services introduced, the value of which exceeds the incremental cost of doing it.

Information technology may also be justified because of its effect on efficiency of the enterprise as a whole, outside the laboratory. Shortened report turnaround time, faster communications, reduction in errors, and production of useful management information may help to reduce the total cost of care in the enterprise or help make it more competitive in the quest for new business. It will certainly help improve patient care. However, if decision makers do not recognize the beneficial effect on the enterprise as a whole and decline to bear the cost of new information technology, old but still desirable services may have to be eliminated or necessary new ones deferred, resulting in a decline in quality and efficiency of the enterprise as a whole, not just in the lagging laboratory.

Efficiency has several aspects. With well-developed information technology, test orders are transmitted with speed and accuracy, work lists are created, specimens are labeled, and tests are done quickly. Communication of results immediately after completion of each test, once too complicated and expensive, now is routine. Maintenance of a large and accessible archive, with rapid retrieval of stored information, once cumbersome and tedious, is similarly a routinely provided service. Workloads can be tracked and the most effective deployment of staff and use of instruments identified without tedious analysis of paper records. Studies of outcomes of therapeutic interventions become feasible and practical.[21]

## Study of Information

The study of information may be divided into three general approaches: information theory, informatics, and information management.

**Information theory** studies information from an engineering perspective, formulating issues mainly in mathematical terms, approaching the subject on the grounds of probability theory and coding theory. This approach is well represented in a number of engineering texts and forms no part of this discussion.

**Informatics** is simply defined as information science; the science of processing data for storage and retrieval. In the laboratory, informatics includes an understanding of the hardware and software that is used to produce and store information, as well as the use of information. "Informatics" is a relatively new word, not found in many modern dictionaries. The *Oxford Dictionary*[22] attributes its origin to the Russian *informatika*, or information, while Collen[23] sees its origin in the French *informatique*. Whichever is the case, the word gradually appeared in several disciplines during the 1970s, mainly in Europe. It has come to mean the study of how information can be collected, represented, stored, retrieved, processed, transformed, used, and applied to sets of problems. Informatics differs from information management mainly in that informatics includes close attention to the technology of information management.

**Medical informatics** has been defined more particularly as "the field that concerns itself with the cognitive, information processing, and communications tasks of medical practice, education, and research, including the information science and technology to support those tasks."[24] Medical information science is oriented toward problems in medical science and uses both methods and technology of computer science. The scope of medical informatics has been defined as consisting of five essential professional activities:[24]

1. Basic research, model building, theory development, exploratory experiments
2. Applied research, including more formal experiments and careful evaluation of effectiveness of approaches
3. Engineering, or tool building and development for specific user needs
4. Deployment, involving practical tasks of putting applications into operation and maintaining and updating them, as well as providing training and support for users

5. Planning and policy development with respect to the role of information technology in health care provision and medical education

   The full range of activities in medical informatics requires knowledge in clinical medicine and basic medical sciences, biostatistics, epidemiology, decision sciences, health economics and policy (including issues of hospital organization, finance and reimbursement), and medical ethics.[24]

   **Laboratory informatics** by this approach comprises the theoretical and practical aspects of information processing and communication, based on knowledge and experience derived from processes in the laboratory and employing the methods and technology of computer systems. In this application, informatics focuses mainly on deployment, planning, and policy development. In addition, utilization review, computer consultation, rules-based expert systems, and decision support are growing areas of attention. Laboratory informatics, reflecting the laboratory's status as a technology center, is more technology-oriented than general medical informatics.

   **Information management** is the organization and use of information. It overlaps considerably with informatics, as defined, but tends not to include the mechanics and technology of information processing. The Joint Commission on the Accreditation of Healthcare Organizations (JCAHO) has promulgated a series of definitions in information management, and since that organization has such a determining effect on medical practice in the United States, their definitions[25] are adopted in the discussions that follow. A JCAHO definition is indicated by an asterisk (*) following the word defined. **Data*** are uninterpreted material facts or clinical observations collected during an assessment activity. **Information*** is interpreted sets of data that can assist in decision making. A **function*** is a goal-directed, interrelated series of processes, such as patient assessment or patient care. **Knowledge-based information*** is a collection of stored facts, models, and information that can *be* used for designing and redesigning processes and for problem solving. It is used to support clinical and management decision making and includes current authoritative texts, journal articles, indices, abstracts, and research reports in print or electronic format. It also includes materials prepared for professional continuing education, performance improvement activities, and patient education.

# Laboratory Information Management

The laboratory typically is a component of a larger entity, such as a hospital or medical care system; if it is a free-standing entity, it offers laboratory information services to clients that may include hospitals, physician offices, clinics, patients, and companies that offer or require laboratory testing of their employees. In any case, clients and professional, federal, and state accrediting and regulatory agencies expect and require certain standards in the management of laboratory information.

Sound information management processes are essential to assure that internal and external information needs are met. Processes must be appropriate to the size and complexity of the services offered by the laboratory. The importance of information processes to the functioning of the laboratory requires that an appropriate share of available resources be devoted to the support of information services. Information management processes must meet minimal standards:

1. Responsiveness to laboratory, institutional and regulatory needs
2. Confidentiality, security, and integrity of records
3. Uniform data definitions and data capture methods
4. Definition, capturing, analyzing, transforming, transmitting, and reporting of patient-specific data and information

## *Responsiveness to Needs*

Laboratories vary in size, complexity, organizational structure, and decision-making processes and resources. Information management processes and systems vary according to a thorough analysis of internal and external information needs. An analysis considers what data and information are required to support the needs of the various activities of the laboratory, the medical staff, and the hospital administration, as well as satisfy outside clients and accrediting or regulatory agencies. Appropriate clinical and administrative staff participate in selecting, integrating and using information technology. Consultation with laboratory staff, medical and nursing staff, administration, and clients ensures that needed data and information are provided efficiently for patient care, management, education, and research. Processes should also provide information needed to justify resource allocation decisions.

## *Confidentiality, Security, and Integrity of Records*

The laboratory builds a record for every person for whom tests are done. The record contains enough information to identify the patient, including age, sex, race, and location, the person or persons requesting the test, and the "normal" or reference range permitting evaluation of the patient test result. The record accumulates results over time, allowing evaluation of changes in physiologic function, disease process, and etiology. **Data accuracy**\* (freedom from mistakes or error), **data reliability**\* (stable, repeatable, precise data), **data validity**\* (verification of correctness; reflection of the true situation) are all assured by appropriate means.

Appropriate levels of security and confidentiality for data and information must be assigned and controlled. **Confidentiality**\* is the restriction of access to data and information to individuals who have a need, a reason, and permission for access. Only authorized individuals are allowed to read or revise the record. Collection, storage, and retrieval systems are designed to allow timely and easy use of data and information without compromising security and confidentiality. Records and information are protected against loss, destruction, tampering, and unauthorized access or use.

Integral to the concept of security of data and information is protection from corruption or loss. Information may be corrupted or lost in a variety of ways, and a formal process must be incorporated into a data management program to prevent or mitigate it happening. **Risk analysis** is the systematic process for evaluating the vulnerability of a data processing system and the information it contains to hazards in its environment. Risk analysis is a necessary part of a risk management and data security program. It identifies the probable result (risk) associated with any given processing and storage environment, thereby allowing the formation of specific program elements that minimize or eliminate the effects of untoward events. Risk analysis provides management with the information needed to make informed judgements about security, system failure, or disaster recovery. Critical program objectives are protected by development of security policies and procedures that prevent loss, corruption, misuse, or unavailability of information. More specifically, the goal of risk analysis is to identify the policies, procedures, controls, and preparations needed to adequately respond to areas of vulnerability and disaster; reduce or eliminate the likelihood of an accident or deliberate act that would result in the loss of data integrity; and reduce or mitigate the effect on the institution of a catastrophic loss of function of the information system. **Risk assessment** requires careful inspection of application systems, data bases, and files to produce a reference base for the system custodians to assess the completeness and quality of the system's backup and recovery procedures. It also suggests the policies, procedures, and controls needed to assure efficient and effective risk management.

## Uniform Data Definitions and Data Capture Methods

**Minimum data sets**\* (collections of related data items), data definitions, codes, classifications, and terminology should be standardized as far as possible. Data must be collected efficiently—in a timely, economic manner, with the accuracy, completeness, and discrimination necessary for their intended use. Records are reviewed periodically for completeness, accuracy, and integrity. The review determines that active or archived patient records are accessible for use and have not been lost or otherwise misplaced, and that if stored electronically, they have not been altered or corrupted, either spontaneously or by some event such as a power surge or failure or a system crash. Those who have custody of records and those who use the data and information contained in them must be educated and trained in the principles of information management. Mechanisms for taking appropriate action to correct and improve the process must be in place. Policies for the length of time records are retained must be specified, based on needs in patient care, law and regulation, research, and education.

**Data transmission**\* is the sending of data or information from one location to another. It must be timely, accurate, and plainly understandable. The format and methods for disseminating data and information are standardized whenever possible and must relate rationally to external information distribution systems. Commonly, this means interfacing with hospital information systems.

## *Defining, Capturing, Analyzing, Transforming, Transmitting, and Reporting of Patient-Specific Data and Information*

**Data definition**\* is the identification of data to be used in analysis. **Data capture**\* is acquisition or recording of data or information. **Data transformation**\* is the process of changing the form of data representation, for example, changing data into information using decision-analysis tools.

To these specific standards are commonly added comparative performance data for quality management and evaluation of efficiency. For this purpose, comparative performance data and information are defined, collected, analyzed, transmitted, and reported. Although some of these measure changes in internal performance over time, the laboratory uses external reference data bases for comparative purposes. It may contribute to external reference data bases when required by law or regulation or to meet requirements for accreditation. In so doing, security and confidentiality of data and information are maintained. When electronic communications are used, they are consistent with national and state guidelines for data set parity and connectivity.

## Laboratory Information System

The term "laboratory information system" should not be confused with the aggregate of computer hardware and software that supports it. The system is a plan expressed in policies and procedures, and implemented in part on a computer. A laboratory information system may at a minimum be expected to lay out and organize work, accumulate data on specimens, report results, maintain a longitudinal patient record, keep audit trails, monitor quality control processes, keep track of workload and distribution, post bills, and keep department policies and procedures on line. Internal communications can be enhanced using electronic mail and bulletin board features. A laboratory system integrated into a larger hospital system may enhance communication with medical and other staff by providing an on-line laboratory guide and by providing patient results electronically. An advanced laboratory system may report results individually, cumulatively as tables of numbers, or graphically. It may allow complex, flexible searches of its database.

An information system is constructed along hierarchical lines, with three main components. The first is the **management system**, which sets the organization's goals and objectives, develops strategies and tactics, and plans, schedules, and controls the system. This is primarily a function of people, who may use machines to help accomplish these tasks. The second component is the **information**

**structure**, consisting of the database, which defines the data structures and to a certain extent defines the organization; procedures, which define data flow; and the application programs, including data entry, queries, updating, and reporting. The third component is the **computer system**, consisting of the central processing unit (CPU), which processes data; the peripheral devices, which store and retrieve data; the operating system, which manages the processes of the computer system; and the interfaces, which connect the system to analytical devices and to foreign computer systems. A more detailed description of the components of a computer system is presented in later chapters.

The hardware and basic programs and software tools used must reflect the needs and objectives of the laboratory and the system it serves. The plan they are intended to support must be coherent, meet the medical service and management objectives of the laboratory, and use the resources of the tangible system efficiently and effectively. These needs require firm central management control, with the authority to command cooperation, internal consistency, and comprehensiveness. Standards and practices are developed with full collegial participation, but their acceptance and implementation leave little room for personal idiosyncrasies that might perturb the smooth functioning of the agreed-on system. It is crucial that the laboratory staff not see the information system as a bureaucratic superimposition or merely another management tool but as supportive and helpful of their professional desires and ethical imperatives to do the best that can be done for patients. It implements a shared goal of improvement of services by organization and documentation of professional practices.

A well-structured system supports practice, but it also limits to some degree individualized approaches to tasks and problems. Even so, no individual or section of the laboratory may be permitted to opt out except for compelling reasons, such as lack of appropriate software support. This does not mean that all users must be on line. It means that the system is coherent and uniformly applicable. Some tests may be better done by a noninterfaced instrument and the data entered by hand. This is a calculated management decision, not an exemption from the information system.

At a minimum, computerization can be expected to standardize procedures, data collection forms, and terminology; simplify and expedite clerical work and eliminate a large amount of transcription error; refine reporting formats; and store, analyze and transform large amounts of data. Computerization alone will improve quality by providing an unchanging, planned structure; i.e., it will go far to "institutionalize good habits."[15] Computerization of a carefully thought-out information management plan will comply with all rational regulations as a matter of course.

## Database

Any business operates from a basic fund of information: its database. The database stores the subjects of a business (master files) and its activities (transaction files). The database is supported by applications programs, manual procedures, and machine procedures. **Applications programs** provide the data entry, updating, query, and report processing. The **manual procedures** describe how data is obtained for input and how the system's output is distributed. **Machine procedures** instruct the computer how to conduct processing activities, in which the output of one program is automatically fed into another program. Processing may be in "real time," that is, concurrent with or immediately after some event, or it may be deferred, with records of events processed together in batches ("batch mode"). Ordinary daily processing is interactive, real-time processing of events or transactions. At the end of the day or other specified period, batch processing programs update the master files that have not been updated since the last cycle. Routinely, reports are prepared for the cycle's activities. Periodic processing in a business information system includes the updating of the master files, which adds, deletes, and changes the information about customers, employees, vendors, and products.

The laboratory database consists of all transactions that take place in the laboratory, such as logging, verifying, reporting, and so on, each linked to an individual, a time, and a place (transaction logging to create an audit trail); a master test list with all reference ranges, critical values, and so on; cost and price information; and patient results. As a rule, all laboratory information should be treated as a single database to permit maximal access and internal communications. This is the reason that acquiring commercial laboratory software for different sections of the laboratory from different vendors should be discouraged.

The database thus arranged can be addressed using a variety of application software products for different purposes. These may come from an LIS vendor or from various commercial sources. The purposes may be managerial, such as budget development, workload comparisons, and so on, or clinical, such as refining normal ranges by age group, development of expert systems, and so on. Data transformation and information extraction may be a major goal.

## Electronic Data Processing

The process of incorporating electronic data processing into a management plan has three main steps:

1. Decide what you want to do.
2. Select the software that will allow you to do it.
3. Select the machine that will run the software.

### Decide What you Want to Do

The management process must be supported by information of all kinds. Data management may be approached in a variety of ways, including the use of expert systems to forecast trends, to develop approaches to lab testing, and so on. An important initial consideration is the marginal utility of the information seeking/processing task. Will it contribute value that exceeds its purchase, installation, training, and operational costs?

**Select the Software That will Allow you to Do it**

Management software can be acquired as individual programs designed for specific purposes or as combined, integrated packages (suites). The major kinds, which will be discussed in some detail in later sections follow:

**Text editors.** Also known as word processors, text editors are used to prepare reports, memos, letters, manuscripts, and so on. A full-featured text editor allows the operator to use preprepared "canned" text, develop footnotes, number pages, count words, verify spelling, provide synonyms (thesaurus), lay out complex equations and place them in text, insert graphical images, and communicate by electronic mail.

**Spreadsheets.** Spreadsheets are programs that simulate the paper spreadsheet used in accounting procedures in which columns of numbers are summed for budgets and plans or otherwise manipulated according to formula. Computer spreadsheets perform otherwise tedious calculations and recalculations that result from entering or changing numbers. They consist of a matrix of rows and columns, the intersections of which are identified as *cells*. The cells of a spreadsheet, which can number in the thousands, can be viewed by scrolling horizontally and vertically. Cells can contain labels or other descriptive text, such as sales or test values. The numbers are the actual numeric data used in a budget or plan. Formulas direct the spreadsheet to do calculations. After numbers are added or changed, the formulas recalculate the data either automatically or on command. Sophisticated multidimensional spreadsheets may be used as analytical database engines, in which data are stored in a separate database apart from the formulas that are stored in a spreadsheet in the usual way. When the spreadsheet is called up, numbers from the database are displayed in the spreadsheet, which functions as a viewer into the database. This strategy allows creation of multiple dimensions in the spreadsheet and development of various business models by varying the database.

**Database programs.** Database programs may be relational, hierarchical, or network. A relational database is an organizational method that links files together as required. In nonrelational hierarchical and network systems, fixed links are set up ahead of time to speed up daily processing. Records in one file locate or "point to" the locations of records in another file. In a business setting, these records might be customers and orders or vendors and purchases. In relational databases, relationships between files are created by comparing data, such as account numbers and names. A relational system can generate a new file from two or more records that meet matching criteria. Common uses in addition to those mentioned are keeping track of personnel files, cataloguing bibliographic references, generating schedules, and so on. Records may also be used to examine relationships among such parameters as patient age, sex, race, laboratory test results, drug therapy, and length of stay, among many others.

**Desktop publishing.** Desktop publishers are programs designed to support the development of documents combining text and graphics, often in multicolumn format, resembling newspapers or magazines. They are used to produce a laboratory newsletter, or a laboratory handbook, for example. New publishers are very sophisticated and can be used in many creative ways, such as developing sites on the Internet and crafting and distributing illustrated reports.

**Process modelers.** Process modeling software is used to analyze and predict the effects of change in one part of a complex process on other parts and the eventual outcome. In the laboratory they might be used to explore the effect of shift changes, volume increments, personnel increments or decrements, or a new analytic process.

**Image analysis.** Image processing and analysis of a picture using digital techniques can identify shades, colors, and relationships that cannot be seen by the unaided eye. Image analysis used in the laboratory to quantify images based on size, shape, and density, mainly to assess the amount of DNA contained in nuclei, but also for more gross structural analysis. Images are represented as **raster graphics**, a technique for representing a picture image as a matrix of dots. Raster display is the digital counterpart of the analog method used in television display. Images are brought into the system by scanning or capture using digital cameras.

**Communications.** Communications software is used to support exploration of the Internet, electronic mail, or facsimile transmission.

**Expert systems.** An expert system, or rule-based system, is a program that uses stored information, based on generalizations and rules, to draw conclusions about a particular case. It differs from a database in that a database stores and presents information unchanged, while an expert system offers "judgments" based on specified facts and rules. An expert system has three parts: a user interface (commands, menus, and so on) a **knowledge base** incorporating stored experience, and an **inference engine**, which draws conclusions by performing logical operations on the knowledge base and information supplied by the user.

### Select the Machine That will Run the Software

Personal computers are now capable of running extraordinarily sophisticated programs, especially when linked into mutually supportive networks. Laboratory operations with requirements for storing and processing very large amounts of information may require a larger ("mainframe") computer system. Computer hardware and associated devices are discussed in later chapters.

## Summary

We can summarize this discussion by comparing the structure and functions of three hierarchical systems that together constitute the laboratory information system. These are the **management system**, the **information system**, and the **computer system**.

- The **management system** includes people using machines. At this level are set the organization's goals and objectives, strategies, tactics, plans, schedules, and controls.
- The **information system** consists of the *database,* which defines the data structures, the *application programs* including data entry, updating, inquiry and reporting, and *procedures,* which define data flow.
- The **computer system** includes the *central processing unit* (CPU) which performs the fundamental computer processes of calculating, comparing, and copying data; the *peripheral devices,* through which data is entered, stored and retrieved; and the *operating system,* which manages the computer system.

# Chapter Glossary

**computer system:** Component of an information system consisting of the central processing unit (CPU) which processes data; the peripheral devices, which store and retrieve data; the operating system, which manages the processes of the computer system; and the interfaces which connect the system to analytical devices and to foreign computer systems.

**confidentiality:** Restriction of access to data and information to individuals who have a need, a reason, and permission for access.

**data:** Uninterpreted material facts, or clinical observations, collected during an assessment activity.

**data accuracy:** Absence of mistakes or error in data.

**data capture:** Acquisition or recording of data or information.

**data definition:** Identification of data to be used in analysis.

**data reliability:** Stability, repeatability, and precision of data.

**data transformation**: Process of changing the form of data representation, for example, changing data into information using decision-analysis tools.

**data transmission:** Sending of data or information from one location to another.

**data validity:** Correctness of data; it reflects the true situation.

**decision support system** (DSS): Information system similar to MIS, but tends to be more analytical, and deal with semi-structured problems using data from both internal and external sources.

**executive support system** (ESS): Information system used at the strategic decision level of an organization, designed to address unstructured decision making using advanced graphics and communication representing vast amounts of structured and processed information.

**function:** Goal-directed, interrelated series of processes, such as patient assessment or patient care.

**informatics:** Information science; the science of processing data for storage and retrieval.

**information:** interpreted sets of data that can assist in decision making.

**information system:** Interrelated components working together to collect, process, store and disseminate information to support decision making, coordination, control analysis and visualization in an organization.

**knowledge based information:** Collection of stored facts, models and information that can be used for designing and redesigning processes and for problem solving.

**knowledge work system** (KWS): Information system used by knowledge workers (scientists, engineers, etc) to help create and distribute new knowledge.

**laboratory informatics:** Field that concerns itself with the theoretical and practical aspects of information processing and communication, based on knowledge and experience derived from processes in the laboratory, and employing the methods and technology of computer systems.

**management information system** (MIS): Information system used to provide current and historical performance data to middle managers who use it in planning, controlling and decision making.

**management system:** Component of an information system which sets the organization's goals and objectives, develops strategies and tactics, and plans, schedules and controls the system.

**medical informatics:** Field that concerns itself with the cognitive, information processing and communications tasks of medical practice, education and research, including the information science and technology to support those tasks.

**information structure:** Component of an information system consisting of the of the database, which defines the data structures, and to a certain extent defines the organization; procedures, which define data flow; and the application programs, including data entry, queries, updating and reporting.

**minimum data sets:** Collections of related data items.

**office automation system** (OAS): Information system used to increase the productivity of data workers (secretaries, bookkeepers, etc), but may also be used by knowledge workers.

**risk analysis:** Systematic process for evaluating the vulnerability of a data processing system and the information it contains to hazards in its environment.

**transaction processing system** (TPS): Basic business systems used at the operations level of an organization to keep track of daily transactions in the course of business. These might include databases and spread sheets.

# References

1. Kazmierczak SC. Statistical techniques for evaluating the diagnostic utility of laboratory tests. Clin Chem Lab Med 1999; 37:1001–1009
2. Aller RD, Balis UJ. Informatics, imaging, and interoperability. In: Henry JB, editor. Clinical diagnosis and Management by Laboratory Methods. W. B. Philadelphia Saunders. 2001:108–137
3. Connelly DP. Integrating integrated laboratory information into health care delivery systems. Clin Lab Med 1999; 19:277–297
4. Forsman R. The electronic medical record: Implications for the laboratory. Clin Leadersh Manag Rev 2000; 14:292–295
5. Becich MJ. Information management: moving from test results to clinical information. Clin Leadersh Manag Rev 2000; 14:296–300
6. Marques MB, McDonald JM. Defining/measuring the value of clinical information. Clin Leadersh Manag Rev 2000; 14:275–279

7. Miller WG. The changing role of the medical technologist from technologist to information specialist. Clin Leadersh Manag Rev 2000; 14:285–288
8. Wills S. The 21$^{st}$ century laboratory: Information technology and health care. Clin Leadersh Manag Rev 2000; 14:289–291
9. Elevitch F, Treling C, Spackman K, et al. A clinical laboratory systems survey: A challenge for the decade. Arch Pathol Lab Med 1993; 117:12–21
10. Miller RA, Shultz EK, Harrison JH Jr. Is there a role for expert systems in diagnostic anatomic pathology? Hum Pathol 2000; 28:999–1001
11. Rashbass J. The impact of information technology on histopathology. Histopathology 2000; 36:1–7
12. Friedman BA, Dieterli RC. Integrating information systems in hospitals: Bringing the outside inside. Arch Pathol Lab Med 1990; 114:113–116
13. Boar BH. The Art of Strategic Planning for Information Technology. John Wiley & Sons, New York, 1993
14. Laudon KC, Laudon JP. Management Information Systems: Organization and Technology. Prentice Hall, Upper Saddle River, New Jersey, 4th ed., 1996
15. Cowan DF. Quality assurance in anatomic pathology: An information system approach. Arch Pathol Lab Med 1990; 114:129–134
16. Friedman BA, Dito WR. Managing the information product of clinical laboratories. (Editorial) Clin Lab Man Rev 1992; Jan/Feb: 5–8
17. Lincoln TL, Essin D. Information technology, health care, and the future: what are the implications for the clinical laboratory? Clin Lab Man Rev 1992; Jan/Feb: 94–107
18. St. Louis, P. Status of point of care testing: Promise realities and possibilities. Clin Biochem 2000; 33:427–440
19. Friedman, BA. Informatics as a separate section within a department of pathology. Amer J Clin Pathol 1990; 94:(Supp 1) S2–S6
20. Buffone GJ, Beck JR. Informatics. A subspecialty of pathology. Amer J Clin Pathol 1993; 100:75–81
21. Friedman CP, Elstein AS, Wolf FM, et al. Enhancement of clinician's diagnostic reasoning by computer-based consultation: A multisite study of two systems. JAMA 1999; 282:1851–1856
22. Oxford Dictionary and Thesaurus, American Edition. Oxford University Press, New York and Oxford 1996
23. Collen WF. Origins of medical informatics. West J Med 1996; 145:778–785
24. Greenes RA, Shortliffe EH. Medical informatics: An emerging academic discipline and institutional priority. JAMA 1990; 263:1114–1120
25. Joint Commission for the Accreditation of Healthcare Organizations. Manual 1997

# 2
# Developing the Laboratory Information System

DANIEL F. COWAN

It was pointed out in Chapter 1 that the term "laboratory information system" means more than an aggregation of hardware and software. The system is a plan expressed in policies and procedures and implemented in part on a computer. Indeed, computers are not necessary parts of information systems, which have existed under one title or another as long as human activities have been organized. Notebooks, card files, ledgers, and indexing systems all are information systems. The hardware and basic programs and software tools used to support a laboratory information system, although provided by a vendor, must reflect the needs and objectives of the laboratory, as defined by the laboratory and developed as an information plan. The information plan must be coherent, meet the medical service and management objectives of the laboratory and the larger institution, if that is the context in which the laboratory operates, and must make efficient and effective use of the resources of the purchased system. Full, inclusive participation of the laboratory staff in the development of standards and objectives for the system is a *sine qua non* for success, as is coherent central management of the system. The information system implements a shared goal of improvement in efficiency and effectiveness of services and must be accepted and used by the entire staff of the laboratory. This means that the information system is coherent and uniformly applicable, although not every aspect of laboratory services must be computerized. Careful analysis of information such as test frequency, keystrokes necessary to order a test on the computer, and other considerations may indicate that some functions should be automated while others are best done manually. This is not an exemption from the information system, only a particular expression of it, based on careful process evaluation.

At the very least, computerization can be expected to standardize procedures, data collection forms, and terminology; simplify and expedite clerical work and eliminate most transcription error; refine report formats; store and analyze large amounts of patient, management, and financial data, and help in compliance with regulatory requirements. Computerization improves service quality and management routines by providing an unchanging, planned structure.[1]

A good vendor system assists management processes and does not require wholesale modification of laboratory policies and procedures to fit the system, although the laboratory staff may elect just such a modification to improve operations to be supported by the computer. After all, there is no point in spending large amounts of money, time, and effort on a computer to continue to do what has always been done in the way it has always been done. Later, after purchase, during installation, many processes that require changing are usually identified, no matter how carefully things were thought out in advance. The purchased system may, by providing a consistent structure, eliminate quirks or incoherence from laboratory operations. It must be so designed as to permit growth and change over time without restructuring the database. A system too precisely tailored to today's requirements may prove to be completely inadequate in the face of volume growth or change in the organization or function of the laboratory, such as might be imposed by the establishment of satellite laboratories or the development of strings of off-site clients. The modern LIS is not like laboratory equipment that has a product half-life, good for only so long and replaced because it is worn out or technologically obsolete. The *hardware may be replaced or components of the software upgraded, but the information system continues.*

## Planning for Purchase of a Vendor-Supplied System

The importance of planning ahead and anticipating developments before buying an LIS cannot be overstated. Commonly laboratories have a plan of organization, a physical layout, and a book of procedures that have been in use for many years. The people who planned the laboratory, both its organization and its physical layout, may no longer work there, and no one can say quite why things are done the way they are except that they have "always been done that way." The laboratory may be based on thinking from the era before computerization, and all practices will probably be manual in concept, based on pencil-and-paper methods. Accommodations will have been made to what was workable at the time, including personnel limitations, testing technology, budget, and personalities. Similar considerations apply to an outmoded computer system that is to be replaced.

The questions "Why do we do what we do?" and "Why do we do it this way and not some other way?" and "How would a computer help us do this process better?" should be applied to every detail of laboratory operations. A more global question would be "If this laboratory did not exist, how would we create it? What would be the ideal size, organization, and scope of a laboratory to support our patients and clients?" There will never be a better time for introspection of this sort. There is no virtue in using a computer to support methods that are manual in concept or philosophy. If the laboratory does not intend to fully exploit the capabilities of a modern computer system and rethink all its processes and change them appropriately, even radically, the costs in time and money to acquire a new system cannot be justified. A new hospital laboratory system will cost more (sometimes much more) than $3000 per bed served by the time it is bought and installed. Many laboratories recognize that this fundamental reengineering is beyond the ability of the staff, not because they lack intelligence or motivation, but because they are too close to the problem and inexperienced in the process. An experienced outside consultant may be invaluable at this point in the study. This period of self-examination is more important than the selection of a particular LIS vendor, since it determines the qualities that will be looked for in a computer system and will fundamentally determine the success of the new information system.

Management processes and control issues must be defined and understood and determined to be consistent with institutional policies and practices, and they must be supported by the vendor's offering. Existing procedures must be identified and understood, not just in their mechanics, but also in their philosophical assumptions, origins, and contribution to operations as they are or ought to be. Work volumes must be accurately determined and changes in volume projected for the future based on experience and on plans for clinical program changes within the hospital or service area. Budgetary limits must be defined and relative priorities established. This process has been well described in a standard text.[2]

# Request for Proposal

A selection process may begin with an informal *request for information*, or RFI. This is a short document that says in a general way what the laboratory is looking for in a vendor, for example, a system for a small hospital, a system for a large hospital, or a system for a laboratory that supports an extensive service network. Because this request is essentially a form letter, it is cheap to send out and cheap for a potential vendor to respond to. The response is likely to be product literature and a letter or call from a sales representative, which will not be adequate unless it has been made clear that a response must provide substantial technical and operational information. The value of the RFI is that it helps to identify a large pool of potential vendors and tends to assure that a company will not be overlooked. The RFI list might be assembled from a list of companies published periodically in *CAP Today*[3] or from advertisements in journals, trade publications, or the Internet.

Detailed review of the department is necessary to develop a study document that may be the basis of a communicative **request for proposal** (RFP). A request for proposal is a statement about the department addressed to vendors, usually organized as a series of questions about the vendor's system capabilities. A good RFP has several important uses:[4]

1. Helps focus the laboratory's goals, plans, and priorities
2. Serves as a guide through the selection process
3. Assists with objective ranking of systems and vendors
4. Helps avoid "specification drift" caused by sales efforts
5. Forms a framework for contract negotiation
6. Screens out vendors that do not address the desired level of function
7. Helps justify selection to management
8. Helps avoid missing candidate vendors

Some institutions require that the RFP process be followed as a matter of routine for all large capital purchases, and may have a prescribed form and process. This is done to avoid any hint of favoritism or impropriety in the purchasing process and to protect the institution and the ultimate user from overenthusiasm for a particular salesperson or presentation materials that may not represent the product accurately. Often the first thing sold by an effective salesperson is the salesperson. It is a good practice to make it clear to all responders to an RFP that statements about functionality and service (for example) will be taken as commitments and incorporated into the final contract.

Considerable care is needed in developing an RFP.[4] First, an RFP is costly to prepare and costly for the vendor to respond to. Many hours of work are involved on both sides. It is time consuming to prepare an RFP, and the laboratory may not have the resources to devote to developing expertise. Outside advice may be needed, and consultants tend to charge by the hour plus expenses. Second, the RFP must not become a list of laboratory idiosyncracies. An overspecified system may discourage vendors from responding. A good system may be lost to consideration because it cannot perform some nonessential function. Valid new functionality not thought of by the laboratory may not be presented by the vendor. Third, an overdetailed RFP may cause delay at the institutional level: it will have to be carefully considered by those who must give approval. Finally, some of the more important characteristics of a vendor, such as reputation, company stability, and quality of service personnel, do not lend themselves to quantitation.

It is important to remember that the RFP prepared by an organization is intended to communicate, and the things communicated may be unattractive to a prospective vendor. If the laboratory presents itself through the RFP as idiosyncratic, focused on minutiae, and obviously wanting to replicate either an existing outmoded process or act out a fantasy, the vendor may not respond to the RFP at all, figuring that if the contract was won, the vendor/client relationship probably would be poor, the installation difficult, and the prospects for a happy client remote. The vendor must always pay attention to the cost of doing business, and the cost of responding to a several-hundred-page RFP is high and the likelihood of success low, especially if the number of negative responses to questions is unacceptably high. The cost of an unhappy client in terms of future lost business may also be unacceptably high.

An RFP should request a client list, with dates and sizes of installations, client references, a list of former clients who have changed to other vendors, and company size (number of employees), history, and goals, as well as specifically product-related responses. The RFP should be organized in a structured question sequence that will permit ready comparison of answers from various vendors. This will facilitate development of a scoring system for ranking vendors.[5]

## Questions to Be Asked in the RFP

Criteria for evaluating vendor offerings (which imply questions to be asked in the RFP) should include three tiers of issues: issues internal to laboratory operations, institutional and other external considerations, and noun for management, including costs of installation and orienting new employees.

### Internal Operations

- Is the system limited to core laboratory functions, or are billing, coding, and so on integral to the system?
- Are all sections of the laboratory, including blood bank and anatomic pathology supported? Does the system support structured or synoptic reports?
- Is the system designed for hospital use specifically, or can it support a multisite facility, such as off-site laboratories or collection centers?
- What analytical instruments have been interfaced to the system (provide a complete list)? How long after the introduction of a new instrument is an interface available? Is there a charge for developing a new interface? How is the change determined?
- What are typical downtime and response-time statistics at a given annual and peak service volume? What is a typical scheduled downtime, and what have other clients experienced in the way of unscheduled downtime (crashes)?
- Does the system include standard, readily available, and readily serviced hardware, network components, and peripheral devices? Is the hardware readily upgradable without prolonged downtime?
- Is system hardware supported by the vendor directly or by a second party? What are the financial arrangements with a second party?
- Does the system conform to general industry standards such as a standard operating system, network and interface protocols, and programming language? Was the system developed in compliance with federal and state manufacturing standards? Specify the standards with which the system is compliant.
- Is the system designed around an open architecture to facilitate incorporation of new technology and interfaces?

- Does the system incorporate a standard database structure, accessible to conventional database tools? Specify the structure and tools. Does the system support encoding systems, such as SNOMED and LOINC?
- What is the vendor's strategy for maintaining accessibility of the data archives over time and as technology changes? Be specific.
- To what degree is the system user-definable? Is customization possible and at what cost? Is the system manager able to define new tests and report formats, enter calculations, and design screen views, or are these vendor services? What are the costs of these services?
- What training manuals are available? Are they intended for system manager use only, or are bench-level versions available?

## External Considerations

- Can the system accommodate physician order entry?
- Is the system user-friendly and easy for the casual user to learn?
- Does the system have a graphical user interface (GUI)?
- With which hospital information systems have successful interfaces been developed? What interface standard is followed? What kind of data traffic is accommodated by the interface?
- Does the system accommodate functions such as reporting by fax, remote reporting by terminal, and radiocommunications?
- Can data and tabulated numbers for clients outside the laboratory be displayed graphically? Can the manner of display be varied for individual clients?
- Does the system provide or support additional services to laboratory client offices, such as on-line laboratory manual, reference (library), management and consultation services?

## Laboratory Management

- Can the system function autonomously, supporting all business functions, or does it depend on or incorporate second-party products?
- Does the system support detailed transaction logging, and can its database track employee productivity and monitor persons accessing records as a security function?
- Does the system track reagent/supplies used in real time and maintain running inventories?
- What administrative and management reports (e.g, turnaround time, workload) are available in the system? Specify in detail. Are they integral or do they depend on or incorporate second-party products? Is management information collected in real time, or must it be back-loaded?
- What provisions are made for initial training of laboratory employees? What provisions are made for new employees in an established system? What is the cost of training, and how is it calculated?

- What is a typical cost of ownership for a system of similar size and complexity? Does the cost include just purchase and installation, or does it include typical upgrades and maintenance? Does it include costs such as telecommunications charges for requested features?

## *User Definability vs. Customization*

In discussions about adapting a vendor-supplied system to a particular site, the terms "user-definable" and "customization" are often used. The terms do not mean the same thing, and the difference should be clearly understood. **User-definable** commonly means that the system provides for individuation or accommodation to the needs of a particular laboratory through the provision of built-in options—menus or tables from which the laboratory selects those that apply. Lengthy menus or tables allow a high degree of individuation without touching the structure of the vendor's product and without revision of computer code. **Customization,** on the other hand, is generally taken to mean that the vendor modifies code or writes new code specifically for the laboratory. This is a costly effort with significant downstream implications. Typically, periodic upgrades or enhancements are, like the basic product, standardized. This means that upgrades assume that the basic structure of the system is the same in every laboratory site, greatly simplifying vendor support. If code is customized—modified—to suit a particular laboratory, someone at the vendor must remember exactly what has been done. Now and in the future, all persons having contact with the laboratory must be aware of the specifics of the modifications. This includes people at help desks attempting to provide support over the telephone. Given the turnover of employees of high-tech industries, it is not good to rely on the vendor retaining this memory. Customization may interfere with upgrades and support. It is best never to customize if there is any workable alternative.

## Functional Requirements of the System

An RFP should focus on critical points, since they will be common to all laboratories with some understanding of information issues. The characteristics required of any computer system intended to support laboratory operations are relatively simple to state. The fundamental features are the heart of the system; that is, the content and structure of the database. A vendor-supplied computer system must be inherently able to capture all important events and to use flexible vendor-provided or user-defined routines to prepare reports. This process is called "transaction logging." The differences among systems become apparent when terms such as "all important events" are defined and when accessibility of the data and the flexibility and power of the software routines are explored. The promises of the vendor's salesperson must be verified by actual use. Another point of difference may be what data is automatically captured in the course of routine work and what must be entered *postfacto*. A good system automatically accumulates necessary data in the course of work and does not require back-loading of data. Back-loading may defeat otherwise well-designed quality improvement and management programs: it will probably be done by a clerk, not the technologist or pathologist doing the work, and important time/event points will be lost. Manual entry is prone to clerical errors that do not occur with automated entry. At a minimum, turnaround time will be extended to no good purpose.

## *Structure of the Database*

In some institutions anatomic pathology is physically, organizationally, and philosophically remote from the clinical laboratories. Under these circumstances, a specialty anatomic pathology-only vendor may be preferred by the anatomic pathology staff. This should be carefully considered before going this route, as there is substantial value in easy access to the clinical laboratory database when evaluating (for example) liver biopsies, bone marrow or lymph nodes. If separate AP and CP systems are to be acquired, great attention should be paid to the ease with which they interface and exchange information. For institutions in which the service laboratories include both anatomic and clinical pathology, there should be a unitary, common, or single database for all laboratory services, anatomic and clinical. A unified laboratory database will become increasingly important as hospitals move toward a totally electronic medical record, but it also has immediate value within the laboratory. It facilitates on-line inquiry from, for example, a surgical pathologist to the chemistry laboratory for serum enzyme levels and to the microbiology laboratory for viral antigen status. The autopsy pathologist has access to the full range of laboratory results for the subject patient. Since LIS file structure is proprietary, at the current level of technology, this database requirement strongly suggests a single-vendor LIS. A heterogenous, multivendor system may have difficulty in coordinated function because of semantic differences in data dictionaries among the components. That is, different components of the system may use words to mean different things, and syntax governing the structure of the language used may not be precisely the same. Upgrades occurring at different times may take the systems out of synchrony. However, recent developments in client/server architecture and open approaches to database design may permit communications among heterologous elements in a coherent information system.

Asynchronous evolution of the software components in a mixed-component system may reveal problems with **record level version control**. Version control is the management of source code in a large software project. It is essential to keep track of the revisions made to a program by all the programmers involved in it; otherwise, inconsistencies and progressive difficulties with clear communication among the software elements may creep in. Each record defines a **data dictionary** with a version number. If data dictionaries are absent, it may be nearly impossible to reference the static database. The implication of these semantic and structural differences is that specialty laboratory systems—stand-alone systems—may not be able to function efficiently as part of a comprehensive computerized data record, decision support, and quality improvement system. Avoiding these problems or resolving them once discovered will require laboratory subspecialists to trade a little autonomy for a share in a greater good. Comparison of the organization of laboratories shows that assignment within a laboratory of where a particular test is done is an artifact of technology and is a management decision that may change with changes in laboratory organization, personnel, or equipment. In one laboratory, flow cytometry, polymerase chain reaction procedures, and gene rearrangement studies may be done in surgical pathology; in another laboratory they may reside in microbiology or hematology; and in yet another they may be done in a special division of the laboratory. The current movement toward open-architecture and client/server systems may obviate the file structure problem in the future. For today, it is a major issue.

## Transaction Logging (Event-Level Processing)

Every event—every user interaction or transaction—that takes place on the LIS is logged or recorded by event, person, place (terminal identification), date, and time. These events can be either WRITE or READ functions. WRITE functions are those that produce **status changes** in the database. READ or **inquiry functions** make no status change. A status change is any action that affects the database: order entry, assignment of an accession number, test performance, result entry, result change, verification, and printing. Some vendors and clients object that this degree of transaction logging is expensive and goes beyond what is needed for the production of laboratory data and basic laboratory management. It substantially increases requirements for disk space and therefore cost. This is true. Restricting transaction logging is one way to keep costs down. It is, however, very shortsighted and can effectively prevent or cripple implementation of a comprehensive quality improvement program, and it may have important ramifications as the laboratory and institution move toward a totally electronic medical record. It certainly interferes with the development of sophisticated laboratory management reports. The value of status change logging may be self-evident. It is important to know who is doing what to the data. The value of inquiry logging may become apparent only when looking to the future when clinical records are entirely on computer. It is a general operating assumption in hospitals that once a paper report has been posted in a chart, the information in it has been delivered to the physician and those who need it. Inquiry logging combined with security hierarchy for access may detect unauthorized approaches to patient information. More important, it may document delivery of laboratory information to the physician. Full inquiry logging is technically feasible and desirable now, but it may not be practical for many institutions. Transaction logging is an effective way to keep track of who is looking at patient records and when. It permits periodic reporting to appropriate authority of summaries of inquiry into the record of any particular patient, and conversely, it may identify someone who habitually browses through patient records without legitimate reason. Knowing that such a record is being kept and will be acted on if abuse is detected may be an effective way to discourage record snooping, and it may be an important contributor to confidentiality in a system of electronic records. This may become mandated under Federal regulations.

To perform some of the tracking mentioned here, all functions have to be logged on as they are done, not backloaded or batched except in small, frequent batches. As each case is accessioned, it is assigned to a particular pathologist, if it is of a kind that requires the personal attention of a pathologist, or assigned to a particular laboratory, technologist, or workstation in the clinical laboratory. Assignment may be made either by kind of case or shift or day, depending on the practice of the laboratory. In anatomic pathology for example, the software should permit date, time, place, and person logging of accessions, grossing in, number of blocks taken as each case is processed, dictation, typing, slide completion, special stains ordered and completed, microscopic descriptions and diagnoses, typing of notes, electronic signature, and printing or release over the system. The system should also know who has corrected typing and any corrections or amendments made after verification (signing) by the pathologist. Provision should also be made for recording the time and/or date the clinical service was provided to the patient, as this may be different from the time the specimen arrived in the laboratory. For example, a biopsy may be done in an office on a particular date (the date of clinical service) but not arrive in the laboratory for accessioning until the next day or even two days later. The implications for billing are important as the date the service was provided must be consistent with the date the patient was seen. All these functions have implications for management of resource utilization, work flow, and medical liability.

Entry of each tissue block or slide specimen creates a new test order, which must be either completed or canceled. Case-by-case and block-by-block entry can produce a complete work list or tally sheet for the histology laboratory, which can be used to account for blocks after processing. Using the list, the technician can indicate the completion of slides (fulfillment of the test order). Because each case has been assigned to a particular pathologist on accession, a physician work list is also created. This should be easy to access each day by each pathologist to assure that all cases are progressing in a timely fashion and none are being overlooked.

Reference ranges must be saved with the test result. Some systems do not save the reference ranges with the test result because it uses up a great deal of disk space. However, the information is historically important and necessary for continuity as when a procedure or analytical instrument change changes the in-laboratory reference value. Also, the reference range for the patient may change for sound physiological reasons, as in the instance of growing infants and children.

Critical data must be held on line for at least five years, the minimum period to comply with current requirements for certain kinds of data. Other data may be available off line if accessible within a short time. In practice, certain information that reflects clinically important characteristics or status changes of the patient, such as sickle cell and other metabolic traits, transfusion history, hepatitis antigen positivity, as well as surgical pathology and cytopathology diagnoses, may be held on line "indefinitely." The American Association of Blood Banks (AABB) requires that records of donors and donor blood be kept indefinitely, while certain other records may be held for five years.[6] Anything beyond the legal minimum is a local option, reflecting the needs and wishes of the medical staff and the availability of money to support their desires. It has been estimated that a typical histopathology laboratory, processing 10,000 cases per year with about 800 characters per report, generates at least 6.5 megabytes per year, or 65 megabytes every 10 years.[7] With storage now available in the multigigabyte range, simply banking data is not a problem. Accessing information from a large database rapidly is a problem in data processing, with costs far surpassing those of storage.

## Evolution of the Database

The vendor system must provide not merely for retention of data over the projected period; it also must be able to accommodate changes in the kind of data and way it is collected. Consistent tracking of a patient by some discrete identifier, linking within a laboratory section and across sections and with previous events over time, is a basic and essential function. Inherent in the long-term storage of data is what may be called "technology drift," analogous to genetic drift. Changes made to data categories must not interrupt continuity of the record. For example, suppose initially patient race is recorded as white, black, oriental, other. After a while, it is decided to elaborate the categories into white, Hispanic, African-American, Japanese, Chinese, Vietnamese, Indian. Can this change be made without loss of access to cases archived in the previous categories? Can report formats be changed over time without impairing review? What provision has the vendor made to assure access to the archives, even though the hardware technology has changed and the software evolved? This problem is familiar to users of personal computers, who have seen problems with the progression of 5.25-inch floppies from standard density through double density to high density and the change from 5.25-inch to 3.5-inch disks, to high-density disks in less than five years. This kind of change continues with the increasing use of writable optical disks and the pending introduction of digital tape for local use.

A rule-based system should be provided for tracking particular kinds of cases or events. The use of rule systems is already established in the clinical laboratory at one level or another. **Routine rules** are those applied to every test and include things such as delta checking and calculation of red cell indices, done according to formulas applied in every case. **Higher-level event rules** selectively apply to all tests in a particular category but are invoked only under specified circumstances. Familiar examples include reflexive cancellation of one component of tests normally ordered together, based on the result of the first, such as bacterial culture and sensitivity, and rules for acceptance of tests, such as time windows to prevent duplicate testing. The highest set of rules is the **clinical action rules** for notification or intervention, e.g., in the case of critical value results or a new diagnosis of a malignancy.

A rules system can be used to develop a great variety of reports intended for management of resource use, for assignment or reassignment of personnel based on work load; and for quality improvement, such as identifying groups or types of cases by pathologist or by resident or by combinations of people, events, places, days of the week, and work shifts. Reports can be useful in identifying points of slowdown when a problem arises with turnaround time, for example.

It is inconvenient and too costly of processing time to address the entire database each time a routine inquiry is made or report written. A badly timed or poorly organized major survey of the database can interfere with the day's work, as it may take hours to do and may degrade system response time to unacceptable levels. The vendor LIS software should be able to develop and maintain secondary databases (extract files or superfiles) drawn from the primary database for defined routine uses, such as preparation of reports, developing purge (or save) extract files, or development of a training database. It should also provide for the downloading of information into a database maintained in a server or personal computer to allow an individual manager or researcher to use the data without involving the LIS central processor.

The vendor should provide a software "tool kit" for use in manipulation of the database. Part of the kit may be standard modular report writers provided to all clients. A flexible and reasonably powerful user-definable program for preparation of routine and *ad hoc* reports should be provided. The report writer, sometimes generically called a structured query language (SQL), must be able to initiate report generation at a frequency and time of day in a format convenient to the user. The SQL implementing specific rule premises may be used to refer particular data to an extract file on the fly or on an event-by-event basis, rather than by retrospectively reviewing and selecting the data from the database, which may take many minutes or hours. A report writer may be useful in the accreditation process for production of paper reports for inspectors who may not wish to deal with computer screens.

Using a system of rules, the SQL can also be the key to adapting to new and unanticipated regulations. Since transaction logging captures all data, new programs can be developed to gather information to meet the new regulation without having to make any other change in the system.

## Encoding

Encoding of procedures and diagnoses should be standard, automatic, consistent, simple, and reliable. No automated system can encode diagnoses that do not include appropriate terms. A minimal level of terminological discipline on the part of users is essential. The trend in cytopathology to use structured report formats such as the Bethesda system allows the building of report screens that assure accuracy in coding. The same is not true in surgical pathology, where variability and ambiguity in wording may be a problem. This is a very important issue, as accurate encoding provides the link for automating comparison of diagnoses from cytopathology with diagnoses from surgical pathology and frozen section reports with final reports. The computer must be able to scan accession lists for a specified time period in one service (cytology) and search for the same patient on a surgical pathology accession list, implying a discrete permanent identifier for every patient. Using an appropriate rule set, if a patient on the cytology list with an abnormal diagnosis fails to appear on the surgical pathology list within a defined time, a reminder letter to the physician, the patient, or both is generated. Having identified the patient on both lists, the computer then compares encoded diagnoses and prepares a report of cases with failure to match to a level defined by the cytologist. This report forms the basis for peer review.

One should expect a vendor of an anatomic pathology system to be licensed by the College of American Pathologists (CAP) to use the Systematized Nomenclature of Medicine (SNOMED) as the basis for coding. SNOMED is the *de facto* standard for diagnostic and procedural encoding. Vendors should not only provide automated SNOMED encoding in their basic system but should also distribute CAP SNOMED changes as part of their software maintenance agreement. Retrieval systems based on free-text search are being offered by some vendors. This is computationally considerably more expensive than searching defined code fields, and it must be shown that text search systems can achieve the links between data files necessary to perform essential quality management.

## Security and Confidentiality

Every vendor of an LIS includes a security system as a basic element. The system must be flexible enough to limit access to patient data to those with a need and a right to know. It must also be able to limit access by category of inquirer (e.g., all physicians) or to specific persons (e.g., admitting physician and designated consultants). Further, it should provide a test-by-test limitation of access; i.e., allow access to all laboratory results except those relating to designated sensitive matters, such as a diagnosis of malignancy or the result of an HIV test or drug of abuse assay. Ideally, it can obscure the result of a test or even that a particular test was ordered from all but those with a need to know. This feature helps to comply with confidentiality provisions in government regulations.

Much of the emphasis of the preceding discussion has been on clinical data management issues. An important by-product of the LIS features described is improved quality of laboratory management. Identification of time and location of orders supports **service-level analysis**. If a terminal is available at a remote site of specimen collection, then the LIS will allow tracking of specimen movement and transit times, which can be of great value in service analyses, especially if specimen containers are individually identified and accessioned. The ability to do segmented turnaround time audits, which allow identifying an individual performing a function and the date, place, and time of day it was performed, helps to focus on (for example) staffing problems, such as scheduling, inadequate numbers, and individual skills. This kind of objective report is helpful in discussions with hospital administration about budgets.

## Site Visit

Under no circumstances should a decision to purchase be made without contacting other clients of the prospective vendor. It is cheap and fast to make telephone inquiries, and they should be made. However, an unhappy client may be unwilling to make negative comments on the telephone or to admit a mistaken selection. There is no substitute for seeing the proposed system in use and talking to the people who actually use it on a day-to-day basis. A client of size and complexity similar to the laboratory considering purchase should be selected for an on-site visit. This client should be using the system as proposed by the vendor, including the current version of the software and all the various laboratory components. Issues for a site visit should include ease of use, opinions about vendor support, flexibility, and any other matters important to the prospective purchaser. Site visits are costly both of time and money, but these costs are trivial in the context of a major purchase and the aggravation and expense of a bad decision.

## Developing a Contract

The process of developing a contract varies with the laboratory. An independent group buying its own system, having made its evaluation and decided that the business will be best served by Vendor X's offering, needs to deal only with its own legal representative and the vendor. Usually, the laboratory is part of a larger institution, such as a hospital or medical center, and will have to comply with all policies and procedures. The laws of the state of the purchaser (or sometimes the state of the vendor) and whether the institution is public or private will influence the contract. It is always wise to specify in the contract which state laws will apply, those of the purchaser or of the vendor.

The process of contracting has been described as a process of consensus building.[8] The consensus begins within the institution, where such matters as cost justification, location of the computer, control of the system, and billing issues must be agreed on. Evaluation of the ability of a vendor to deliver on the contract, in terms of both company viability over the long run and client satisfaction with the vendor's product and service, should include expert evaluation of financial statements, usually over five years, résumés of owners and key personnel proposed to work with the laboratory, and client information provided in the response to the RFP. More specifically, the contract will answer the following questions:[8]

- What is being bought?
- How much will it cost, and what are the terms of payment?
- How will it be installed and who will install it?
- What are the installation costs and how much time will installation require?
- What are the physical requirements for the computer room?
- What electrical services are required?
- Who will do the training, where and how will training occur, how much does training cost, and who pays for it?
- Who will operate the system?
- How should the system perform?
- What is the definition of system acceptance?
- Who maintains the system, and who repairs it?
- Who upgrades the system?
- What are the rights and obligations of the laboratory?
- What are the rights and obligations of the vendor?
- What are the penalties for failure of the system to perform to specification?

Perhaps the most important safeguards that can be built into a contract are **event-based payment,** and **guaranteed response times.** Payment terms and events may vary, but often specify include 25% due on contracting, 25% due on delivery of equipment, 25% due on go-live, and 25% due on 60 days of satisfactory performance in use. Sometimes vendors will "lowball" the offering price by underspecifying the hardware, then later offer additional hardware to bring performance up to desired (but uncontracted for) levels. This ruse is eliminated by specifying a performance level at a service volume in the contract and holding the vendor liable in the contract for meeting that level. We have found it useful to specify experienced installers by name in the contract in order to avoid being the training site for new vendor hires.

# Problem Resolution

Large computer systems are well described as complicated, expensive, and cranky. The same may be said about large laboratories. It is not to be expected that a major computer system will be installed in a complex laboratory without some difficulties with software, hardware, or personnel. The installation process requires the participation and cooperation of, at a minimum, laboratory staff, vendor staff for software issues, usually hardware vendor staff, and often institutional information services staff. The best preventive of problems and misunderstanding is a carefully constructed, unambiguous contract, preferably with performance and penalty clauses, a detailed installation plan deemed workable to all parties, clear communication among all concerned, and patience and forbearance. A periodic meeting among the principals is advisable, even if no problems are on the table, to establish and maintain a cordial working relationship to be exploited when problems arise.

It may be worthwhile to employ an experienced consultant to help develop the installation plan and in time of need to mediate and translate between the laboratory and the vendor. The vendor must provide a competent staff with an experienced project manager. The laboratory must also provide a high-level person as project manager, empowered to inflict pain on persons in the laboratory who foot-drag or otherwise fail to follow through on obligations. Medical and nursing staffs and important clients must be kept apprised of progress, and a clear, detailed, and thorough training plan must be established and fulfilled for all concerned.

Even with the best of plans and preparation, things may happen. Delivery of essential items of hardware may be delayed. The system may not perform in test runs. It may not perform to expectations in acceptance trials. Any of a number of issues may appear. When problems arise, it is essential to formulate problem-directed questions and establish facts to provide the basis of problem resolution sessions with the vendor. Careful analysis may help to characterize the problem and identify any contribution to it of the laboratory or laboratory staff. Is the cabling and computer environment provided by the laboratory a contributor? Are all the laboratory people involved carrying out their responsibilities? Is the installation plan appropriate and realistic? Why is the hardware late? Has there been a change in availability on the part of the hardware vendor? Is delay related to introduction of a new (possibly better) product? What part of the system is not working? What is the nature of the failure? Is it a failure of system performance or of installation? Is the hardware appropriately configured? Are people appropriately trained? Do the operators know what they are doing? Is a performance failure due to design, software defect, deficiency, or integration?

Design flaws may be **patent** (obvious or readily discoverable) or **latent** (subtle or not easily discoverable). Because the appropriate solution, including the buyer's rights to recourse under the law, depends on the nature and seriousness of the problem, it is important to identify it and register a point with the vendor as soon as possible. If the problem is due to some inherent deficiency of a software module, it may be best to reject the system quickly to minimize loss. The longer the laboratory tries to use a less-than-satisfactory system, the more difficult it may be to reject it. The laboratory's lawyer should be brought in for advice at appropriate times to be sure nothing is being done (or not being done) that might compromise rights under the contract or the law.

When a proper analysis and marshaling of facts has been done and the nature of the problem defined, one of a number of approaches may be used. Always notify the vendor of the problem, and request that they be part of the analysis and solution. They probably have seen the problem (or one like it) before and may have a ready answer.

- If the problem is a repairable bug or installation glitch and is annoying but not critical, fix it and go on. Such an incident may help to establish a closer and more confident relationship between the vendor and the laboratory, if timely and appropriate steps are taken.
- If the problem is serious, obtain a written commitment from the vendor to fix it within a specified period of time. Assure yourself that the vendor can actually do it.
- If the system works but fails contracted performance specifications, such as response time under a particular test volume load, demand that the vendor upgrade the system at no cost to you until the performance criteria are met.
- If the problem is very serious, preventing use of the system, and you are not convinced that the vendor can fix it, consider rejecting the defective component or the entire system. Give the vendor a reasonable period of time to make good, but do not pay for any components not yet delivered, even if payment is specified in the contract. After all, the vendor has not upheld his end of the contract, and every bit of leverage helps.
- Consider replacing the defective component with a unit from a different vendor. This may be next to impossible unless the software is open-architecture or the hardware modules are compatible.
- Consider termination of the contract. (Be sure a termination clause has been written into the contract!) Demand refund of any money paid, and keep all delivered components until the money is refunded.
- With apparently unresolvable issues, such as whether the laboratory has contributed significantly to the vendor's problems or about an amount to be paid or refunded, consider an arbitrator. Binding arbitration may be written into the contract for just this purpose and to avoid the trouble and expense of a lawsuit.
- When all else fails, consider a lawsuit either to void the contract and get a refund or to compel the vendor to make good. When deciding between voidance of a contract or compulsion, also consider the desirability of a

long-term relationship with a vendor who must be sued to make good on a contract.

It is always desirable to maintain a businesslike posture when problems with a vendor arise. There must never be a question as to whether or not a vendor will be required to perform to contract any more than a question whether the buyer will be required to pay for equipment and services received. Hostility, threats, insults, and personal recriminations are to be avoided. Satisfying as they might seem at the moment, all they do is add static to an already charged situation. Most problems, especially technical problems, can be resolved by discussion. The vendor is not in business to make enemies nor to earn a reputation for failure to meet client expectations. Also, it is important to be sure that the laboratory is not the problem in an unsuccessful installation, as word will get around the industry, and the laboratory may earn the reputation as a client not worth the trouble and cost to a vendor.

## Build or Buy?

Occasionally it will be proposed that an institution or the laboratory build its own system, rather than go to the market. It might be feasible to build if the local organization contains experienced developers and understands project managment at the level required. Also to be considered is the ability of the local organization to maintain the product they have built. Most who have considered this option have decided against it. Arguments in favor of it usually cite the possibility of developing a perfect system tailor-made for the users, the high up-front cost of a vendor system, and high costs of continuing service. Also to be considered is the fact that for most large institutions the proposed expenditure of several million dollars on a vendor system necessarily involves the legal and purchasing departments, who may tend to make the project theirs, not the laboratory's. Home building tends to avoid this development. Building your own system is not to be taken lightly, and a protracted period of prayer and meditation is advisable before the decision is made.

## Application Service Providers (ASP)

Application service providers are companies that rent software functionality over a network; either a private network or the Internet. An application service provider has been defined as "any third party whose main business is providing a software-based service to multiple customers over a wide-area network in return for payment".[9] The software that is the basis of the services resides on the ASP company's computers. It is usually accessed through Web browsers (see Chapter 7). ASPs appeal to small businesses that want minimally customized, standard applications, to vertical industries that need specific software functionality, to business-to-business electronic commerce applications, and to large organizations needing complex niche applications that would not be cost-effective to develop and maintain in house. Technical support is provided by the ASP. Software can be modified only by the ASP technicians.

A few definitions are needed for the following discussion. A **vertical industry** is one in which all participants are in the same business, large or small, such as medical, legal or engineering and architectural practices, funeral services, and the like. **Horizontal** refers to a function that is similar in diverse industries, such as truck fleet management, tax preparation services, and so on. A **portal** is an Web site or service that offers a broad array of resources and services, such as e-mail, discussion forums, search engines, and on-line shopping. The first Web portals were on-line services, such as AOL, that provided access to the World Wide Web, but by now most of the traditional search engines have changed themselves into Web portals to attract and keep a larger clientelle.

Types of applications provided by ASPs include the following:

- Minimally customized, packaged applications, such as small-business software, or larger-enterprise resource planning packages
- Vertical industry applications such as documentation and software for medical practice management
- Vertical industrial portals, which host business-to-business (B-to-B) electronic commerce and provide industry-specific software functionality
- Horizontal portals, which provide specialized "niche" functionality that can be shared by companies across many different industries

## Risks of Using an ASP

The subscriber loses control of the timing of software upgrades. Most ASP companies are new (under two years old), and the business is very volatile. The ASP provider may fail or may be acquired by another company. Clients may not trust sending valuable and sensitive client information to a third party, the ASP, over the Internet. This is especially a concern when the data to be sent is medical record information. Potential clients may feel that the industry is too new to be trusted, since the providers have not been in business long enough to have a track record and to demonstrate company viability.

## Benefits of Using an ASP

The ASP may offer specific expertise in an application not available through local sources. The subscriber avoids the expense of buying, installing, supporting and upgrading costly software applications. An application can be brought up and running for little money outlay, with little delay. Resources are not diverted from the core business. A multi-site user may use an ASP as a central computing and data storage focus, enhancing standardization and communication, saving in the process the cost of setting up the physical infrastructure at each office.

## Types of ASP

ASP services generally include the following:

**Application outsourcing.** Functions as simple as billing and quality management services or as complex as most or all of the applications used in a small laboratory

**Application hosting.** Web sites that are interactive with their clients and provide transaction handling, i.e., run applications for clients

**Web sourcing.** Provision not only of software applications but population of the applications with data that might be difficult or inconvenient for the user to access on his or her own. E-trade is an example of a Web source

Using an ASP must be considered very carefully. It is possible that an effective, time- and money-saving service may be aquired, or it could result in confusion and loss of important elements of control, such as medical records. Viability of the ASP provider and legal liability issues must be carefully considered.

## Summary

The characteristics of the vendor-supplied LIS that add up to a good system are not always obvious. Good systems tend to cost more than lesser systems, relating to fundamental issues such as software complexity and hardware requirements. Budgetary constraints may force the choice of a limited system, but considerable thought must be given to investment in basic operations. It may be better to begin with a well-structured system with relatively few software applications, with the expectation of adding applications as money becomes available, rather than to accept one that offers a wider array of applications packages for the same money but at the cost of more important fundamentals.

Acquisition of a commercial LIS requires several steps, which must be taken in order. The first is to define the needs of the laboratory, which include medical service and management objectives. Among the objectives must be the meeting of current regulatory requirements. Potential vendors are identified through a structured process, and their systems are evaluated in terms of their ability to support the service and management objectives. Key questions for the vendor are the structure of the database and the kind of data recorded for each service encounter, as the answers predetermine the kinds and quality of information that can be drawn from the data. The vendor must provide specific report writer modules that address the defined management and regulatory issues and also provide the means for the user to create *ad hoc* reports to meet new or unanticipated needs.

# Chapter Glossary

**ASP** (application service provider): Third party whose main business is providing a software-based service to multiple customers over a wide-area network in return for payment.

**customization:** Modification or creation of case specifically for a particular client.

**data dictionary**: In essence, a database about data and databases, which holds the name, type, range of values, source, and authorization for access for each data element in the organization's files and databases. It also indicates which applications use that data so that when a change in a data structure is made, a list of affected programs can be generated.

**extract file:** Subfile or extract (sometimes called a superfile) of a larger database focused on a particular topic, series of issues, group of patients, or type of data.

**horizontal function:** Function that is similar in diverse industries, such as truck fleet management, tax preparation services, and so on.

**LOINC** (Logical Observation Identifiers Names and Codes): Database providing a standard set of universal names and codes for identifying individual laboratory results and diagnostic study observations. Developed and copyrighted by The Regenstrief Institute.

**open architecture:** Computer system in which the specifications are made public to encourage or permit third-party vendors to develop add-on products.

**portal:** Web site or service that offers a broad array of resources and services, such as e-mail, discussion forums, search engines, and on-line shopping.

**RFI** (request for information): Document that invites a vendor to submit information about the hardware, software, and/or services it offers.

**RFP** (request for proposal): Document that invites a vendor to submit a bid to provide hardware, software, and/or services.

**SNOMED** (Systematized Nomenclature of Medicine): Encoding system developed by the College of American Pathologists that assigns discrete numbers to components of a dianosis, procedure, or etiology.

**SQL** (structured query language): Software tool or language used to interrogate and process data in a relational database. The term is used both generically to refer to such a tool and specifically to refer to the product developed by IBM for its mainframes and variants created for mini- and microcomputer database applications.

**semantics**: Study of the meaning of words. See **syntax.**

**status change:** Action that affects a database, such as entry of an order, assignment of an accession number, entry of a test result, and so on. Contrasted to viewing, which makes no change.

**syntax**: Rules governing the structure of a language statement. It specifies how words and symbols are put together to form a phrase.

**transaction file:** Collection of transaction records. Data in transaction files are used to update master files, which contain the subjects of the organization. Transaction files can be used as audit trails.

**transaction log:** Running record of every event transpiring on a system, including who, what, where, and when, at a minimum.

**user definable:** Applied to the software of a system, allowing for individuation or accommodation to the needs of a particular laboratory through the provision of built- in options—menus or tables from which the laboratory selects those that apply.

**version control:** Management of source code in a large software project in a database that keeps track of the revisions made to a program by all the programmers involved in it.

**vertical industry:** An industry in which all participants are in the same business, large or small, such as medical, legal, or architectural practices, funeral services, and the like.

# *References*

1. Cowan DF. Quality assurance in anatomic pathology: An information system approach. Arch Pathol Lab Med 1990; 114:129–134
2. Aller RD, Balis UJ. Informatics, Imaging, and Interoperability, In Henry, JB, edition. Clinical Diagnosis and Management by Laboratory Methods, Ch 6, pp. 108–137 W. B. Saunders, Philadelphia, 20th ed., 2001
3. *CAP Today*. College of American Pathologists. Northfield, Illinois
4. Weilert M. What's right and what's wrong with laboratory information system requests for proposals. Clin Lab Man Rev 1992; Jan/Feb:9–16
5. Rose R, Maffetone M, Suarez E, Whisler K, Bielitzski. A model for selecting a laboratory information system. Clin Lab Man Rev 1992; Jan/Feb:18–29
6. AABB standards for blood banks and transfusion services, 17th Edition. American Association of Blood Banks, Bethesda Maryland
7. Travers H. Quality assurance indicators in anatomic pathology. Arch Pathol Lab Med 1990; 114:1149–1156
8. Elevitch FR. Negotiating a laboratory information system contract Clin Lab Man Rev 1992; Jan/Feb:30–38
9. Wainewright P. ASP insider: An application service primer. 1990. http://www.aspnews.com/news/article/0,,4191_373981,00.html

# 3
# Validation of the Laboratory Information System

DANIEL F. COWAN, R. ZANE GRAY, BEVERLY C. CAMPBELL

The use of computer systems and computerized devices in the laboratory is becoming nearly universal, and increasingly processes once performed by people are being transferred to machines, the inner workings of which may be only dimly understood. The task of the people managing the work of the laboratory is to comprehend the processes by which the computerized laboratory information system (LIS) in use, usually acquired as a package from a vendor, may be shown to be doing the job it is expected to do. The functions of the system must be validated. Useful discussions of regulation[1] and inspection and accreditation[2] of laboratory information systems are available. However, despite its importance there is remarkably little published outside the blood bank literature about the validation of laboratory information systems that is accessible to general users of the systems, that is, addresses specifically laboratory issues in terms and concepts familiar to the laboratorian. Our intention here is to discuss LIS validation as it applies in the laboratory in general, to define the issues related to validation, and to suggest an approach to dealing with them.

Validation of the laboratory information system is the continuing process of proving the system fit for its intended use, initially and over time. Validation consists of defining, collecting, maintaining, and independently reviewing evidence that the system is consistently performing according to specifications. This is no small task, as many parts of a vendor-supplied LIS are proprietary, and some are so complex as to be beyond the ability of a user to evaluate in detail. Validation is resource intensive, and while certain aspects of validation testing are increasingly done with the support of automated utility programs, it remains a mainly manual operation involving many work hours. Difficult or not, this task must be undertaken, because it is an essential component of a quality management system, and the laboratory has a legal and ethical responsibility to assure itself and its clients that data

Modified from an article published in Arch Pathol Lab Med 1998; 122:239–244.

provided through the LIS are accurate, consistent, and reliable. Various professional accrediting associations require validation of the laboratory computer system, including the College of American Pathologists (CAP), the American Association of Blood Banks (AABB), and the Joint Commission on the Accreditation of Healthcare Organizations (JCAHO). The federal Department of Health and Human Services claims an interest, and the Food and Drug Administration (FDA) asserts jurisdiction under the Safe Medical Devices Act of 1990 over a computer system supporting the operations of a blood bank that produces blood products.[1] The FDA in effect holds that such a blood bank is in fact a manufacturer of biologicals and is to be held to the same current good manufacturing practices (cGMP) as any such manufacturer. Computer systems must be validated to the FDA standard when they are used in conjunction with manufacturing, storage, or distribution of biologicals and drugs. Blood products are deemed to be biologicals. This introduces a new way of thinking into the laboratory, even for those used to meeting the highest standards of the laboratory peer group. Regulation concerns not only the clinical laboratory and the LIS more generally but also applies to *in vitro* medical devices, of which computerized cytology instruments are a prime example.[3] Hence, regulation will be addressed along with the general issue of LIS validation.

# General Validation Issues

## *Validation for Quality Assurance and Improvement*

A quality management system addresses four questions: What is it that I do? How do I know that I do it well? How can I convince others that I do it well? How do I get better at what I do?[4] While these are familiar in the context of the clinical and anatomical laboratories, they apply equally well to the LIS. What the information system does is collect, process, store, and distribute information. Validation is directed at the next three questions. It demonstrates to all concerned, in and outside the laboratory, that the LIS manages information well, with the expected accuracy and reliability, file integrity, auditability, and management control. Validation also identifies weak points or areas for improvement and, with proper planning and documentation, can show that the LIS has in fact gotten better or warn that adverse trends and conditions are developing in time to prevent them. It is important to recognize that system failure does not necessarily mean loss of operation; it can mean failure to provide expected services in a timely manner.[5]

A laboratory information system is a specific application of a planned system of processes, operations, and procedures, part of which is supported by a computer system.[6] A computer system includes not only the core computer, consisting of the hardware and its controlling software, but also people, peripheral equipment, documentation and defined procedures that relate to it. The central questions in validation are "**Does this complex system work?**" and "**Do you control it?**" A computer- based system acts with nearly incomprehensible speed, handles enormous volumes of information, can broadcast it widely almost instantaneously, and must store it indefinitely in electronic form, not readable until it is displayed on a screen or as a printout. Validation of the system poses special problems that must be addressed by very carefully structured, highly documented processes.

It is important to recognize that computer programs, except for the most simple, no matter how carefully written and tested, are always defective to some degree. All software contains errors, or "bugs," that may or may nor be evident in casual use but will inevitably show up with use of the program over time. It is also important to understand that programs do not deteriorate spontaneously or wear out. They stay the same until they are changed by some exogenous factor. However, under conditions of use, deeply buried flaws may surface, or a once functional program may not integrate well with newly added functions. The implication for validation is that **a program is always suspect** and must be tested in use under varying conditions and load over a long time, and the process and results of testing must be documented—an unending process.

In contrast, hardware may leave the manufacturer working perfectly as far as it can be ascertained, and the user may be satisfied by a routine of acceptance testing that it functions according to all specifications. Unlike software, some hardware deteriorates with use over time, and therefore a device that was at one time fully functional may become unreliable and even fail. The implication for validation is that hardware must be under a program of testing that will predict failure before it occurs, and in the event of a crash, data in process at the time will not be lost or corrupted and can be recovered with full confidence.

The process of validation naturally divides into developmental validation, acceptance validation, and retrospective validation. **Developmental validation** is integrated into the process of customizing, configuring, adapting, or inventing a new system or component. It is the responsibility of the vendor who offers the product for sale or license. **Acceptance validation** or acceptance testing is the initial approval process for live use of the system by the user. **Retrospective validation** is the determination of the reliability, accuracy, and completeness of a system in use. While this process is actually concurrent with use, the term "retrospective" is used by the FDA, we have adopted it to avoid confusion. Ideally, validation begins before the system is acquired by development of a plan and by systematic evaluation of the vendor and the vendor's system of validation. The reality of the situation is, however, that as the process of validation becomes better understood, it is applied to systems in use. This raises an important question: If the system is working well and has given no problems, why do we have to go through the process of validation? One answer is that if you prepare blood products, the FDA says you have to validate. A better answer is that computer systems are constantly being revised or adjusted and are therefore actually evolving systems, and not as static as they might seem. An appropriate process of validation prevents problems, and, if one does occur, mechanisms are in place to identify it and its cause, and to prevent a recurrence. Also, a proper process of validation identifies objectively when it is time to upgrade the system or its components.

## Vendor Validation Testing

As part of the presentation of a product to a prospective client, a system vendor must document and attest that an appropriate program of validation has been carried out. No single agency regulates the development of computer-supported information systems, and there is no universal industry standard. Therefore, the user must have a reasonably clear idea of the validation processes used by a prospective vendor and must demand appropriate documentation. Although not required, some vendors have adopted the ISO 9000 standards of the International Organization on Standardization.[7] The ISO is not a certifying body. If a vendor claims to follow ISO standards, the claim has to be certified by a third party.

The validation processes used by a vendor may be extremely detailed and organized at stages or hierarchical levels in the system. The same processes also apply to locally written systems. While the details are highly technical and beyond the scope of this discussion, they may be summarized briefly. The lowest level is proving that a single function within a program works as intended. This level is referred to as **string testing,** a string being a continuous set of alphanumeric characters that does not contain numbers used in calculations. An example of this level is the printing of a label. The next level up is testing of a functional module or unit (**unit testing**) of some complexity, such as accessioning of a specimen. Above that is the level of **module testing,** in which a product function as a whole is evaluated. Last is **system testing,** in which the performance of functions and modules working together as an integrated whole is proven. The methodologies used include testing the internal workings of code and individual statements and conditions within the program. As these are all known to the developer, this process is called "white box testing," in contrast to "black box testing," user-oriented testing of observable input and output from a process not known to the user. Specific test methods include equivalence class partitioning, boundary value analysis, and error guessing, used to validate the limits of a program or product, including expected and unexpected conditions, to assure that appropriate actions are taken. Regressive validation ensures that changes have no unexpected effect on existing functions.

It is difficult for a person not involved in the development of complex software products to comprehend the amount of specification documentation that lies behind the product. One vendor describes ring binders occupying

200 square feet, floor to ceiling, relating to blood bank products alone.[8] The only really practicable approach to assess the developer's validation practices is to include questions on these practices and any formal certification of them in a request for information (RFI) or request for proposal (RFP) and to include the vendor's responses as a commitment in a final contract. Close examination of site-preparation manuals and technical manuals may give some insight, and, if finances permit, engaging an expert consultant to report on the prospective vendor's practices may be valuable. An arm's-length approach to the vendor's source code may be a wise policy, as too close an inspection may imply in the minds of some regulators a duty to review it in detail, a task usually well beyond the ability of a laboratory staff.

# General Process of User Validation

The general process of user validation includes several steps.

## Identification and Description of the System to be Validated

To address identification and description issues, the intended functionality of the system must be specified and documented for reference. Identification of the system by name specifies and limits the scope of validation. The description of the system should include the primary functions of the system and the service needs it is to meet. It includes a statement about the functional environment of the system, that is, the systems that interface or communicate with it, and it specifies the users of the system. This includes other systems (e.g., a hospital information system) and instrument interfaces. It specifies the names of the component hardware and software vendors, the names of the persons responsible for operating and maintaining the hardware, the operating system, and the applications software, and the name of the custodian of the data. Hardware components are specified by name, model number, and vendor or supplier, and software components are specified by module name, version, or release and vendor. The description also includes software specifications; an estimation of the user, workstation, terminal device, memory, and storage requirements, and a description of each functional module; the interaction of the modules, and the interaction of the system to be validated with other systems. A graphical depiction of the system and its modules and interfaces is a useful summary document.

## Specification of the Stage in the System Life Cycle

A computer system can be thought of as having a life cycle consisting of several stages. A stage in a system life cycle can be any one of a sequence of events in the development process of an information system. It will be bought, used, upgraded, and perhaps eventually replaced. Validation tasks depend on the cycle stage of the system and include definition of requirements, system design specification, implementation, testing, checkout, and operation and maintenance. Specifying the stage in the system life cycle allows testing and validation to be conducted at distinct points of development of the information system.

## Formalization of the Process for Prioritizing and Deciding

Validation of software is done according to priorities established in the laboratory reflecting perceived need. Setting of priorities may depend on whether the FDA has an interest in the laboratory. Ordinarily, the core operational components have highest priority, as their function is to capture, store, and make available common patient information such as demographics, order and specimen collection data, and charges. General laboratory functions also hold high priority but in most cases only for immediate patient care. If the laboratory operates a blood bank that processes blood products, the blood bank donor module is the primary concern. Blood bank modules also have the long data storage requirements, along with anatomic pathology and microbiology.

## Development of Hazard Analyses

Hazard analysis is determination of the potential degree of human harm that might result from the failure of a device or system; i.e., specification of the penalty for failure. Failure may be as serious as issuing bad data or as minor— but annoying—as printing poor-quality paper reports. A hazard analysis is part of every procedure.

## Identification of Regulatory Concerns

Pinpointing regulatory concerns will determine which regulatory agency, if any, will claim jurisdiction, and which set of standards will apply to the operation of the system and the validation process. The agencies may include the FDA, state health departments or licensing bodies, and professional accrediting organizations, such as the CAP, AABB, and the JCAHO.

## Documentation

Validation of a system produces a large volume of documentation, including not only the general statements about validation and test plans but also test scripts and attached listings, screen prints, and test reports. A document must include an explicit statement of pass/fail status, the signature of the person conducting the test, and the person reviewing the test status and disposition.

The documentation must be compiled, organized, and kept in a designated location for management and regulatory review.

# Validation Plan

The first step in user validation is the development of a validation plan that implements in a very specific way the general issues already specified. A validation plan defines the initial and continuing program to be followed by the laboratory and specifies the documents needed to support it. Some LIS vendors may participate actively in post-acceptance validation, and others may offer useful advice.

## *Initial Validation Program*

### Compile all Documentation of Functional Needs and Specific Plans for the System

Define the testing and operating environments and all system interrelationships, the size (capacity) of the system, and the data and samples to be processed. Include existing evidence of validation of components by the vendors of software and hardware. Specify the events and criteria for selective revalidation. Define significant hardware and software updates and a schedule for revalidation in the absence of change. Develop a plan to discover error and institute corrective action. Assign areas of responsibility to named individuals. Develop a cross-referenced filing system so that all interrelated documentation is available on short notice.

### Review the Vendor's Record

The vendor must present evidence that it has followed established standards for system development and maintenance. Attestation and evidence of vendor validation is an essential component of documentation. If a recommended standard (e.g., ISO 9000) has been used, then a third-party certification must be provided. The validated processes must be pertinent to the system under consideration. Reviewed vendor records, in addition to validation documents, may include licenses and agreements among component vendors, system documentation, system management, and operator and user manuals. Evidence of product support by the vendor, such as approach to problem reporting and resolution, the system used for assignment of priority to requests for assistance, and system for follow-through on reported problems should be presented. Review of vendor source code is seldom feasible, as it may be extremely voluminous, may require expertise not available to the buyer, or may be proprietary. The implications of too intimate a familiarity with the vendor's source code have been touched on.

## Review Vendor-Supplied Documentation
## for Software and Hardware

The vendor is expected to supply full documentation of the product supplied, including system specifications, technical manuals for the operators of the system, and applications manuals for the users, but not including the documents accumulated during the process of product development. Part of the validation process includes determining that all necessary manuals are available, useful, and on hand. As vendor-supplied documentation of the system as a whole may be excessive for the user in the laboratory, it may be supplied to the system manager, and operational summaries such as bench-level operator manuals may be provided or developed, which are reviewed for accuracy and completeness. Maintenance and error logs are kept. The existence and use of appropriate vendor-provided materials, operator manuals, and maintenance and error records is specified in standard operating policies and procedures (SOP), periodically reviewed and documented.

Review and documentation of source code is primarily a matter of concern to regulatory agencies, who hold the user responsible for the validity of the code. For reasons already given, code review is vicarious, and depends on certificates and attestation statements.

## Decide Which Subsystems Must Be Validated
## and Prioritize the Systems to be Validated

While all systems should be validated to some degree, not every component must be validated to the style and standard of a regulatory agency. Some validation is done by the hardware vendor and the system vendor and reported to the user. It may be convenient to validate all components to the most rigorous standard to avoid confusion arising from parallel and unequal standards. Not every task can be done at once. Some are more critical than others, so rational priorities must be established, based on hazard analysis.

## Review Laboratory-Developed Standard Operating
## Procedures and Maintenance and Error Logs

SOPs are procedural instructions, written in a standard form, that specify the steps required to perform tasks. The manual of SOPs includes the procedures for handling all operations, from normal events to recovery from catastrophic interruptions by any cause. It should include detailed descriptions of all validation protocols, routine operating policies and procedures, and disaster recovery procedures with detailed documentation of all test results, events, and actions taken and the results of tests and actions. Personnel qualifications and responsibilities are also included. SOPs are written to a level of detail that allows an appropriately trained person to execute the procedure as defined. All SOPs are initially authorized by a designated competent authority, written by a knowledgeable person, and reviewed regularly. Review and the results of review are documented. Since a large number of SOPs are created, it is recommended that a "rolling review" be instituted; for example, one twelfth of the procedures are reviewed each month to avoid an unwieldy and hasty annual review.

## Design Test Plans and Document Results

Test plans are designed to prove that a system functions to the extent that its components work according to expectation and design. They identify requirements that assure that the systems perform as expected running in the installed environment. **Test scripts** identify the exact procedures for testing and documenting a successful or unsuccessful test. They are developed in conjunction with the test plan and must indicate the action taken when a test is not successful. Test plans and scripts should have corresponding numbering systems to facilitate cross-referencing. The elements of a test script include the **functional area** under test, the **specific program** or module under test, usually designated by a mnemonic, a **validation scenario,** which says exactly what is being done, **criteria for acceptance,** an **acceptance statement,** i.e., whether the tested element is accepted or not, and an **approval statement.**

## Develop a Security Plan

A security plan defines the level of security for each user, typically by functional category, i.e., clerk, technician, physician. Security level and access are tightly controlled by the LIS administrator. Security level defines the functions that a user is allowed to perform and reflected in the security level assigned to the unique user identification number and password. Security is assigned according to a hierarchy, the most fundamental functions being READ and WRITE. READ means that a user can view but not change data. WRITE allows change of data. Further, a security level may allow a clerk to read and write demographics and read but not write test results. A pathologist may read and write, but other physicians may read only.

Apart from the issue of security and confidentiality of patient information is the security of the operating system and applications software and the hardware itself. Physical access to the computer and to stored tapes and other archival systems must be limited to appropriate people, who are identified in the SOPs. To keep unauthorized users out of the system software as well as away from patient information, policies and procedures are defined to prevent access to the software either inadvertently or by crackers gaining entry over network and modem lines.

As part of the vendor's program of maintenance and support, it may be necessary for the vendor to log on to the system from a remote site over telephone lines. This capability must be controlled and documented as part of the overall system of security. At one extreme, the vendor calls the system administrator for access each and every time access is needed. At another, the vendor has direct dial-in access, according to a defined plan. Each dial-in must be logged by time, date, and reason for the call; the person logging in, the action taken, and the results of the action recorded.

### Develop a Plan for Change Control

Change control refers to keeping track of all revisions, alterations, and fixes applied to a hardware or software component. All changes made in a computerized system are formally authorized and documented. "Changes" include any replacement, alteration, or enhancement of the hardware or software or important operational routines. Procedures governing change should specify the need for change and identify the authorizer of the change, the various validation protocols to be followed, the process of change, including the module affected, the person making the change, the tasks needed to effect it, the date they are performed, the result of the change, and recognizing that change, however carefully planned, may have unanticipated effects, how much revalidation is necessary following the change.

### Provide and Maintain an Appropriate Safe Environment for the System

Vendors of computer equipment generally define the environmental conditions necessary for optimal functioning of the equipment, including temperature and humidity and the amount of floor space necessary to allow access for maintenance and upgrade. Usually, warranties depend on the vendor's prior evaluation of the proposed space. Periodic measurements of temperature and humidity are made and documented. The period is defined by the stability of the measured parameter over a length of time. Highly stable environments are measured less often than volatile ones. An alarm system warns of incidents. The alarm system most practically displays alert or alarm messages to an operator working at a computer console, who takes whatever action is specified by procedures. A hierarchy of warnings may be established, whereby a duty operator at a console is authorized to handle incidents of relatively low import, while more serious happenings are reported immediately to a manager. Alert buzzers or other noisemakers are usually neither needed nor appropriate if an operator is more or less continually at a console or frequently checks a display. They may have a use when a displayed notice is not acknowledged within a specified time period.

### Develop a Disaster Plan

A disaster plan is a group of detailed instructions formulated as SOPs that define what is to be done in the event of a major malfunction or a catastrophic interruption of function. The first part of a disaster plan is a definition of a disaster and specification of the kind of occurrence likely to befall the facility. The definition varies depending on the physical location of the computers and the history of the geographical region, including exposure to such events as blizzards, power outs, earthquakes, hurricanes, or tornadoes. The plan indicates what provisions are made for preservation of the record, including archives; how services will be supported during the period of downtime, how they will be brought back up, and who will perform each task. Any significant uncontrolled downtime must be followed by a period of selective revalidation to ascertain that all systems are working according to specification. Full documentation of the event and of all steps taken in the recovery period is mandatory. It is prudent to maintain a duplicate archive in a place not likely to be affected by the same catastrophic event. Currently, some laboratories are developing provisions for a "hot backup," an alternative computing site to which operations are shifted in the event of catastrophic failure of the primary system. This may become a requirement for accreditation of a laboratory by the College of American Pathologists.

## Conduct Stress Testing

In testing the system as a whole, it is important to know how the system performs within the extremes of its rated capacity. Commonly, a system is designed and implemented at a level of capacity well within the workload expected to be placed on it, and an expectation for growth is built in. It is not enough to show that a system is functioning reliably at the middle of its rated capacity, since sooner or later system work will approach the specified limits of capacity. A system designed to accommodate 150 concurrent users may be initially installed with only 100 users, but eventually, 150 users may have to be accommodated. Similarly, the number of tests or procedures put through a system may rise from a comfortable level to one that approaches or reaches the system's design limits. It is expected that as capacity is reached, response times will be degraded; the system will slow down. It must be shown that the system functioning at its limits will not lose or degrade stored data. This is analogous to the idea of linearity in a clinical laboratory test. The process for evaluating this scenario is called *stress testing*. Since it is not feasible to load an operational system with data and users to stress-test it to the point of failure, various approaches are used. Some system vendors and after-market vendors offer testing programs to address this issue. Other strategies involve the use of vendor-supplied utilities delivered with a computer's operating system, software scripting products, or simply putting enough extra people on line to approximate the rated capacity of the system. It is important to test loading situations with several or many staff members attempting to modify the same patient record at the same time to be sure that the record is not garbled or otherwise compromised.

Data is intended to be stored for a long time in the system. It must be shown that there is no loss of integrity of stored data over time. Integrity of the archive can be tested by creating one or more test patients for whom each and every test offered by the laboratory is ordered and resulted. Thereafter, the records of these test patients are printed and compared with the reference record, i.e., the data as entered, to identify any loss or corruption of data. This test is run at designated intervals, and the results of the comparison are documented. A comparison study is done every time the system hardware or software is upgraded and at least quarterly. An upgrade includes introduction of new laboratory test procedures, installation of new software error correction routines or patches, and addition of new disk storage space or random access memory. Integrity testing is also done on recovery from an unscheduled downtime occurrence.

It is very important to demonstrate that after an unplanned, uncontrolled interruption in function (crash), the system, when brought back up, has neither lost or corrupted data as a result of the crash. A typical way of assessing the integrity of the archive is to print the test result records of the test patients and compare them with the reference records. Combined with tests of other more dynamic functions, such as entering orders, printing labels, entering results, and transmitting results, this procedure gives a quick sample of every function in the laboratory, including the ability to print records in the specified format.

## Continuing Validation Plan

### Maintain an Inventory of Hardware and Software

An inventory is a complete listing of all components of the system and the source and date of acquisition.

### Create and Maintain SOPs

This task is familiar to managers of clinical laboratories. Knowledgeable individuals draft policies and procedures, which in effect define the information system. The SOPs are authorized, reviewed, and approved by competent authority in the laboratory. They are reviewed, changed, or continued as often as necessary, and at least once a year. Review is documented by signature, and the reasons for change, if any, are specified. Outmoded procedures are retired but maintained in an archive file.

### Test the Hardware and Software, and Document the Results

All hardware and software are tested before acceptance and periodically thereafter. All such testing is according to plan as defined in the SOPs, and the results are documented. These tests, run under the general heading of system qualification, are done in three parts: on installation (installation qualification), at start, restart, recovery, and maintenance (operational qualification), and in performance of the procedures for which the system was acquired (performance qualification). A master test results file is maintained in a designated office. While parts of the documentation may be kept for convenience in sections of the laboratory, the master file governing all sections of the laboratory is kept in a single place.

## Maintain Current Hardware and Software Documentation

Vendors provide elaborate volumes of documentation of both hardware and software. While duplicate volumes relating to particular functions may be kept in laboratory sections or a computer room, a complete master set is maintained in a designated office.

## Ensure That System Procedures Are Followed

A comprehensive set of SOPs and vendor-provided user reference guides describe system procedures to be followed. It must be ascertained and documented that these procedures and guidelines are in fact followed. An automated operations cycle, which includes various tasks and activities to be completed on a scheduled basis, is used for the core functions of file and queue management, report and chart generation, and foreign system and instrument interfaces. The operations processes are most often performed in the background as computer-driven operations, ensuring that procedures are consistently the same. Procedures not carried out as part of operations cycles are documented and reviewed by supervisors at an appropriate level.

## Monitor Performance and Problem-Reporting Procedures

Records of problems and steps taken to identify their cause and to fix it are kept. System administration assures that these records are kept.

## Run Backup and Restore Programs in Accordance with Procedures and Documentation

Some of these programs are run as part of routine operations, according to a schedule. Others are run following unscheduled downtime. The performance of these procedures is documented.

## Maintain, Test, and Ensure Compliance with the Disaster Recovery Plan

Disaster drills should be run periodically to ensure that all persons understand their responsibilities and that all systems function as they are supposed to. The results of these tests are documented.

## Train Personnel for Job Requirements, Including Familiarity with Policies and Procedures

Training is crucial if a system is to be used appropriately and if all policies and procedures are to be followed. A formal training program, or at least a program that orients new employees to the system and documents training in their areas of responsibility, is mandatory.

Record retention and organization is a very important issue, based on the principle that if you haven't documented it, you haven't done it. Validation records must be organized and accessible. This usually means cross-referencing test panels and test results, maintaining logs of maintenance and software changes, and the like. How long records must be kept is not all that clear. Some say two years, and we advise five years to meet the requirements of the most demanding agency.

**Validation for Regulatory Requirements**

Regulated systems are those that impact product safety and/or reliability and those that generate data or reports for submission to regulatory agencies. While we believe that our recommendations will validate a laboratory information system to a level that will attain the objectives of assuring that the system will consistently perform according to specification, we do not pretend to say that following our recommendations will automatically satisfy FDA standards for validation. That is for the FDA to determine. The FDA has provided some guidance in the matter.[9,10] The FDA guideline definition says: "Process validation is establishing documented evidence providing a high degree of assurance that a specific process will consistently produce a product meeting its predetermined specification and quality attributes."[11] Although the vendor of a system should play a role in the complex and expensive task of product validation at the user's site, because the FDA does not regulate every aspect of a vendor's production, the agency assigns responsibility to the user to comply with cGMP relating to the production of biologicals. In practice, the user must ascertain and verify the vendor's compliance status as part of the overall validation plan.

# Chapter Glossary

**acceptance validation** (acceptance testing): Initial approval process for live use of a system by the user.

**change control:** Process of tracking all revisions, alterations, and fixes applied to a hardware or software component of a computerized system; all changes are formally authorized and documented.

**developmental validation:** Validation procedures integrated into the process of customizing, configuring, adapting, or inventing a new system or component; the responsibility of the vendor who offers the product for sale or license.

**disaster plan:** Group of detailed instructions formulated as SOPs that define what is to be done in the event of a major malfunction or catastrophic interruption of function.

**hazard analysis:** Determination of the potential degree of human harm that might result from the failure of a device or system, i.e., specification of the penalty for failure.

**hot back-up:** Alternative computing site to which operations are shifted in the event of catastrophic failure of the primary system.

**module validation** (module testing): Testing of the function of a product as a whole.

**process validation:** Establishing documented evidence providing a high degree of assurance that a specific process will consistently produce a product meeting its predetermined specification and quality attributes.

**regressive validation:** Testing process that ensures that changes in a system have had no unexpected effect on existing functions.

**retrospective validation:** Determination of the reliability, accuracy, and completeness of a system in use (same as concurrent validation).

**SOPs** (standard operating procedures): Procedural instructions, written in a standard form, that specify the steps required to perform tasks.

**stress test:** Form of testing in which a load approximating the maximum designed work capacity is placed on the system to determine whether a system operates with expected reliability at the limits of its capacity.

**string:** Continuous set of alphanumeric characters that does not contain numbers used in calculations.

**string testing:** Proving that a single function within a computer system works as intended.

**system validation** (system testing): Testing of the performance of functions and modules working together as an integrated whole.

**test script:** Description of the exact procedures followed for testing and documenting a successful or unsuccessful test. Scripts are developed in conjunction with the test plan and must indicate the action taken when a test is not successful.

**unit validation** (unit testing): Testing of a functional module or unit of some complexity.

**validation:** Continuing process of proving an information system fit for its intended use, initially and over time.

## *References*

1. Brannigan VM. Regulation of clinical laboratory information systems after the 1990 amendments to the Food and Drug Act. Clin Lab Man Rev 1992; 6:49–57
2. Aller RD. The laboratory information system as a medical device: inspection and accreditation issues. Clin Lab Man Rev 1992; 6:58–64
3. Brindza LJ. FDA regulation of computerized cytology devices. Anal Quant Cytol Histol 1991; 13:3–6
4. Cowan DF. Implementing a regulation-compliant quality improvement program on a commercial information system. Anal Quant Cytol Histol 1992; 14:407–414
5. Winsten DI. Taking the risk our of laboratory information systems. Clin Lab Man Rev 1992; 6:39–48
6. Cowan DF. Quality assurance in anatomic pathology: An information system approach. Arch Pathol Lab Med 1990; 114:129–134
7. International Organization for Standardization. 1, Rue de Varembé casse postale 56 CH-1211, Geneva 20, Switzerland
8. McNair, D. Group Vice President, Regulatory and Government Affairs, Cerner Corporation, Kansas City, Missouri. Personal communication, 1997.
9. Draft Guideline for the Validation of Blood Establishment Computer Systems. (Docket No. 93N-0394) October, 1993. Food and Drug Administration, Center for Biologics Evaluation and Research, Rockville, Maryland
10. Guideline for Quality Assurance in Blood Establishments. (Docket No. 91N-0450) July 1995. Food and Drug Administration, Center for Biologics Evaluation and Research, Rockville, Maryland

11. Guideline on General Principles of Process Validation. May 1987. Food and Drug Administration, Center for Drugs and Biologics and Center for Devices and Radiological Health, Rockville, Maryland

# 4
# Security and Confidentiality on Laboratory Computer Systems

DANIEL F. COWAN

The issue of computer system security has changed somewhat over the years, as technology has evolved from reliance on inaccessible, large, centralized mainframes to the use of distributed, linked or networked systems. Modern computer technology based on microcomputers and on-line access and broader use of powerful and user-friendly programs has put computer applications and other data-processing functions previously done only by computer operations experts into the hands of users. This improvement in efficiency and effectiveness presents, however, a serious challenge to achieving adequate data security. Progress in distribution of computer technology has not been accompanied by an increase in the knowledge of users about the vulnerability of data and information to such threats as unauthorized deliberate or accidental modification, disclosure, and destruction. Perhaps the greatest challenge is for all users to be aware of the possible ways that the integrity of a computer system can be compromised and to understand that full and confident use depends on the integrity of the system.

This discussion is intended to make the reader aware of some of the bad things that can happen to data and information, and it will offer some practical solutions for reducing exposure to threats. The first part of the discussion speaks about computer system security in a very general way in a variety of settings; the second section specifies how security is maintained in our own laboratory as an example of an operational security system. The final section discusses computer viruses and Internet security.

## Objectives of a Security System for Patient Records

Following are the objectives of information security for patient records:[1]

- To ensure the privacy of patients and the confidentiality of healthcare data (prevention of unauthorized disclosure)
- To ensure the integrity of healthcare data (prevention of unauthorized modification of information)

59

- To insure the availability of healthcare information to authorized persons (prevention of unauthorized or unintended withholding of information or resources).[2]

## Security Interests

Broadly, two spheres of interest relate to security of health records, patients and institutions. Patients have the right to expect that information about them or provided by them in confidence will be recorded accurately, held in confidence, used for their benefit, and not released or disclosed without their permission. Records cannot be disclosed to third parties without informed consent, a precisely defined concept. Informed consent requires that the patient is made aware of what is to be disclosed, understands what is to be disclosed, is competent to provide consent, and consents freely, without coercion.

Institutions, as holders or custodians of the records, desire privacy of business data and protection from liability. Much important business information, such as costs and services provided, can be gleaned from patient records.

## Protecting Data and Information

Protection of data and information and the technology that underpins an information system is everyone's responsibility. Owners, developers, operators, and users of information systems each have a personal stake in protecting these resources. System and network managers must provide appropriate security controls for any information resources entrusted to them. They must understand the sensitivity and criticality of their data and the extent of losses that could occur if the resources are not protected. They must also understand that for a laboratory system to be successful it must be accessible. Managers must ensure that all users of their data and systems know the practices and procedures used to protect information resources. In turn, users must know and follow prescribed security procedures. Any question or doubt should be resolved by the system manager or other responsible person.

## Sensitive Data

All data is sensitive to some degree; exactly how sensitive is specific to each business environment. In the U.S. government, unauthorized disclosure of personal information is prohibited under the Privacy Act of 1974. In some cases, data is far more prone to accidental errors or omissions that compromise accuracy, integrity, or availability than to deliberate disclosure. For example, in a hospital information system, inaccurate, incomplete, or obsolete information can result in bad patient management decisions that could cause serious injury and require time and money to rectify. Data and information critical to an institution's ability to perform its mission must be both reliable and available for use. Some data may be manipulated for personal gain. Fraudulent exploitation of systems that process electronic funds transfers, control inventories, issue checks, control accounts receivable and payable, and so on can result in serious losses. One way to determine the sensitivity of data is to do a risk analysis. Ask "What will it cost if the data is wrong? Manipulated for fraud? Not available? Given to the wrong person?" If the damage is more than can be tolerated, then the data is sensitive and should have adequate security controls to prevent or lessen the potential loss. "Adequate" is defined by the degree of hazard or possible loss. Elaborate, overly rigid controls to maximize security of trivial data will be ignored or subverted by users if they find them to be unwarranted and will tend to discredit the security system.

## *Risks Associated with Computerization of Records*

In recent years, computers have taken over virtually all major record-keeping functions. Personal computers and user-friendly applications programs have made it cost-effective to automate many office functions. While computerization has many obvious advantages, automated systems introduce new risks, and steps must be taken to control them. Many of the same risks existed when manual procedures were used but in different form. One risk is the concentration of patient information in a single location. A record room full of paper records is vulnerable to fire and flood, as are electronic records on tape or disk, which are, in addition, susceptible to electromagnetic influences that can damage or corrupt them. Electromagnetic records do not last forever; there is a certain attrition of electrons from the medium over time. New risks are created by the unique nature of computers. One is the ability of computer users to access information from remote terminals not under the eye of a record librarian. We must be able to positively identify the user, as well as ensure that the user is able to access only information and functions that have been authorized. News accounts of computer "hackers," computer virus attacks, and other types of intrusions emphasize the reality of the threat to government, commercial, medical, and private computer systems. Another risk is the gradual, spontaneous degradation of information stored on electronic media over a period of years. Change in format of electronic records over years of operation may make archives nearly as inaccessible as if they had been destroyed.

## *Limits of Security*

No matter how many controls or safeguards are used, total security cannot be attained. Risk can be decreased in proportion to the stringency of the protective measures, recognizing that each measure costs ease of access and usability for legitimate operators. The degree of protection used is based on the value of the information; that is, a judgment is made about the gravity of the consequences if a certain type of information were to be wrongfully changed, disclosed, delayed, or destroyed and about the need to keep it readily available for users. This is especially true in hospital systems, where large amounts of information must be kept secure, safe, and confidential but readily available to support patient care decisions.

## *Security in Systems and Networks*

Ideally, a computer system recognizes individuals uniquely and without ambiguity. Recognition may be based on one or more of three characteristics: what you know (e.g., passwords), what you have (data cards, and so on), and who you are (a personal, physical characteristic). It is well within the limits of existing biometrics technology to identify individuals by voice characteristics, palm or thumb prints, or the pattern of vessels on the retina. These "who you are" technologies are, however, both expensive and probably excessive in the context of most medical-related computer applications. Also, they do not adequately address the problems of interconnected computer systems.

Almost all computer systems that support more than one user, such as those supporting organizations, are governed by a user-ID and password-based security system. Access to such systems must be granted by a central security authority within the organization. Before access is granted, the owner of the data must review each user's request for access and legally authorize access to the information. Once access is granted, the new user is assigned a user ID (or user name) and a temporary password with which to log into the computer system. Passwords assigned to the user are stored in the system in a one-way encrypted format. This means that it is computationally impossible to turn the encrypted password back into the real password. For this reason, any password in most computer systems is unknown to anyone except the user. Not even the security administrator for the system in question can ascertain the real password for any user. On extended networks, such as the World Wide Web (WWW), the standard user name/password system is used, but unlike purely local systems, transfer of information across what may be vast distances through hundreds of systems places that information at risk of being intercepted or tapped. If a site on the network or Web contains sensitive information, the information is usually encrypted before transmission from the source (the Web server) and decrypted after reception at the destination (the Web browser). The encryption mechanisms are fairly complex and very difficult to defeat, ensuring that the information cannot be acquired by anyone other than the authorized user.

A typical encryption device involves the use of a *key*, a string consisting of numbers, letters and symbols used by an algorithm to create a code for encrypting data. The key is known to the sending device and to the receiving device or devices. It precedes a message. If the key strings do not match, the message cannot be decoded. The security of the key is related to the length of the code string. Running through all possible combinations in a code string 20 characters long requires a long time—weeks to months—even for a very powerful computer, and most times, it is just not worth it to a hacker.

## Practical Security Measures

Security measures must be effective but neither so complex nor so secret that they become problems in themselves. Superficially, it might seem that a security system is most secure if only a few people understand it and aspects of it are hidden in files known only to the few. Arcane and obscure systems are risky. The problem here is dependence on a few individuals who may die, retire, or be lured away without informing successors of the way the system works. The organization could be crippled by being denied access to its own files. A good security system must be comprehensible to informed users and system managers. It must be described in policies and procedures, which are themselves made available to a limited group. To a degree, they are generic and therefore readily understood by the trusted managers who must make them work. The essence of a good security system is its logical basis, defined procedures, an effective monitoring operation, and above all, the sense of responsibility of the users to the system and the information it contains. An analogy may emphasize the point. Bank funds are not embezzled by strangers off the street. Embezzlers are trusted insiders who have betrayed their trust. Embezzlement is detected by systems of cross-check and audit. The armed robber off the street is recognized as such and dealt with by different means. It is largely the same in computer systems. Trusted employees who fail their trust are like embezzlers; crackers are more analogous to armed robbers.

The basis of a secure system is trustworthy users. This is not enough, however, as any electromechanical device can fail and data repositories can be damaged from a variety of causes, so system security must employ appropriate backup, and fail-safe recovery and validation procedures.

## General Security Responsibilities for the User

All institutional computer system users must understand and comply with certain general principles of information resource protection. The following considerations apply.

### Information Is a Valuable Asset

One does not walk away from a desk leaving cash or other valuables unattended. The same care should be taken to protect information. Questions about the value or sensitivity of the various kinds of information handled are resolved by a manager or supervisor.

## Institutional Computer Systems Are Used Only for Authorized Purposes

The computer systems used in daily work should be applied only to authorized purposes and in a lawful manner. Computer crime laws prescribe criminal penalties for those who illegally access federal or state computer systems or data. Also, the unauthorized use of institutional computer systems or use of authorized privileges for unauthorized purposes could result in disciplinary action, often summary dismissal or severe curtailment of privileges, which separate the offender from his or her job. The employer or institution has often invested large sums of money in equipment and services and has a right to expect that they will be used for business, not personal matters or play.

## Follow Established Policies and Procedures

Specific requirements for the protection of information have been established, based on years of experience in prevention of computer security breaches. These requirements are found in policy manuals, rules, and procedures, and if they are not understood, they can be explained by the system manager.

## Recognize Accountability for Use Made of Computer Systems

A person who receives authorization to use any institution-owned computer system is personally responsible and accountable for his or her activity on the system. Accordingly, use is commonly restricted to those functions needed to carry out job responsibilities. In systems that log all transactions, security audits can reveal exactly who did what, when, and from which terminal or station.

## Report Unusual Occurrences

Many losses could be avoided if computer users would report any events that seem unusual or irregular. These might include such things as unexplainable system activity not initiated by the user, data that appear to have been changed or wrong, and unexpected or incorrect processing of results. Anything peculiar should be followed up. Some incidents may represent intrusion, while others may signal impending equipment failure.

## Keep Passwords Secure

The password used to verify identity is the key to system security. Passwords are never revealed to anyone. Passwords are not written down to be found by passers-by or interested others. This implies that passwords should be easy to remember (more about this later). Typically, security systems do not display the password on screen as it is being entered to prevent it being observed by others during the sign-on process. In Texas and other states, disclosure of a password is a prosecutable offense under the penal code. Most computer systems require periodic password changes. It is not the user's choice as to when this occurs. Periodic password changes keep undetected intruders from continuously using the password of a legitimate user. After log-on, the computer attributes all activity to the identified user. Therefore, a terminal is never left unattended—even for a few minutes—without logging off.

## Security and Control Guidelines

The essence of security is the selection and maintenance of an appropriate and workable security philosophy. Perfect software, protected hardware, and compatible components don't make for security unless there is an appropriate and enforced security policy. Users should understand the security system. An excellent password mechanism is not very effective if users select silly or obvious passwords.

Security reflects a set of policies and the operation of a system in conformity with those policies. Some common-sense protective measures can reduce the risk of loss, damage, or disclosure of information. Following them assures that the system is properly used, resistant to disruptions, and reliable.

### Safeguard Sensitive Information

Sensitive reports or computer disks should not be left unattended on top of desks or in unlocked storage where they can be read or stolen. Organizational policies and procedures should specify which information is locked up when not in use. Working arrangements should be such that over-the-shoulder viewing is discouraged or prevented. Patient records and other sensitive information should be deleted or discarded in such a way that it cannot be recovered. The "delete" command merely removes pointers, allowing data to be written over. An expert can recover the data even when it does not appear to be there. The safe way to clear a floppy is to reformat it. Printed reports should be finely shredded. Password encryption can block access to data stored on a hard disk. A power lock allows only key-holders to turn on power to the personal computer. Specific files shared by several users on a single computer or on a LAN can be encrypted to make them unintelligible to unauthorized people. Access-control software can divide storage space among several users, restricting each to his own files.

### Look After the Equipment

Cover machines when not in use. Back up files frequently. Provide proper environmental conditions and battery backup power supplies to minimize equipment outages and information loss. Be sure the power source is clean and steady. A dedicated computer circuit, an in-line power conditioner and an uninterruptable power source (UPS) are not luxuries.

Theft of computer equipment is a chronic problem, especially in low-security offices. Physical security devices or password-locked software on personal computers are useful. Relatively cheap devices such as lock-down cables or enclosures that attach equipment to furniture can be very effective in preventing theft, as are lockable cabinet workstations.

### Back up Data

Complete system backup should be done periodically, determined by how quickly information changes or by the volume of transactions. Backup to disk, backup to server, but backup. Backups should be stored in another location so that both original and backup are not lost to the same disaster. Do not introduce unauthorized hardware or software. Follow house rules at all times. Be wary of public access or "free" software. Shareware may share a virus as well as the program. Do not use pirated software. It is illegal as well as foolish, as it might well be contaminated. Installation of unauthorized hardware can cause damage or invalidate warranties. Support could be a major problem. Use only hardware or software that has been bought through normal channels and complies with all software licensing agreements. Some organizations impose drastic penalties for use of pirated or unauthorized software.

## Types of Security Deficiencies or "Holes"

### Physical Security Holes

Security fails when unauthorized persons gain physical access to the machine, which might allow them to do or see things they shouldn't be able to do or see. A good example would be a public workstation room where it would be simple for a user to reboot a machine into single-user mode and enter the workstation file store if precautions are not taken. Another example is the need to restrict access to confidential backup tapes, which may (otherwise) be read by any user with access to the tapes and a tape drive, whether they are meant to have permission or not.

### Software Security Holes

Security fails when badly written items of "privileged" software can be induced into doing things they shouldn't do, such as delete a file store, create a new account, or copy a password file. This kind of hole can appear unexpectedly, so certain procedures should be followed.

1. The system is designed so that as little software as possible runs with privileges and the software that does is robust.

2. Subscribe to a service that can provide details of newly identified problems and/or fixes quickly, and then act on the information.

### Incompatible Usage Security Holes

Security fails when the system manager inadvertently assembles a combination of hardware and software that, when used as a system, acts in unexpected ways. The security hole is created by the attempt to do two unconnected but useful things. Problems like this are hard to find once a system is set up and running, so it is better to anticipate and test the system with them in mind.

## *Selecting Good Passwords*

Prevent impersonation by maintaining password security. Avoid passwords with obvious personal associations, such as the name or birthday of a spouse or child. Don't select one that is very simple or short. For example, "mypassword" is not a good password. The aim is a password that is easy to remember but difficult to guess or derive. Passwords should be changed frequently, at least as often as required by the system.

A well-chosen password makes it as hard as possible for a hacker to make educated guesses about the choice. Lacking a good educated guess, the hacker has no alternative but a brute-force search, trying every possible combination of letters, numbers, and punctuation. For example, a real word chosen at random may seem to be impossible to identify. However, if a hacker uses an electronic dictionary and instructs his computer to try every word in it, sooner or later the search will succeed, more likely sooner than later when searching for real words, which are limited in number. A random combination search of apparently irrational combinations of numbers, letters, and symbols is a different matter. A search of this sort, even done on a machine that could try a million passwords per second would require, on the average, over a hundred years to complete. Most machines can try fewer than a hundred combinations per second.

Experienced hackers know that people tend to be a bit lazy in selecting passwords and choose something easy to remember. They tend to begin with the obvious. How hard they work at it depends on the potential rewards. Since no one is likely to be very titillated by perusing a list of serum glucose values, sophisticated passwords might seem to be less an issue in the laboratory than they would be in a bank. However, we cannot know who is trying to get into the system or why, so it is better to take password security very seriously. Malice can be hard to understand, but it underlies a lot of hacking. Experienced and equipped crackers are likely to use a computer to run through number combinations, names, or words. They might also go to the trouble of looking up facts about a targeted person, often readily available from public records or from personal knowledge.

**Bad passwords** include your log-in name in any form (as is, reversed, capitalized, doubled, and so on); your first or last name in any form or a spouse's or child's name; other information easily obtained about you, such as license plate number, telephone number, social security number, the brand of your automobile, the name of the street you live on; and so on. A password of all digits or all the same letter significantly decreases the search time for a cracker. A word contained in English or foreign language dictionaries, spelling lists, or other lists of words is readily found with the aid of a relatively simple program. A password shorter than six characters makes random searches much simpler than a password of six or more characters.

**Good passwords** include a word with mixed-case alphabetics; a word with nonalphabetic characters, e.g., digits or punctuation; a word that is easy to remember so that it does not have to be written down; one that can be entered quickly, without having to look at the keyboard, making it harder for someone to steal the password by watching over the shoulder.

The idea is to select something irrational and impersonal so that there are no clues or logic trees that might help in deciphering it. Sing-song or otherwise rhythmic words are easy to remember and can readily composed. Pronounceable nonsense words can be made by alternating consonants and vowels. This makes easily remembered words such as "mooloogoo" or "roadagoad." Another device is to combine short words with illogical symbolic or numerical connectors: 1cat2bat, 5+minus, and so on. A more elaborate way is to take a line or two from a song, poem, or saying and use the first letter of each word and the punctuation. For example, "Save your Confederate money, boys, the South will rise again" becomes "SyCmb,tSwra"; "The eyes of Texas are upon you" becomes "TeoTauy." The perfectly clear logic here is inaccessible to all but the inventor.

## Summary

Ultimately, computer security is the user's responsibility. The user must be alert to possible breaches in security and adhere to the security regulations that have been established. The security practices listed are not inclusive but rather are designed to raise awareness about securing information resources.

### Protect Equipment

Keep hardware and peripherals in a secure environment. Keep food, drink, and cigarettes away from it. Know where the fire suppression equipment is located and know how to use it.

### Protect the Work Area

Keep unauthorized people away from equipment and data. Challenge strangers in the area.

**Protect the Password**

Never write it down or give it to anyone. Don't use names, numbers, or dates that are personally identified with you. Change it often, but change it immediately if compromise is expected.

**Protect Files**

Don't allow unauthorized access to files and data. Never leave equipment unattended with a password activated. Sign off!

**Protect Against Viruses**

Don't use unauthorized software. Back up files before implementing any new software.

**Lock up Storage Media Containing Sensitive Data**

If the data or information is sensitive or critical to the operation, lock it up!

**Back up Data**

Keep duplicates of sensitive data in a safe place out of the immediate area. Back it up as often as necessary.

**Report Security Violations**

Report any unauthorized changes to data. Immediately report any loss of data or programs, whether automated or hard copy.

**Adopt a Sensible Security System**

Do not allow security to become so over-riding a concern that it impedes work. Discriminate between concern and paranoia. Understand that the information system serves the business purposes of the enterprise, and must remain an agile servant. Security is cooperative, not adversarial. Secure a system according to its needs, neither more nor less, and if its needs are great enough, isolate it completely.

# Laboratory Information System Security at UTMB

The approach to LIS security at the University of Texas Medical Branch is standard and incorporates the principles outlined in this chapter. It can be taken as representative of systems widely used in laboratories. Security of the LIS may be divided into two global issues: security of the core system, including the computer, its operating and applications software, discussed above, and the integrity of the recorded data and maintaining limited access to the recorded data in the interests of confidentiality of the medical record.

## Confidentiality: Patient Privacy

As a general matter, the information in the medical record belongs to the patient, while the paper on which it is written belongs to the doctor or the institution. Only those with a need to know are supposed to be able to see the record. Maintaining a medical record on a computer raises the prospect that anyone with access to the computer can see, without anyone else knowing, information about a patient that is none of the viewer's business. Revealing confidential information about a patient, if it includes such things as the results of drug screening or tests for venereal disease, can subject the patient to gossip and opprobrium. Concerns about patient privacy are rational and require an answer.

Experience seems to teach that most breaches of confidentiality arise from abuse of authorization; for example a laboratory employee sneaks a peek at the results of a neighbor's biopsy or at the results of tests done on a daughter's boyfriend. Celebrities are also at risk, even if they are only local celebrities, such as a prominent member of the hospital community or a local politician or businessperson. The best defense is for the hospital community to know that there is a security system in place that detects breaches of confidentiality and that someone caught doing so will be fired. It must be understood that a look at a paper record when no one else is around may go undetected, but the computer system tracks *all* use whenever and wherever and can ferret out unauthorized access.

Before looking at the issue of privacy of the electronic record, it might be helpful to look at access to the paper record of a patient on a clinical service in a teaching hospital to get a little perspective. Assume that the nursing unit on which the patient is staying is staffed by 10 nurses and aides on the day shift, 7 on the evening shift, and 3 on the night shift—20 persons with legitimate access to the information in a chart. They cannot be denied access if they may be called on to care for the patient. Actually, more nurses are involved, since staffing a job for 24 hours a day, 7 days a week, or 3 shifts a day for 7 days (21 shifts of 8 hours each) requires 168 work hours, or 4.2 people working 40 hours a week. Actually, it requires more than that, since staffing must allow for vacation and sick time. A typical figure would be 5.2 FTE per 24-hour-per-day, 7-days-per-week position. Let's round it to 25 nurses with legitimate access. Add 3 ward clerks, 4 residents, and 10 medical students plus 3 assorted therapists and social workers, and we are up to 45 people before the chart gets to medical records for review. Add clerks and chart reviewers, and we are probably near 60 people, without yet including the patient's doctor and medical consultants. The true situation is more complex than the hypothetical but plausible scenario just given. As part of an intensive internal review leading toward introduction of an institution-wide electronic medical record at the University of Texas Medical Branch, a detailed study of current security access was made. The object of the study was to identify people who had legitimate, job-related access to some aspect of a patient record under the existing paper-based system and who would have to be incorporated into a security matrix for the electronic record. The study identified 289 separate job categories as having legitimate access to some part of a patient record, however narrow. The number of people was not determined. The categories included everyone from primary physician to billing clerk. Add to this subtotal unknown numbers of auditors, billing clerks, and reviewers in the offices of government and other third-party payers. There is no reason at all to think that UTMB is in any way different from any large academic center. This is the level of "privacy" to which privacy of the electronic record should be compared.

## Access to the Laboratory Record

Access to the laboratory is defined in the context of a general security plan. A laboratory system must recognize security levels for users, typically by functional category. Thus a physician would have greater access to a record than would a clerk or technician. Security levels define the functions that a user is allowed to perform. Assignment of security levels in the system is tightly controlled by the LIS manager, who assigns a level according to a categorical list defined in the manual of LIS policies and procedures on notification by competent authority. For example, the medical staff office notifies the LIS manager that a particular physician has been approved for practice privileges in the hospital, or the laboratory manager sends notification that a particular person has been employed in the laboratory at a certain level of responsibility. At notice of termination, the LIS manager cancels access privileges.

On notification, the LIS manager assigns a new user an identifying number and enters into a table in the system an assignment of functional access level associated with that number. The user number is not a guarded secret, but neither is it widely published. A temporary password is assigned. The new user initiates a first transaction with the LIS, which recognizes him or her based on the assigned number and temporary password but does not allow access until a new secret password has been agreed on. The user selects a password, either a word or a combination of letters and numbers, depending on the inclinations of the individual, and enters it when prompted to do so. The computer scans its list of previously assigned passwords, and if it is not already in use, assigns it to the new user. Thereafter, the user signs on by entering the user number and then the password. Once admitted, the user can perform whatever functions are allowed by the assigned security level.

The most fundamental computer functions are READ and WRITE. READ means that the user can view data but cannot change anything. READ may mean to see on screen or to cause a printout to be made. WRITE allows the user to enter or change data. According to security level, a clerk may enter demographic information but not laboratory results, a technician may enter a result but not verify it, while a supervisory technologist may review the entered result and approve (verify) it for release. A pathologist may both read and write, with verification authority, while a nonlaboratory clinician may read but not write. As a rule, none but the LIS staff may enter any function of the LIS software. All changes made by others are limited to the database only. Even access of the LIS staff is limited according to function. Assignment of security is a very guarded function, as are changes in the operating software or basic system operations.

Every test done in the laboratory is assigned an access security level when the test is set up. Since the general purpose of a laboratory is to provide and not hide information, all tests are given a low-access security level. At a low security level, any person authorized to log on to the LIS can see the result. This is appropriate for the great majority of tests. When it is indicated, we can, as we have done in the past for HIV results, assign a high-access security level to the test. The result is not available to someone who has a low-security access assignment. The fact that the test was ever ordered at all can also be hidden from unauthorized users.

Every person granted sign-on privileges is assigned a security access level. Typically, physicians are assigned a level that allows access to all patient results. A clerk might be assigned a low access. Laboratory technicians doing the test must have a high access level.

Assuring privacy of an HIV result was accomplished by our assigning the test a high security level so that only high-access persons (physicians) can see the result. This can be done for every test done in the laboratory. Therefore assuring privacy is not a technical problem; it is a medical staff policy issue.

The implications of a policy decision to obscure a test result must be fully understood. For a physician to see the result of an obscured test, the physician must log on the LIS personally using his or her individual password. An agent lacking the appropriate security level, such as a nurse, student, or physician's assistant, cannot get the information for the physician on his or her own password. Considering the sites at which care is given (e.g., emergency room) and especially if the test involved is for a drug, attaining a high level of privacy for the patient may prevent efficient team response to an emerging medical problem.

Continuing with the example of a drug of abuse, if the highest privacy level is assigned, then the result will be available only from the toxicology laboratory, not from any other part of the laboratory.

Finally, everything said here applies only to the LIS. There is no such security hierarchy on the HIS. Anyone with authorization to access the HIS inquiry function, which includes just about everybody on the hospital and clinic staff, can see the results of any test on any patient. The only way this can be prevented is by LIS blocking transmission of a result to the HIS, which is what was done in the case of HIV results. The drawback is that no one, no matter what his or her security level may be, can see the blocked test result, because it just is not there. A person would have to log on to an LIS terminal to see the result. Again, whether this practice is acceptable in all care sites is a policy decision. Whatever electronic measures are taken, the blocked test result will appear on the printed record, an entirely different security issue.

# Medical Information on the Internet

The Internet is fast becoming a dominant telecommunications medium. It is logical to incorporate the Internet or some segment of it ("intranet") into the system for communicating medical information, especially among the sites in a distributed-service network, such as a string of clinics or client physician offices using the services of a central laboratory.

The Internet is a vast TCP/IP-based network connecting users worldwide. It is composed of standard communications protocols, routers, servers, WANs, and LANs. Its essence is its openness, redundancy, and ease of use. An intranet is an organization's private internal network composed of standard communications protocols, routers, servers, WANs, and LANs—essentially the same as the Internet. The difference is that an intranet is available only to internal company users. This limitation is accomplished by the use of firewalls and other security strategies. A firewall is a perimeter security computer device that links an organization's TCP/IP network to the Internet and restricts the types of traffic that will pass. Simple firewalls may be implemented in routers (**packet-filtering firewalls**) that filter information packets based on defined criteria, such as time of day, source or destination IP address, direction of traffic (whether from within or from outside the firewall) and type of access, such as e-mail or telnet. More complex firewalls (**application level gateways**) authenticate outside users, using tokens or some other electronic device carried by an authorized person; encrypt data and conduct encrypted conversations with other firewalls; limit access to a specific set of IP addresses; filter traffic based on the content of the message (e.g., block any message containing the words "secret" or "confidential"; and create user logs and audit trails.

## *Legal Protection of Information on the Internet*

The **Health Insurance Portability and Accountability Act** (HIPAA) of 1996 (PL 104- 191, the "Kennedy/Kassebaum law") contains important provisions relating to patient privacy and electronic communication of medical-related information, including over the Internet or an intranet. This Act is implemented by the Health Care Financing Administration (HCFA).

**Standards for Privacy of Individually Identifiable Health Information** (45 C.F.R. Parts 160–164), pursuant to Sec. 264, HIPAA (Summary prepared by the Joint Healthcare Information Technology Alliance[3]), are intended to protect the privacy of individually identifiable health information maintained

or transmitted electronically in connection with certain administrative transactions or maintained in a computer system.

## Information Protected

Information that relates to an individual's health, healthcare treatment, or
payment for health care and that identifies the individual is protected from
the time it becomes electronic, either by being sent electronically as one of
the specified administrative simplification transactions or by being maintained in a computer system. This protection continues as long as the data is
in the hands of a covered entity. Paper versions of the information, such as
computer printouts, are also protected.

Covered entities are encouraged to create deidentified health information by
removing, encoding, encrypting, or otherwise concealing 19 potential identifiers, including name, address, health plan number, zip code, and so on. An alternative method of deidentification is permitted to entities with appropriate statistical
experience and expertise that can certify that the chance of reidentification of
data is low. Deidentified data can be used and disclosed freely.

## Covered Entities

Provisions of the proposed regulation apply to healthcare providers who transmit
data electronically, health plans, and healthcare clearinghouses. Covered entities may disclose identifiable health information to contractors and business
partners, including auditors, consultants, claims clearinghouses, and billing firms,
for the performance of specific functions. Except when the business partner is
providing a referral or treatment consultation, the covered entity must enter into
a contract requiring that identifiable health information be kept confidential.

Because HIPAA does not provide authority to regulate directly many of
these business partners, this contracting requirement is meant to extend the
reach of the regulation. Business partners would not be permitted to use or
disclose health information in ways that the covered entity could not.

## Individual Rights

Individuals would have the following rights:

- The right to receive a written notice of information practices from health
  plans and providers. (This notice must detail the types of uses and
  disclosures the plan or provider will make with protected health
  information.)
- The right to access their own health information, including a right to
  inspect and obtain a copy of the information.
- The right to request amendment or correction of protected health
  information that is inaccurate or incomplete.
- The right to receive an accounting (audit trail) of instances when protected

health information has been disclosed for purposes other than treatment, payment, and healthcare operations. (Healthcare operations include activities such as quality assurance, utilization review, credentialing, insurance rating for individuals enrolled in a health plan, and other activities related to ensuring appropriate treatment and payment for care. It does not include marketing or the sale of protected health information.)

**Obligations of Healthcare Providers and Plans**

Following are the requirements for healthcare providers and plans.

- Develop a notice of information practices. Providers would provide this notice to each patient at the first service after the effective date of the rule, and they would post a copy of the notice. Plans would provide the notice at enrollment and at least every three years thereafter.
- Permit individuals to inspect and copy their protected health information at reasonable, cost-based copying fees.
- Develop a mechanism for accounting for all disclosures of protected health information for purposes other than treatment, payment, and healthcare operations.
- Permit individuals to request amendments or corrections to their protected health information. Such requests would be accommodated if information created by the provider or plan were determined to be erroneous or incomplete.
- Designate a privacy officer who will be responsible for all necessary activities.
- Provide training to all staff or others who would have access to protected health information in the entity's policies and procedures regarding privacy.
- Establish administrative, technical, and physical safeguards to protect identifiable health information from unauthorized access or use.
- Establish policies and procedures to allow individuals to complain about possible violations of privacy.
- Develop and apply sanctions, ranging from retraining to reprimand and termination, for employee violation of entity privacy policies.
- Have available documentation regarding compliance with the requirements of the regulation.
- Develop methods for disclosing only the minimum amount of protected information necessary to accomplish any intended purpose.
- Develop and use contracts that will ensure that business partners also protect the privacy of identifiable health information.
- Be prepared to respond to requests for protected health information that do not require consent, such as for public health, health oversight, and judicial activities. Entities must have reasonable procedures for verifying the identity and authority of persons requesting such disclosures.

## Disclosures Without Patient Authorization

Covered entities could use and disclose protected health information without patient authorization for purposes of effecting treatment, payment, and healthcare operations. Individuals must be informed of the right to request restrictions concerning the use of protected health information for treatment, payment, or healthcare operations. The rule does not require a covered entity to agree to such an "opt out", but the entity is bound by any restrictions it agrees to. Under specific conditions, covered entities are permitted to disclose protected health information for federal, state, and other health oversight activities; for public health activities and emergencies; for judicial and administrative proceedings; to a law enforcement official with a warrant or subpoena; to next of kin; to coroners and medical examiners; for government health data systems; for purposes of hospital and other facility directory listings; for certain banking and payment processes; and for health research.

Extending the reach of the "common rule," the regulation requires that disclosure of protected health information without patient authorization for research, regardless of funding source, be approved by an IRB or equivalent privacy board. Beyond the existing criteria of the common rule, IRB review must include judgments that the use of protected health information is permissible for the following reasons:

1. The research would be impractical to conduct without it.
2. The research is of sufficient importance to outweigh the intrusion into individual privacy.
3. There is an adequate plan to protect identifiers from improper use or disclosure.
4. There is a plan to destroy identifiers at the earliest opportunity.

## Uses and Disclosures with Patient Authorization

Covered entities could use or disclose protected health information with the individual's consent for lawful purposes. If an authorization permits the covered entity to sell or barter information, that fact would have to be disclosed on the authorization form. Authorizations must specify the information to be disclosed, who would receive the information, and when the authorization would expire. Individuals could revoke an authorization at any time.

Covered entities would be prohibited from making treatment or payment conditional on an individual's agreeing to authorize disclosure of information for other purposes.

## Minimum Necessary Use and Disclosure

With or without patient authorization, the rule requires covered entities to make all reasonable efforts not to use or disclose "more than the minimum amount of protected health information necessary to accomplish the intended purpose of the use or disclosure, taking into consideration practical and technological limitations."

## Scalability

The Department of Health and Human Services (HHS) intends that these new privacy standards be flexible and scalable, taking into account each covered entity's size and resources. Thus, each entity is expected to assess its own needs and implement privacy policies and procedures appropriate to its business requirements.

## Costs

HHS estimates the five-year cost of compliance for covered entities as at least $3.8 billion. This estimate includes development of policies and procedures; issuing notices to patients; providing for inspection, copying, and amendment of records; development and implementation of authorizations; and paperwork and training. Not estimated are the costs of developing mechanisms for "minimum necessary disclosure," internal complaint processes, sanctions, compliance and enforcement, and additional requirements for research.

## Enforcement

For each provision violated, the Secretary of HHS can impose a penalty of up to $25,000 in any calendar year. Criminal penalties include fines of up to $50,000 for violations of the privacy regulation, even more if an action involves "malicious harm" or selling data for commercial advantage. The regulation does not include a "private right of action"; that is, patients cannot sue entities for privacy violations.

## Preemption

The regulation establishes a "floor" of privacy protections. State laws that are "less protective" of privacy are preempted, but states are free to enact "more stringent" statutes or regulations.

HCFA has no jurisdiction over many of the entities that are considered "business partners" of covered entities. It asserts control by pass-through; that is, it holds covered entities responsible for the actions of business partners. This means that hospitals, as originators of an individual's medical data, are responsible for certifying that any business partners with whom they share data (including insurance companies, bill collectors, researchers, and state and local government agencies) comply with security and privacy regulations, all of which have not as yet been issued. Compliance may not be workable.

Certain clauses in the rules, specifically "in the public interest," have been questioned as providing a window for abuse of privacy. Cited are employers, healthcare researchers (including pharmaceutical companies that fund research), federal, state, and local governments, and law enforcement personnel, any or all of whom could make a plausible case of acting "in the public interest".[4]

## Security Considerations for the Internet

The Internet poses its own set of security issues. The U.S. Health Care Financing Administration (HCFA) has issued a detailed Internet Security Policy,[5] which covers Internet communications security and appropriate use policy and guidelines for HCFA Privacy Act-protected and other sensitive HCFA information. Since this agency of the federal government asserts authority over many areas of medical services, it is worth citing the essential points of its policy. The policy is issued under the authority of the Privacy Act of 1974, which mandates that federal information systems protect the confidentiality of individually identifiable data. The act requires (Sec. 5, U.S.C, §552a(e)(10)) that federal systems "establish appropriate administrative, technical, and physical safeguards to insure the security and confidentiality of records and to protect against any anticipated threats or hazards to their security or integrity which could result in substantial harm, embarrassment, inconvenience, or unfairness to any individual on whom information is maintained." This is HCFA's responsibility, which applies to contractors acting as HCFA agents. This means that it flows through state agencies or other government organizations acting as contractors, as well as any other entity authorized access to HCFA information resources.

"HCFA Privacy Act-protected and other sensitive HCFA information" is held to mean data that, if disclosed, could result in harm to the agency or individual persons, including individually identifiable data held in systems of records, information used to authorize or make cash payments to organizations or individuals, proprietary information, and sensitive or critical correspondence that must not be altered or disclosed without authorization. The policy covers all systems or processes that use the Internet or interface with the Internet, but it applies to Internet transmission data only. The essential features of the applied methodology include proper identification of users (authentication or identification) and encryption. In addition, the system must incorporate effective password/key management systems.

**Authentication** refers to generally automated and formalized methods of establishing the authorized nature of a communications partner over the Internet communications channel itself, generally called an "in-band" process. Authentication approaches include formal certificate authority, based on use of digital certificates, locally managed digital certificates, self-authentication by the use of symmetric private keys, and tokens or "smart cards."

A digital certificate is an electronic file issued by a trusted third party, the *certificate authority*. Digital certificates are based on public/private key technology. Each key is a unique encryption device, and no two keys are identical. This uniqueness allows positive identification of the owner. They are tamper-proof and cannot be forged. Digital certificates do two things. They authenticate that a holder (person, Web site, router, and so on) is who it claims to be. Also, they protect data exchanged on line from tampering or theft. Certificates may be personal, identifying an individual, or they may identify a server. Server certificates identify a particular Web site, permitting an organization to accept personal information, such as medical or other personal information, credit card numbers, and so on, free from interception or tampering by encrypting transmitted data.

A symmetric private key (secret key) is a single key used to both encrypt and decrypt a message. An asymmetric key system has one "public" key used for encryption and a secret key for decryption, held only by the intended recipient. The holder of the private key distributes public keys to anyone wishing to communicate with him. Only the private key can decode the message encrypted by the public key. A "smart card" is a credit card-like device with a built-in microprocessor and memory used for identification.

**Identification** refers to less formal methods of establishing the authorized nature of a communications partner, which are usually manual, involve human interaction, and do not use the Internet data channel itself but another "out-of-band" path such as the telephone or postal service. Acceptable identification approaches include telephone identification of users and/or password exchange by telephone, Certified Mail, or bonded messenger; personal contact exchange of identities or passwords; and tokens or "smart cards."

As of November 1998, the minimally acceptable encryption system was specified as providing protection equivalent to that provided by an algorithm such as triple 56-bit DES (defined as 12-bit equivalent) for symmetric encryption, 1024-bit algorithms for asymmetric systems, and 160 bits for the elliptical curve systems. Encryption may be based on hardware, using private key devices, or on software, which may employ one of several approaches, including off-line systems that encrypt and decrypt files before entering the data communications process; in-stream systems such as agreed-on passwords, and standard commercial systems that involve the transport layer or the e-mail layer.[5]

Anyone attempting to use the Internet for the transmission of information covered under this policy must have a security plan and be prepared for audit. HCFA must be notified of intent to use the Internet.

# E-Mail Communication of Health Information

Increasingly, patients and doctors communicate by e-mail. It is fast and efficient, and the patient may feel that the doctor is more accessible by e-mail than by telephone. Because e-mail is neither very private nor secure, no communications intended to be private should be sent by e-mail. Criteria for e-mail messages must be set, and the patient should be required to give informed consent for e-mail to be used, even if the patient is the initiator. The University of Texas Medical Branch has established an e-mail policy for doctor/patient communications that is cited here as an example of permissible and nonpermissible uses. The following topics are appropriate for e-mail communication:

• Prescription refills
• Scheduling appointments
• Confirming appointments
• Laboratory test results
• Medical advice and request for additional health information
• Clarification of treatment plans
• Authorization for release of medical records

Certain topics, such as discussion of HIV status, workmen's compensation claims, psychiatric disorders, and urgent matters, are not appropriate for e-mail communication.

# Computer Viruses

"Security" encompasses the preservation of the integrity of information as well as privacy. A computer **virus** is a program written to insert itself into an existing program and, when activated by execution of the "infected" program, to replicate and attach copies of itself to other programs in the system. Infected programs copy the virus to other programs. The writer of the virus may mean to play a harmless prank, such as popping up a message, or to actively destroy programs and data. In either case, the best that can be said for it is that it is malicious mischief, and the worst that it is under some circumstances a criminal offense. The economic impact of viruses is great. One computer consulting firm (Computer Economics, Carlsbad, California) estimates that virus attacks cost businesses around the world $12 billion in 1999. These losses result from lost productivity, network downtime, and the expense of getting rid of the virus. A survey conducted by *Information Security* magazine found that 77% of information technology managers regarded viruses as their number-one problem.

A virus is attached to an executable program that is downloaded from a network or incorporated into shareware or to programs passed from one computer user to another, often written by amateurs but sometimes commercially distributed. Most viruses are passed by the sharing of infected floppy disks, often associated with pirated software, such as games. It has not been common for infection to come from networks, as networks typically contain detection and cleanup programs. Read-only programs can be infected on hard drives or floppy disks that are not write-protected, since the read-only function is controlled by the operating system. Virus infection of the operating system may allow access to read-only files. CD-ROMs are read-only, as are write-protected floppy disks, and cannot be infected.

A virus must be attached to a program that has to be executed to activate the virus program. Most older viruses cannot be attached to data files; however, a relatively new group, the **macro viruses,** can. Macro viruses appear to be targeted at Microsoft word processor and spreadsheet programs.

Recently, delivery of viruses has begun to change. E-mail systems have been clogged by viruses. In the past, viruses were spread via attachments, and the e-mail itself was considered safe, but a new virus, "Bubbleboy," was activated by opening infected e-mail. Earlier viruses were designed to attack operating systems. Current viruses are more directed at applications, which may help them escape various filters placed on networks. The latest way of delivering a virus is to attach it to downloadable music files.

Several kinds of viruses are recognized under a variety of names. Some are intended to permeate a program subtly, eventually having its effect. A **worm,** in this context, is a destructive program that replicates itself throughout disk and memory, using up the computer's resources, eventually causing the system to fail. A polymorphic or **stealth virus** is one that changes its binary pattern each time it infects a new file to keep it from being identified. A **logic bomb** is a program intended to destroy data immediately. In contrast to a virus, it may insert random bits of data into files, corrupting them, or it may initiate a reformatting of a hard drive.

To understand the way in which viruses affect programs, it is helpful to know a few elements of the structure of programs and storage strategies. A **header** is the first record in a file, used for identification. It includes the file name, date of last update and other status data. A **partition** is a part of a disk reserved for some special purpose. A **boot sector** is the area on a disk, usually the first sectors in the first disk partition, used to store the operating system. When the computer is started up, it searches the boot sectors for the operating system, which must be loaded into memory before any program can be run.

Viruses can be grouped into several classes based on the specific point of attack or mode of action. An **executable virus** is one that attaches itself to the file's header, located at the end of an EXE file or the beginning of a COM file. The virus corrupts the header, either changing the command that initiates the program or simply preventing it from working. A **partition table virus** either moves or destroys the computer's partition table information and loads the virus code in place of the partition table. A **boot- sector virus** overwrites the sector with bad information, preventing the computer from booting.

Various antivirus detection and cleaning programs have been developed to remove these viruses. Since the virus is located in a particular part of the disk, it is relatively easy to detect. **Memory resident viruses** avoid detection by placing their code in different areas of memory, to be activated when an application program is launched. Depending on the location of the virus it may cause problems ranging from annoying messages to system crash. Viruses hidden in the COMMAND.COM region frequently cause crashes. To hide out in the disk, in essence masquerade as application code or data, the virus may occupy unallocated space; that is, space the computer has not assigned to data. In these instances, the virus code stands a good chance of being overwritten. Some viruses are hidden in the upper part of resident memory, near the 640K limit; others are hidden in video card buffers.

A Trojan horse is, as the name implies, a program designed to be attractive to a potential victim; it may represent a game or some desired application. The target voluntarily takes the Trojan horse into his system. The application is just a cover for the "real" program, which is designed not to wreck the host system, which it may do, but to cause it to respond to the attacker, perhaps by transmitting passwords, the content of files, and various other information out of the system.

Reliance on e-mail communication has become a fact of life in many if not most enterprises. This evolution is itself vulnerable to attack. A **denial-of-service attack** is one in which a mail server or Web server is deliberately overloaded with (usually computer generated) phony communications to prevent it from responding to valid ones. A line of defense is to identify the IP address of the sender and refuse to accept any communication from that address. A **distributed denial-of-service attack** is one in which the attacker recruits a large number of machines, often using Trojan horses, requiring the target to block a very large number of IP addresses, thus interfering with the very purpose of e-mail in an organization that depends on rapid communication with clients.

To summarize:

- Viruses are passed by people sharing infected floppy disks containing games and other passed-around software. Some are acquired by downloading files from the Net or from bulletin board services (BBSs).
- Viruses can infect data files as well as EXE and COM files.
- Viruses are contained in programs and files that are loaded into your computer. They are not (at least currently) acquired by viewing or connecting to the Net.
- Viruses cannot infect read-only files on a CD or a write-protected disk.
- Viruses can infect programs flagged read-only on a hard drive or a floppy disk, since a virus infecting an operating system can turn read-only flags off.
- "Weird things" like letters sliding down the screen or intrusive messages are probably virus induced; however, most computer malfunctions are not virus related.
- Rarely, viruses have been acquired from retail commercial software.

Avoiding virus infection is a matter of using only virus-scanned applications and avoiding use of pirated software. The best protection is to use a frequently updated virus scanning program, such as (but not limited to) F-Prot, Norton Anti-Virus, Central Point Anti-Virus or McAfee Scan. Given the rate at which viruses are introduced, estimated at three per day, scanners must be frequently updated. A scanner more than a few months old may offer no real protection against the current crop of viruses.

Preventive measures for the individual user include the following:

- Run only virus-scanned applications. Lock up the computer and disks when not in use.
- Boot only from write-protected, virus-scanned disks.
- Scan frequently for viruses using an updated scanner.
- Write-protect stored floppy disks.
- Scan every disk that has been run in someone else's machine before running it in yours.
- Flag and set file attributes of EXE and COM files to be read-only and execute-only.
- Back up files frequently, and back up in more than one way (e.g., to a server and to a floppy)
- Make and keep handy a bootable, write-protected disk containing the scan program.

# WEB Crackers

Not every person who seeks unauthorized access to computer systems does it with intent to violate patient privacy, insert viruses, or otherwise destroy files. With the Web have come Web crackers, people who seek to gain personal entry into a system or Web site rather than send in a virus. There appear to be three broad groups of Web crackers. One, who may be likened to adolescent graffiti "artists," is a vandal who seems content to strew obscenities and otherwise deface a Web site. These people are not necessarily very expert, but they can nevertheless cause considerable damage and expense to the owners of the sites. Others, who may command a high level of expertise, aim higher and attempt to enter high-security sites as a demonstration of prowess, not doing any particular damage except perhaps to leave some evidence behind as a sort of signature. Their reward seems to be the approbation of their peers. Crackers in the third group appear to be motivated by greed or malice or both; their aim may be to convert or transfer assets, steal credit card numbers, steal or destroy business files, or the like. These individuals may not want their presence known at all. There would seem to be little point in any of these crackers working to gain access to clinical laboratory computer systems. Unlike public sites, there would be little exposure for the graffitist to display talent, the systems present no challenge to the talented amateur compared with the FBI or Pentagon secure systems, and it is not clear what crackers might gain from destroying or altering patient records or browsing columns of chemistry results. The risk of prosecution for a felony would seem to outweigh any potential for gain. However, one should never underestimate the human potential for mischief, malice, and stupidity, and it is necessary that all people working with systems related to patient care be careful, systematic, and thorough in their approach to system security.

# Chapter Glossary

**authentication:** Generally automated and formalized methods of establishing the authorized nature of a communications partner over the Internet communications channel itself (an "in-band" process); may include formal certificate authority, based on use of digital certificates; locally managed digital certificates; self-authentication by the use of symmetric private keys; and tokens or "smart cards."

**biometrics:** Method of identification based on a physical characteristic, such as a fingerprint, iris pattern, or palm print.

**boot sector:** Area on a disk, usually in the first sectors in the first disk partition, used to store the operating system. When the computer is started up, it searches the boot sectors for the operating system, which must be loaded into memory before any program can be run.

**boot-sector virus:** Virus that overwrites the boot sector with bad information, preventing the computer from booting.

**certificate authority:** Third party providing digital certificates for the purpose of validating a certificate holder's identity.

**cracker; computer cracker:** Person who gains illegal entry into a computer system.

**denial-of-service attack:** E-mail system attack in which a mail server or Web server is deliberately overloaded with (usually computer-generated) phony communications to prevent it from responding to valid ones. A line of defense is to identify the IP address of the sender and refuse to accept any further communication from that address.

**distributed denial-of-service attack:** E-mail system attack in which the attacker recruits a large number of machines, often using Trojan horses, to send false messages, requiring the target to block a very large number of IP addresses.

**digital certificate**: Secret, tamper-proof electronic file issued by a third party, the certificate authority, for the purpose of verifying the identity of the certificate holder. They may permit or restrict access to specific files or information.

**encryption:** Using an algorithm—a conversion of original plain text into a coded equivalent ("ciphertext")—to provide security for transmission over a public network.

**executable virus:** Virus that attaches itself to a file header, located at the end of an EXE file or the beginning of a COM file. The virus corrupts the header, either changing the command that initiates the program or simply preventing it from working.

**firewall:** Network node set up as a boundary to prevent traffic from one segment to cross over into another.

**gateway:** Computer that performs protocol conversion between different types of networks or applications. For example, a gateway can connect a personal computer LAN to a mainframe network. An electronic mail, or messaging, gateway converts messages between two different messaging protocols.

**HIPAA:** Health Insurance Portability and Accountability Act of 1996 (PL 104-191, the "Kennedy/Kassebaum law"). Regulates patient privacy and electronic communication of medical-related information, including over the Internet or an intranet. This act is implemented by the Health Care Financing Administration (HCFA).

**hacker:** Person who writes programs in assembly language or in system-level languages, such as C; term implies very tedious "hacking away" at the bits and bytes. Increasingly, the term is used for people who try to gain illegal entry into a computer system.

**header:** First record in a file, used for identification. It includes the file name, date of last update, and other status data.

**identification:** Methods of establishing the authorized nature of a communications partner, which are usually manual; involve human interaction and use not the Internet data channel itself but another "out-of-band" path such as the telephone or postal service; may include telephone identification of users and/or password exchange by telephone, certified mail, or bonded messenger, personal contact exchange of identities or passwords, and tokens or "smart cards."

**IP** (Internet protocol) address: Part of the TCP/IP used to route a message across networks. It identifies the sender or the recipient.

**key:** Numeric code used by an algorithm to create a code for encrypting data for security purposes.

**logic bomb:** Program virus that is intended to destroy data immediately. In contrast to a virus, it may insert random bits of data into files, corrupting them, or it may initiate a reformatting of a hard drive.

**macro virus:** Virus that can be attached to data files.

**memory resident virus:** Virus that avoids detection by placing its code in different areas of memory, to be activated when an application program is launched.

**packet:** Frame or block of data used for transmission in packet switching and other communications methods.

**partition:** Part of a disk reserved for some special purpose.

**partition table virus:** Virus that either moves or destroys the computer's partition table information and loads the virus code in the place of the partition table.

**public domain software:** Any program that is not copyrighted and can be used without restrictions.

**scalability:** Ability to expand with minimal change in current procedures to accommodate growth.

**security:** Protection of data against unauthorized access.

**security hole:** Point of deficiency in a security system.

**shareware:** Software distributed on a trial basis through BBSs, online services, mail-order vendors, and user groups. A fee is due the owner if the software is used beyond the trial period.

**surge protector:** Device between a computer and a power source used to filter out power surges and spikes. A voltage regulator maintains uniform voltage during a brownout, but a UPS keeps a computer running when there is no electrical power. UPS systems typically provide surge suppression and may also provide voltage regulation.

**stealth virus** (polymorphic virus): Virus that changes its binary pattern each time it infects a new file to keep it from being identified.

**Trojan horse:** Program designed to be attractive to a potential victim who voluntarily takes it into his system. The program is designed to cause the system to respond and cede some level of control to the attacker.

**UPS** (uninterruptable power supply): Alternative power source automatically accessed when primary electrical power fails or drops to an unacceptable voltage level. A battery-based UPS provides power for a few minutes allowing the computer to be powered down (shut off) in an orderly manner.

**virus:** Program written to insert itself into an existing program and, when activated by execution of the "infected" program, to replicate and attach copies of itself to other programs in the system. Infected programs copy the virus to other programs.

**worm:** Destructive program that replicates itself throughout disk and memory, using up the computer's resources and eventually causing the system to fail.

# *References*

1. Barrows, RC Jr, Clayton PD. Privacy, confidentiality, and electronic medical records. J Am Med Inform Assoc 1996; 3:139–148
2. Behlen, FM, Johnson, SB. Multicenter patient records research: Security policies and tools. J Am Med Inform Assoc 1999; 6:435–443
3. Joint Healthcare Information Alliance (JHITA) http://www.jhita.org/hipprs.htm
4. CIO, 2000 CIO Magazine, January; wysiwyg://content/7/http//wwwcio...1/ procedures_sidebar1_content.html
5. HCFA Internet Security Policy, November 24, 1998. Health Care Financing Agency (HCFA), Baltimore, Maryland

# 5
# Total Cost of Ownership

Daniel F. Cowan

It seems to be well known that a computer-based information system is costly to acquire. Less well understood are the costs associated with maintaining and operating a system over time. Several large laboratory information system vendors had no ready answer, even in general terms, to the question "Do you offer any advice to potential clients about the costs of ownership of your system?" This is not very surprising, as even large, computer-dependent industries often have only the vaguest notion of the true costs of ownership of their systems. According to one estimate, each Microsoft NT workstation typically costs an organization $6,515 per desktop per year,[1] of which capital hardware and software costs account for only 25%. Some of the remaining 75% of costs, which may be overt or hidden, are associated with management and technology support.[1] The Gartner Group, a consulting firm, says that the five-year cost of a personal computer is $44,250.[2] Vendors not are generally expected to provide much information about cost of ownership beyond the services they provide under contract, as costs are mainly related to how owners choose to use and support their system rather than to any particular computer characteristic.

**Total cost of ownership** (TCO) is an accounting method or model used to understand and control computing costs while maintaining the productivity of the information system throughout its life. There is surprisingly little written about TCO in comparison to other management issues, especially as they relate to the laboratory. Most discussions of TCO focus on the computer itself, in particular the desktop workstation and network. This approach seriously underestimates the TCO of a functioning laboratory information system, so the discussion that follows goes considerably beyond those limits. TCO should be understood to encompass all costs of owning and operating an LIS. By collection and organization of fiscal data, the manager of a computer-supported information system is enabled to understand and control the direct (budgeted) and indirect (unbudgeted) costs incurred by owning and operating it. All costs of acquisition and operation are determined for the system throughout its life span. Assessing TCO is an important function of system management, the more so as information systems are increasingly based on networks, and a progressive shift toward complex client/server systems is taking place. The fundamental questions are "Where does all the money go?" and "Are we getting a reasonable added value for dollars spent?"

System managers must be able to proactively monitor and maintain all the hardware, software, and peripheral devices in the technology that supports the information system, as well as identify personnel and other costs of operation needed to produce the information product. This task has become much more complex since the time when systems were based on inflexible host mainframes and dumb terminals. Relatively little continuing oversight was needed, as the mainframe and its dumb devices was what it was, with little opportunity and typically little need for "management." This means not that owning a mainframe is cheap but that the costs, which are high, are generally easily recognized. The idea of TCO, of course, contains a certain element of fantasy, as operating costs can never be predicted with certainty; they can only be estimated based on experience. Few business operations do analysis in the depth needed to understand TCO, and analytical tools are not well developed, although several workstation and network management software products have appeared on the market. Many of the more important considerations, such as access to professional services, vendor's market position, service-level agreements and availability of applications, as well as other intangibles like effect of innovation on consumer satisfaction, are not really quantifiable.

It is also important to recognize and accept the mind-set that the information system is a business-driven activity, not primarily a technology function. That is, all decisions made by IS managers must be based primarily on the needs of the business the information system serves, not on the desires of the technical staff to be state-of-the-art. The ability to relate IS activity directly to business and service needs greatly improves the IS group's ability to compete for capital and personnel resources in the enterprise. Also, seeing the information system as an integral component of an enterprise's success tends to shift focus from the cost of the system to the comprehensive and long-term value added by it. From a business perspective, in the long run it doesn't matter much if the system costs a lot so long as the value it adds substantially exceeds its cost. In hospitals and laboratories however, in which operating margins are narrower and narrower and capital resources increasingly constrained, close scrutiny of costs and recognition of opportunities for improved efficiency will always be an important issue.

# Types of Costs

## Direct and Indirect Costs

Understanding direct costs ought to be relatively simple, as they tend to be specified in budgets. However, the budgets may not accurately reflect inventory, personnel costs, and items such as repair rates. One suggested model[1] for identifying direct costs uses five categories:

- Hardware and software, including capital purchases and lease fees
- Management (network, system, and storage administration, labor and outsourcing fees, management tasks
- Support (help desk, training, purchasing, travel, maintenance contracts, overhead)
- Development and customization
- Communications fees (lease lines, server access)

The Gartner Group's analytical model,[2] accepted by many as the industry standard uses four categories:

- Capital costs
- Administrative costs
- Technical support
- User operations

Each of these categories is further divided into discrete cost items, with information provided by clients and by the group's own research.

Indirect costs are much harder to quantify than direct costs, as they are not budgeted in ways attributable to an information system or may not be budgetable at all. They include costs incurred by users who do their own support or provide help or advice to peers, time spent learning applications, and unauthorized time spent playing games, surfing the Internet, and so on. Productivity lost to either scheduled or unscheduled downtime is also an unaccountable indirect cost. It is important to understand that since they are unaccounted for, indirect costs tend to grow with little or no control. It is reported[1] that more than 50% of cost growth is off the formal IS budget. It is also important to understand that excessive and ill-advised efforts to control budgeted costs by reducing support services will surely result in an increase in indirect costs, as users spend more and more time trying to support themselves, probably not nearly as well and efficiently as a professional support group could. One study suggests that budgets for hardware exceed budgets for support by 4 to 1,[3] while the real life cycle cost of a personal computer in a business operation is closer to 10 times its purchase price.[4] Productivity lost to downtime will also increase as IS management and support personnel become increasingly overextended.

While TCO is a relatively recent introduction, applied mainly to personal or desktop computers and their network linkages, the ideas incorporated into the cost analysis can be applied to mainframe-centered systems as well. It is almost immaterial whether the LIS is based on a mainframe and terminals, or is a complex mix of servers, personal computers, and networks. TCO thinking is applied mainly to systems already in operation. A more global approach to TCO suitable for the laboratory includes three categories: selection, purchase and installation, and operation. Few laboratories are still not computerized to some degree, so selection from scratch is increasingly unusual. However, selection processes might apply in a computerized laboratory considering major system revisions, such as changing vendors, integrating several laboratories, or other, nonroutine operations that involve the participation of nonmembers of the LIS staff who can be considered fixed costs of operation.

Attribution of costs depends on the philosophy of the larger organization. For example, it makes sense for all computerization projects, no matter which part of the organization is involved, to be allocated against an institutional information services cost center. It makes equal sense to allocate all costs of laboratory computerization to the laboratory. So long as the issues of decision and control are not involved, it really makes no difference where on the ledgers the costs appear. Some aspects of laboratory computerization—for example, cabling—may be allocated to institutional IS, as the cables may carry traffic for other services, such as radiology and pharmacy, while others that are more function-specific might be allocated to the laboratory. Cost shifting is common, although cost shifting is of course not cost avoidance, a point that may not be appreciated at the lower levels of an organization.

## Selection

The costs of selection include the salaries of the people who devote time to the process of identification of potential vendors; preparation of RFI and RFP and the evaluation of vendor responses; the time devoted to preparation for meetings and participation in meetings, meetings with vendors; and travel for site visits (fares, hotel and subsistence, hours spent). The process of in-depth review of laboratory operations has been described earlier (see Chapter 2). This kind of review should be done periodically, whether or not an LIS is in development, as laboratory missions and resources evolve. It may be convenient to allocate all or part of these costs of review to the development of an LIS. A relatively simple method for determining these costs is to have all participants keep time logs of all activities relating to system selection and multiply hours spent by salary per hour. Typically, these salary costs far exceed costs of travel and other expenses. Some institutions employ a consultant to help plan the selection process, develop the RFP, evaluate responses, and construct and negotiate the contract. Consultants may be retained for the selection period at a flat rate or, more commonly, at an hourly rate, with compensation for all expenses incurred. Rates begin at about $200 an hour. The selection phase of the process is completed on the signing of a purchase agreement.

Recognizing that the most costly aspect of the selection process is the accumulated hours of time spent examining laboratory operations and identifying and studying the offerings of potential vendors, it seems reasonable to involve only a few people in it. This could be a serious mistake, as few in the laboratory and certainly no one outside the laboratory have both the breadth of vision and the depth of detailed knowledge needed to properly study laboratory operations and identify vendors who can best meet the needs of the laboratory. These studies have to be inclusive, not only because of the amount of knowledge and experience that must be brought to bear on the problem but also to foster a broad sense of "ownership" of the computerization project. There is too much disruption, too much work, and too much aggravation involved in computerization for the laboratory staff to feel that something has been foisted off on them by people who don't understand laboratory operations. Certainly administration has the legal authority to make decisions with little input from the people most affected, but the distinction between that which is legal and that which is accepted as legitimate is an important one. It can mean the difference between success and failure of the project.

The problem, then, is not whether to be inclusive or not but rather how to manage meetings, organize information flow, and provide appropriate staff support for the participants. All meetings should be called for specific reasons, follow set agendas, be held to scheduled times, and be properly minuted. All opinions must be considered, but rambling monologues should be controlled. During the course of the study and selection process, certain individuals will emerge as leaders; some will prove to have a knack for the particular logical approach needed for the details of computerization. These are the people who are prime candidates for a site visit team and for future membership on the LIS staff.

## Purchase and Installation

Purchase and installation costs include the price of the hardware, which becomes the property of the purchaser as a capital asset; preparation of the location in which the computer is to be placed and wiring of the facility, which include labor costs both inside and outside the laboratory; training of the staff; development of tables and other applications functions; and instrument interfaces. Installation costs may recur if new analytical instruments requiring new interfaces are brought into the laboratory. After the initial setup period new instrument interfaces can be thought of as either extended installation costs, as part of the capital cost of the new instrument, or as part of continuing operations, as suits laboratory management.

While the hardware devices become the property of the laboratory, operating systems and applications software remain the property of the vendors who permit use in return for licensing fees. Fee structures vary with vendors, but a common arrangement is for there to be an initial licensing fee, with continuing maintenance charges, which may come due monthly, quarterly, or annually, depending on the terms of the contract. Maintenance includes periodic modifications or upgrades of the performance of the applications and vendor support in the event of a problem with the hardware or software. License and maintenance fees may be scaled to reflect such features as the volume of the laboratory, the number of peripheral devices supported, the number of service sites, and other components of use. These are all specified in the initial contract, so some estimation, often quite accurate, can be made.

Actual installation requires many hours of time from laboratory personnel and vendor engineers alike. Vendor charges for installation may be a single package cost or may be calculated by the hour; the charges, of course should be defined in the contract.

Development of SOPs (operations, validation, applications, and so on) was discussed in Chapter 3. In a large, complex laboratory, upwards of 100 LIS-related SOPs are needed to cover installation, validation, and operations both in the central LIS area and in the laboratory. Time logs may be helpful in calculating the cost of production of SOPs.

Training is an essential component of the operation of an information system. If training is deficient, things will not work right, and therefore it is a false economy to underfund training. Exactly how much training will be needed by each employee depends entirely on the complexity of the work the employee does on the LIS and the frequency with which equipment and operating procedures are changed. Training costs should be budgeted up front. If they are not, they will be incurred as indirect costs of self-instruction, peer support, and inefficiency.

## Operation

Operation of the laboratory information system requires a dedicated staff, a budget for maintenance and operations, and capital costs. Organization of the LIS-related staff can vary widely depending on management philosophy. Some laboratories have all LIS-related people in a separate division; others keep the central group small by design. The central group works on system issues. Laboratory section-specific operations may be the purview of specially trained technologists (sometimes called database coordinators) who work in the specific laboratory sections. The philosophy here is that people who are closest to the work understand it better and will therefore support it better. Also, time not spent on specifically LIS issues can be used in other division-related business. A technologist's time can be allocated for budget purposes between LIS and the division, depending on actual hours worked.

Unlike selection, purchase, and installation costs, operational costs continue throughout the life of the information system. In general, operating costs include the salaries of the information system staff, maintenance fees, office supplies, utilities, paper and electronic media, and replacement, repair, or upgrade of equipment. In many businesses and industries, the cost of warding off or repairing the damage done by crackers is a significant, if unbudgeted, expense. Also, an educational program for laboratory staff must be planned and carried out, and the LIS staff must have their skills maintained. Typically, this means either bringing in vendor trainers to conduct classes or laboratory staff traveling to the vendor's training site. In either case, travel costs (time, transportation, maintenance) must be included. All these costs are budgeted and readily accountable.

# Ways to Manage TCO

It is important to keep a broad view when managing TCO. Remember that the TCO is the total of all costs, direct and hidden, associated with the information asset over its life cycle. If a broad view is held, it will become easier to recognize that shifting costs from one center to another usually does not result in savings; indeed, it may require additional outlay of money, time, or effort. Develop an asset management program.[4] As far as possible, recognize costs and build them into the budget. Be attentive to four issues:

**Know** what you have. Develop and maintain an inventory of all hardware and all applications software. Understand who is doing what. Identify which assets are owned, which leased. Determine what is being used and how it is being used.

**Understand** how information assets are being managed, and plan for improvement. Be able to predict what will be needed and when.

**Determine** which assets must be tracked, and decide which are not worth the cost of tracking them. Develop a multiyear asset replacement plan.

**Identify** sources of potential savings. Avoid paying for things that are not used, and don't overpay for things of marginal value. Compare the costs of service contracts with the cost of in-house support.

Details follow.

## *Standardize*

Limit the system to machines and software from as few vendors as possible to take advantage of economies inherent in standardization. This allows support staff to concentrate in depth on a few items rather than maintain a shallow acquaintance with a large number of items. Require all vendors to follow industry standards for hardware, software, and communications devices. Several vendors provide management tools. Simple Network Management Protocol (SNMP) is one widely used network monitoring and control protocol. In the SNMP, protocol data is passed from hardware and/or software processes (SNMP agents) that report activity in each network device (hub, router, bridge, and so on) to the workstation console used to oversee the network. This information is captured in a management information base (MIB), a data structure that defines what can be obtained from the device and which processes can be controlled, e.g., turned on or off. Microsoft offers a product, SMS, with many of the same functions as SNMP.

Desktop Management Interface, or DMI, is a management system for microcomputers initiated by Intel that provides a bidirectional path to interrogate all the hardware and software components within a computer system. A memory-resident agent works in the background. The agent responds to queries by sending back data contained in management information files (MIF) or by activating MIF routines. Static information in an MIF includes items such as model and serial number, memory, and port addresses. Active MIF routines can report errors to the management console as they occur or report on the content of ROM or RAM chips.

While DMI is designed to be a complete management system, it can work with SNMP and other management protocols. DMI can be used to fill and update an SNMP MIB with data from its MIF. A single work station or server can contain the SNMP module and service an entire LAN segment of DMI machines. One very practical and cost-avoiding feature of a system in which all microcomputer components are DMI enabled is the ease of adding new devices such as adapters and controllers. DMI-enabled devices can report their status and conflicts can be identified on installation.

One important way costs may be reduced is to identify a standard software load—a group of programs used throughout the operation that can be collated to a CD for simplified loading. The initial software load can be followed up by an automated upgrade system. Application installation managers keep all users at the same upgrade level automatically. Whenever a workstation is turned on, it goes to the network manager for an automatic download of upgrades. This kind of system works best in an environment in which all participants are supported by the same software. Other strategies have to be developed for persons whose work requires specialized, nonstandard software.

## Maintain and Upgrade

Keep the system components as up to date as possible. Newer machines may be more capable of carrying out tasks and are likely to require less maintenance and repair. Personal computers (microcomputers) should be regarded as disposable devices with a finite, usually short, life expectancy. While they may formally be counted as assets, they really are expense items, equivalent to paper, toner cartridges, and the like, since they have a short life and little or no value when replaced. Electromechanical devices wear out and must be replaced. Using standard releases of software throughout the laboratory simplifies support and reduces the likelihood of incompatibilities.

However, avoid fads, and do not be the first to try something new just because it is available. Do not upgrade any more often then is necessary. If the system is functioning well and business needs are relatively flat, there is little point in accepting the costs of upgrading, as compared to maintaining equipment at the current level. Following are the essential questions:[4]

- What do I need to know about my IT assets to make rational business decisions?
- How am I managing assets, and what can be improved?
- What assets should I track and at what cost?
- What is the payback, and where will savings come from?

The need to keep system components as up to date as possible does not justify using untested technology. The decision to engage with a vendor in developmental work (alpha or beta site testing) should be taken only after careful consideration of time and aggravation costs. An agreement with the vendor about cost sharing and compensation to the laboratory for helping develop a salable product is always in order.

One strategy to consider is leasing all or most of the system's hardware. Leasing has the advantage of assuring upgrades under the contract. It also has the effect of moving hardware from capital budgets to operating budgets, which may be an advantage in a system in which capital dollars are increasingly constrained.

## Plan Support Carefully

Keep the support structure slim by using vendor on-site support programs and by limiting the use of older machines, even if they are capable of carrying out routine tasks. The more standard the machines, the smaller the parts inventory must be and the more expert support staff can be. Use applications software (if not supplied by the primary LIS vendor) for which there is on-line help from the manufacturer. Develop "help desk" functions in order to make contact of support personnel more efficient. Develop a library of help scenarios or algorithms for common problems.

## Systematically Replace Manual Systems

Use software (e.g., relational databases) to replace manual inventory systems, not only of personal computers, other terminal devices, and software but also laboratory equipment and supplies. Electronic inventory systems will relate the cost of ownership of the information system to a wider functionality in laboratory management and can help to reduce costs in other areas of the laboratory. Concentrate cost reduction efforts on the existing installed base of hardware and software, and do not pursue unproven solutions that require fundamental changes in either.

## Maintain Openness

Avoid closed, proprietary single-vendor systems if at all possible, since they tend to lock into narrow solutions and limit choices. When you are locked into a single vendor, you lose bargaining power.

## Exercise Good Routine Business Practices

Build business practices around a management information system that keeps important inventory, contract, warranty, expiration date, and other important information organized and readily accessible. Develop an early warning system that will prevent being taken by surprise, especially by matters such as contract expirations that will take a long time to resolve.

**Identify invoice errors.** Invoice errors are common and may result from changes in the vendor's organization, ownership, or accounting systems. Be especially attentive to fees for software use and maintenance, as they are not matched by the delivery of physical assets.

**Avoid penalties for late payment and for violation of other contract provisions,** such as use of the product beyond the contracted limits. The time for a change of mind is before, not after, a contract is signed.

**Periodically evaluate the vendor's prices and terms of sale.** Special offers may have lapsed, and other vendors may offer a better product at a lower price. Do not allow friendship with a sales representative to influence business decisions.

**Pay close attention to lease expiration dates.** If taken by surprise when a long-term lease expires, one may be faced with high month-by-month payments while processing a renewal.

**Identify underused hardware and software.** Eliminate, replace, or consolidate to achieve more efficient use.

**Do not overpurchase equipment.** Evaluate equipment being replaced for reassignment to a lower-demand use within the department, providing maintenance and support are not major considerations.

**Do not spend time evaluating hardware or software when there is little chance of a purchase within a reasonable time.** Save that effort when actual purchase is pending.

# Justifications Based on Value Added

Laboratory information systems should never be justified as cost-savings devices. There is no convincing evidence that, if properly accounted, computerization of a laboratory will save the hospital money. Jobs that go away in one area because of automation usually reappear somewhere else, usually relating to support of the LIS. Our own LIS operation employs nine people, none of whom were needed in their current jobs before the advent of the system. Computerization is justified on the basis of **value added** to the operation of the institution. More work can be done with the same number of people (improved efficiency, not lower costs). The generation and reporting of laboratory results can be speeded up, effectively limiting the process from the time the specimen arrives in the laboratory to the time the analytical process is completed, eliminating time spent in generating, delivering, and posting paper reports. Data is better organized and more accessible. Consumers of the service are better served. An extremely refined management system can be developed without reliance on large numbers of people doing things by hand.

In summary, the issue is not whether an LIS is cheap, because it is not, but rather whether it is worth what it costs to acquire and to operate.

# Chapter Glossary

**desktop management interface** (DMI): Management system for microcomputers that provides a bidirectional path for interrogating all the hardware and software components within a computer system. A memory-resident agent works in the background. The agent responds to queries by sending back data contained in management information files (MIFs) or by activating MIF routines

**direct costs:** Recognized, budgeted costs of operating an information system. Different models are used. One uses five categories: hardware and software, including capital purchases and lease fees; management (network, system, and storage administration, labor and outsourcing fees, management tasks); support (help desk, training, purchasing, travel, maintenance contracts, overhead); development and customization; and communications fees (lease lines, server access). Another model uses four categories: capital costs; administrative costs; technical support; user operations.

**indirect costs:** Unbudgeted and therefore largely unaccountable costs associated with operation of an information system. They include costs incurred by users who do their own support or provide help or advice to peers, time spent learning applications, and unauthorized time spent, for example, playing games; productivity lost to either scheduled or unscheduled downtime.

**management information base** (MIB): Data structure that defines what can be obtained from a computer or peripheral device and which processes can be controlled; e.g., turned on or off.

**TCO:** Total cost of ownership is the total of all costs, direct and hidden, associated with the information asset over its life cycle.

# *References*

1. Microsoft TechNet document Total Cost of Ownership (TCO) Overview. Feb 1998
2. Hildebrand C. The PC price tag. CIO Magazine, Oct 15, 1997. CIO.com/archive/enterprise/101597_price__content.html
3. Sherry D. The total cost of ownership. Summit OnLine Internet document, 1998 summitonline.com
4. Shoop K. Asset management demystified. Internet document, 1998 supportmanagement.com

# 6
# Computer Basics

Daniel F. Cowan

The computer has become the indispensable instrument in the laboratory. Not only are computers necessary for management and the communication of information, but they are usually the core of analytical instruments. No one can claim to be conversant with the production and communication of information from the clinical laboratory without a basic knowledge of the workings of computers. This discussion is an overview of computer systems, architecture, and programs, first focused on the small microcomputer or "personal computer," then commenting on larger systems and the newer client/server systems. Some of this information will be old to some readers and quite new to others. Bear with us; our objective is to bring all readers to a level of familiarity with computer organization, components, and limitations that will enable them to follow discussions about system selection, integration, and validation, among other topics. Many books have dealt with topics mentioned here in passing, and we do not pretend to be (and feel no obligation to be) comprehensive or exhaustive in this discussion. Topics have been selected for elaboration based on their relevance to computer issues met in the laboratory. The discussion ends with a glossary of terms that must be assimilated if one wishes to follow any discussion of computer systems.

## Definitions and Descriptions

A **computer** is an electromechanical device used to process data according to a set of instructions or **programs** that do particular tasks. The computer and all equipment attached to it are **hardware,** and the programs that tell it what to do are **software.** Computers do three things, all involving data. The computer processes data by performing mathematical calculations with it, by comparing it with known sets of data, and by copying it, that is, moving it around in any order to create a report or listing. The functional components of a computer that support its work are **input, output, processing, storage,** and **control.**

Computers are integrated into **computer systems,** complexes made up of the central processing unit (CPU), the operating system, memory and related electronics, and all the peripheral devices connected to it (such as monitors and printers). A **computer environment** is a computer configuration that includes the CPU model or variation and all system software. A computer environment sets the standards for the applications that run in it. Occasionally the term "environment" refers only to the operating system used in the computer. It may also include the programming language used.

Computer systems generally fall into three classes or size ranges: **microcomputers** (small personal computers), medium-sized **minicomputers,** and large **mainframes.** Very large mainframes with great processing power are called **supercomputers.** A **workstation** is a single-user microcomputer or minicomputer, commonly configured for high performance—that is, specialized for scientific, graphics, or computer-assisted design (CAD) applications. The functional difference among the systems is in the amount of work they do within the same time. Computer power is based on many factors, including word size and the speed of the CPU, memory, and peripherals. This distinction among computer sizes, never very neat, is at best a convenient fiction, as there is considerable overlap in computing capacity, and as innovations appear, functions that once required a mainframe come to be within the capability of a minicomputer, while minicomputer functions migrate to the microcomputer.

Computer systems are configured for the total user workload based on the expected number of simultaneous (concurrent) users, which determines the number of terminals required; the type of work performed; and the amount of data expected to be maintained in active use, or "on line." The design of a system, the **computer architecture,** is based on the expected use of the system—e.g., whether it will be used for business, science, engineering, or graphics—which in turn determines the type of programs that will run and the number of programs that will be run concurrently. Architecture sets the standard for all devices that connect to the computer and all the software that is run on it. It specifies how much memory is needed for tasks and how memory is managed. It specifies register size and bus width and how concurrent use is handled. A **register** is a small, high-speed computer circuit that holds information about internal operations, such as the address of the instruction being executed and the data being processed. An **address** is the location or reference number of a particular memory or peripheral data storage site. Each element of memory and each sector of a magnetic storage disk has a unique address. Programs are compiled into **machine language**, which references actual addresses in the computer. A **bus** is a connection or conduit over which information is passed between computer components. A **clock** is a circuit that generates a series of evenly spaced pulses. All switching activity occurs when the clock is sending out a pulse. The faster the **clock rate,** the more operations per second can be carried out. Clock speeds are expressed as megahertz (MHz), or millions of cycles per second, and gigahertz, billions of cycles per second. The original IBM PC ran at 4.77 MHz. Clock speeds of over 1.5 gigahertz are now routine in microcomputers, even higher in mainframes.

Performance rate or execution speed of a computer is commonly expressed in terms of **millions of instructions per second** (MIPS). Microcomputers and workstations perform in the 20–50 MIPS range. The processor in a minicomputer might perform in the neighborhood of 400 MIPS. MIPS rates are only one aspect of performance, which is influenced by the efficiency with which instructions are implemented. System software, bus and channel speed and bandwidth, and memory speed and memory management techniques also affect performance. Large modern machines may be expected to have execution speeds measured in BIPS (billions of instructions per second).

A computer board, or **printed circuit board,** is a flat board made of reinforced fiberglass or plastic that holds and interconnects chips and other electronic components via copper pathways. The copper circuit, so thin as to appear "printed," is etched in copper foil. To make the circuit, the foil is put on the glass or plastic base and covered with light-sensitive "photoresist," a film used in photolithography. This material hardens when exposed to light and becomes resistant to an acid bath that is used to wash away unexposed areas. A negative image of the designed circuit, which is extremely small and generated by a computer, overlays the foil and its covering photoresist. Light shining through the negative image hardens exposed areas that remain after etching. On washing in acid, the unhardened areas and the underlying foil are removed. The main printed circuit board in a system is called the **system board,** or **motherboard**, while smaller ones that plug into **connector slots** in the motherboard are called **add-on boards,** or **cards**. Cards connect to peripheral devices and may incorporate electronic elements for special purposes, such as increasing memory.

A computer is directly controlled by its native language **instruction set,** the repertoire of machine language instructions that it follows. This set defines what functions the computer performs and how instructions are written to perform them. The instruction set is a major architectural component built into either the CPU or into microcode. It determines how programs will communicate with it in the future.

**Programs** are collections of instructions that tell the computer what to do. Programs are written in a programming language comprehensible to the programmer, and in operation they are converted into a language comprehensible to the machine. This translation from programming language to machine language is done by intermediate programs called assemblers, compilers, and interpreters.

**Assembly language** is a programming language one step away from machine language. Each statement in assembly language is translated into one machine instruction by the assembler. Since a specific assembly language is hardware dependent, each CPU series has its own assembly language.

**Machine language** is the native language of the computer. For a program to run, it must be in the machine language of the computer that is executing it. An **assembler** is a program that translates assembly language into machine language. A **compiler** translates a high-level language into assembly language first and then into machine language. An **interpreter** translates and runs a program at the same time. It translates a program statement into machine language, executes it, then goes to the next statement.

A program uses three components: machine instructions, buffers, and constants and counters. **Machine instructions** are the directions or logic that the computer follows. **Buffers** are reserved space, or input/output (I/O) areas, that accept and hold the data being processed. They receive information needed by the program. **Constants** are fixed values against which data is compared, such as minimums and maximums and dates. **Counters** or variables, are spaces reserved for calculations relating to the work being done and for keeping track of internal operations, e.g., how many times a function is to be repeated.

A typical program accepts data in a reiterating input-process-output sequence. After data has been entered into one of the program's buffers from a peripheral device, such as a keyboard or disk, it is processed. The results are then sent to a peripheral display device—the terminal screen, a printer, or another computer. If data has been changed, it is saved into memory on disk.

Any computing process is an interaction between the **application program**, which does the actual data processing, and the computer's **operating system**, which performs basic functions such as input or output of data, display control, and other routines. All operations of the machine are conducted in **binary code.** Machine instructions vary in length and follow their own logic path. Some instructions cause a sequence of operations, while others (GOTO instructions) refer the process back to the beginning of a routine or to other parts of the program. What may appear to be a very routine task, such as displaying a record, may actually require hundreds of thousands to millions of discrete machine steps.

Programs may reside permanently within the computer, built into its components, or may be installed from a source such as a program disk when they are needed. The computer's ability to call in instructions and follow them is known as the **stored program concept.**

A program that remains in memory at all times is a **resident program**. Certain programs that are used frequently may be brought into RAM (random access memory), closed (terminated), but held in memory so that they can be activated over the application currently in use. These **terminate and stay-resident** (TSR) programs give ready access to such things as dictionaries, calendars, and calculators.

To be followed, program instructions must be copied from a disk or other storage source into **memory,** the computer's working space. The first instruction in the program is copied from memory into the machine's control unit circuit where it is matched against its built-in instruction set. If the instruction is valid, the processor carries it out. If for whatever reason the instruction is not read as valid, the program will not run, and the system may fail to function at all. It may fail by simply locking up, or it may display error messages. The essential point is that the programs must work with the operating system, which may be tied to a particular hardware architecture. For programs to run in a particular machine, the machine must operate in a manner very similar to the machine for which the programs were designed. Proprietary rights do not permit competing manufacturers to produce precisely identical devices, so the focus is on developing products that, while not identical to the reference product, behave in operation as if they were. This similarity in operation is called **compatibility.**

If the initial instruction is read as valid, the computer executes instructions in order until it reaches a branch point, a GOTO instruction that sends it to a different place in the program. In following the program the machine can execute millions of instructions per second, tracing the logic of the program over and over again on each new set of data it brings in. Each single operation may be simple; the great number of instructions to be followed makes for great complexity. Early computers could follow only one set of instructions at a time. Modern computers are able to **multitask**—to follow more than one program at a time. Thus a document may be printed while another is being worked on. Large computers may allow inputs and outputs from different users to be processed simultaneously.

## Bits and Bytes

In a computer, information is represented by the presence or absence of an electrical charge. It is there or it is not. This basic unit is the binary digit, 0 or 1, or **bit.** A bit in a computer is a pulsing voltage in a circuit, a location on a magnetic tape or disk, or in a **memory cell,** the elementary unit of data storage, in a transistor or capacitor. Bits are usually manipulated as groups, such as the **byte,** a group of 8 bits that represent one letter or symbol character, a single decimal digit (0–9), or a binary number from 0 to 255. This system of binary digits is called **binary code.** The byte is the basic unit that can be held in the computer's registers and processed at one time. This fundamental unit of 8 recurs as its multiples in referring to computer power. Thus the designation of machines as 8-bit, 16-bit, or 32-bit indicates progressive processing power. Microcomputers are rated by the number of bits each register can contain. **Bit specifications** are the size of the computer's internal word size or register size, which is the number of bits of data the CPU can work with at the same time. The early Apples and IBM PCs were 8-bit machines. The 80286 processor manufactured by Intel was a 16-bit device. The 80486 is a 32-bit device. If the clock rates and basic architecture are equal, a 32-bit computer works twice as fast internally as a 16-bit computer. The Pentium chip series was introduced by Intel in 1993. The first version of the Pentium chip had 64 I/O pins, meaning that it could move data 8 bytes at a time, and because of other design features, could process two instructions at a time. The Pentium II chip (1996) incorporated design features relating to the way it connects with other components of the computer. The Pentium III, adds new sets of instructions for higher performance.

Use of byte (or megabyte) to refer to both the machine processing capacity and the storage capacity of a disk can result in some confusion for the user. One megabyte of **memory** indicates the ability of a machine to store and process 1 million characters of data or instructions; megabyte applied to a disk simply implies the ability to store 1 million characters of data or instructions. Processing memory, or RAM, is electronic, temporary, fast, and relatively small in capacity, while disk storage is physical, permanent, slow, and great in capacity. Because of the use of 8 rather than 10 as the unit of multiplication, the prefixes kilo-, mega- and giga- do not have precisely their usual values. A **kilobyte** (KB) is 1024 bytes. A **megabyte** (MB) is 1,048,576 bytes, or 1024 KB. A **gigabyte** (GB) is a billion bytes. For perspective, 20 MB is the equivalent of 10,000 typed pages. Therefore, vast amounts of data can be held in storage, while only a fraction of it can be processed at any one time.

## Memory

Computer memory is organized according to a hierarchy: bits, bytes, words, double words, paragraphs, banks, and pages. The **bit** is the basic unit of binary code—1 or 0, on or off. The **byte** is 8 bits, the **word** usually 2 bytes or 16 bits, and the double word 32 bits. A paragraph, in DOS programming, is a 16-byte block of data. Banks may be logical, a 64-KB region of memory, or physical, referring to an arrangement of identical hardware components (memory locations) supplied by chips massed together when reading from one memory location. In virtual memory systems, a page is a segment of the program that is transferred into memory in one operation.

## Codes

The symbols used in communication do not exist inside a computer. What is there is a coded version of them. Since coding takes place in groups of 8, a coding system using a base 10 would be awkward. **Hex** or **hexadecimal** (meaning based on 16) is a numbering system used as a shorthand to represent binary numbers. The hexadecimal system uses the numbers 0–9 and the letters A–F in sequence. Thus A is equivalent to 10, B to 11. Each half byte (4 bits) is assigned a hex digit. Two hex digits make up one byte. The decimal (dec), hex and binary equivalents are as follows:

| Dec | Hex | Binary | Dec | Hex | Binary |
|-----|-----|--------|-----|-----|--------|
| 0 | 0 | 0000 | 8 | 8 | 1000 |
| 1 | 1 | 0001 | 9 | 9 | 1001 |
| 2 | 2 | 0010 | 10 | A | 1010 |
| 3 | 3 | 0011 | 11 | B | 1011 |
| 4 | 4 | 0100 | 12 | C | 1100 |
| 5 | 5 | 0101 | 13 | D | 1101 |
| 6 | 6 | 0110 | 14 | E | 1110 |
| 7 | 7 | 0111 | 15 | F | 1111 |

In a hex number, each digit position is 16 times greater in value than the one to its right.

The **American Standard Code for Information Interchange,** or **ASCII** (pronounced "ask-ee"), is a binary code for data used in communications, all microcomputers, and most minicomputers. ASCII is a 7-bit code providing 128 character combinations, the first 32 of which are control characters. Since the common storage unit is an 8-bit byte providing 256 combinations and ASCII uses only 7 bits, the extra bit is used differently depending on the computer. For example, IBM-compatible microcomputers use the additional bit for graphics and foreign language symbols. In Apple Macintosh machines, the additional values are user-definable.

## *Chips*

The development of the modern computer began with the invention of the **transistor** in 1947 in the Bell Laboratories of the American Telephone & Telegraph Company (AT&T). A transistor is a solid device made of materials that change electrical conductivity when a charge is applied. A transistor is used to open or close a switch or amplify a signal. In its normal state, the transistor is nonconductive. When voltage is applied, it becomes conductive, and a charge can flow. Transistors, diodes, capacitors, and resistors make up **logic gates.** A group of logic gates is a **circuit,** and a group of circuits is a **system.**

Originally, transistors were handled like the vacuum tubes they replaced: each one was soldered individually onto a circuit board that connected it to other transistors, diodes, and resisters. Eventually, a set of interconnected transistors and resistors was placed together on a silicone wafer in a structural unit called a **chip** or **integrated circuit.** Chips were much smaller than the aggregate of transistors they replaced and much more efficient in the speed of transmission of electrical impulses and the power required to operate the chip. The shorter the distance an energy pulse has to travel, the shorter the transit time and the faster the operation. Switch times are measured in trillionths of a second. Chips are made progressively smaller with advances in technology; most are now less than 1/16 to 1/4 inch on a side and less than 1/

30 inch thick. A chip may contain from a few dozen to millions of transistors, resistors, and diodes.

Chips are categorized by function. A **logic chip,** or **processor,** carries out the logical functions of a circuit. An entire processor contained on a single chip is a **microprocessor.** Depending on requirements and size limitations, a computer may contain one or thousands of logic chips. Memory chips come in two basic forms, both of which store memory in storage cells, or **bits.** The essential difference between them is the ability of the chip to store data (as electrical charges) with or without power. **Random access memory** (RAM) chips are working storage, used when computing functions are being carried out. They store charges only when powered. **Read-only memory** (ROM) chips store charges in the absence of power and thus can retain memory in the form of programmed routines. ROM are chips usually programmed at the time of manufacture and cannot be changed by the user; hence "read only." Because of this function, which is somewhere between the hard-wiring of the machine and the operations of the coded software, they are also called **firmware.** Also included under firmware chips are PROM, a form of ROM programmable by the user; EPROM, an erasable reusable PROM; and EEPROM, an electrically erasable ROM. EEPROM chips can be erased many times and are used in applications where data must be updated frequently and held when the device is turned off. They can be erased either inside the computer or after removal. EPROM chips are erased using ultraviolet light and have a relatively short life span. They are gradually being replaced by **flash memory,** a memory chip that is erased not byte by byte but in fixed blocks that range from 512 bytes to 256 kilobytes. The name is meant to suggest its ability to be erased quickly. Flash memory chips are cheaper than EEPROM chips and can hold more data.

**Logic array** and **gate array** chips contain assemblies of separate logic gates that have not been tied together. The chip is completed to perform its special function by application of a thin metal top layer, designed to tie the gates together in a particular pattern. This form of component assembly obviates the need to design a chip for a new application from scratch. The **application-specific integrated circuit** (ASIC) is a custom chip that integrates standard cells from a library of units with defined, reliable functions. As it combines proven components, it is faster than design from scratch and easily modified.

While memory chips are very reliable, occasionally an error occurs. A charge may appear where it should not be or may be absent when it is supposed to be present. Detection circuits are built into the memory circuits to protect against this error. Detection circuits are standard in IBM-compatible microcomputers. **Parity checking** is the error detection technique used to test the integrity of digital data in the computer system or on a network. Parity checking uses an extra ninth bit, the **parity bit,** that holds a 0 or 1 depending on the data content of the byte. Every time a byte is transferred, the parity bit is tested. Parity systems may be "even" or "odd." In even systems the parity bit is 1 when there is an even number of 1 bits in the byte. In odd systems the bit is 1 when there is an odd number of 1 bits in the byte.

Specialty limited-function chips are often used in low-cost consumer products, such as analog-to-digital signal conversion in telephones, and in calculators, watches, and certain automobile function controls. An entire system, including RAM, ROM, processor, timing clock, and input/output controls can be put on a chip for more complex operations.

# Hardware

A computer consists of a **basic input /output system** (BIOS), a **central processing unit** (CPU), **mass data storage devices,** and **input /output** (I/O) **devices.** Mass storage devices include the floppy disk, hard disks (hard drives), tape drives, and optical disks.

A BIOS or ROM BIOS is instructions incorporated into a ROM chip that control interactions with peripheral devices and applications programs. The BIOS includes routines for the keyboard, terminal, and communications ports and for keeping the time and date. It also executes start-up functions that test internal systems and prepare the computer for operation. It surveys control cards (plug-in boards) related to peripheral devices and establishes communications with them. Finally, it loads the operating system from memory and passes control to it. It should be evident that the BIOS limits the freedom with which newer (more advanced) peripheral devices may be incorporated. The BIOS must be upgraded periodically to maintain **compatibility** with various peripherals and software.

The basic I/O devices are a keyboard for input and a video display terminal (VDT), which may be a bulky cathode ray tube (CRT) in desktop machines or some other technology in flat-screen displays, for output. Other I/O devices are printers for producing paper copies and modulators-demodulators or **modems,** for telephone and facsimile communications with other computers and printers. In the laboratory, analyzers, which are actually dedicated microcomputers, may be connected to the computer (interfaced) as input devices. One computer may be connected with another through an **interface,** consisting of a wire connection, plus communications software.

The CPU is the part of the computer where all logical and arithmetic operations are decoded and carried out. A **bus** is an internal physical connection that connects the CPU to its main memory and the memory banks located on the cards that control peripheral devices. It is a common pathway linking hardware devices, and it is available to all devices. An **address bus** carries information identifying memory location, and a **data bus** carries signals to that location. The expansion slots into which peripheral device controllers are plugged connect with the data bus. Data buses have different **bit specifications,** or sizes, referring to the number of bits carried. If bus clock rates are equal, a 16-bit bus transfers data twice as fast as an 8-bit bus. Address buses are also rated by bit specification, which determines how much memory the CPU can address directly; for example, 20-bit buses address 1,048,576 bytes; 24-bit buses address 16,772,216 bytes.

An **expansion bus** is a series of slots into which expansion boards for peripheral devices (including the monitor) are plugged. Expansion buses have a relatively low rate of clock speed, owing to the necessity to connect with peripheral devices that operate at speeds lower than the CPU's speed. It is therefore a bottleneck limiting the performance of a computer, even though the CPU may operate at substantially higher speeds. This limitation is overcome with the use of a **local bus,** a connection from the CPU to peripheral devices, that runs at higher clock speeds than the expansion bus. A **network bus** is a cable that connects all devices in a network. A signal is transmitted to all network devices simultaneously, but only the addressed device responds.

For a peripheral device to be used, it must be physically connected to the computer and must be able to communicate with it. The computer's **operating system** must be aware of the device, control it, and receive signals from it. This is done by means of a **driver,** a program routine that links a peripheral device or internal function to the operating system. The driver contains the precise machine language necessary to activate all device functions. It includes detailed knowledge of its characteristics, which in the case of a video monitor would be the number of pixels of screen resolution, in the case of a disk drive the number of sectors per track. Basic drivers for standard components of a system (e.g., mouse, disk drive, monitor, printer, keyboard) are provided with the operating system and are supplied with new peripheral devices or certain software applications. For example, graphics, word processing, and desktop publishing applications include drivers (routines) for many popular displays and printers.

**Communications ports** are the pathways into and out of the computer. External sockets for plugging in communications lines, modems, and printers are provided. The rockets consist of **serial ports** and **parallel ports,** controlled by interfaces. A **serial interface** is a data channel that transfers digital data serially, one bit after the other. Communications lines are usually serial, and for this reason communications devices such as modem, mouse and scanner are connected to the computer via serial ports. Serial interfaces have multiple lines, but only one is used for data; the others are for control functions and communication. A serial port is an I/O connector used to attach a modem, mouse, scanner, or other serial interface device to the computer. The typical serial port uses a 9- or 25-pin connector (DB-9 or DB-25) connected to wires that plug into the target device. Serial transmission between computers and peripheral devices is governed by an industry standard (Electronic Industries Standard/Telecommunications Industry Association-Recommended Standard-232) variously abbreviated **EIA/TIA-232, EIA-232,** or **RS-232.** Communication over the serial cable is limited to from 50 feet to several hundred feet, depending on the quality of the cable. RS-232 defines the purpose and signal timing for each of the communication lines, not all of which are used in every application. An RS-232-compliant device transmits positive voltage for a 0 bit, negative voltage for a 1.

The universal serial bus (USB) is a 12-MB daisy-chain bidirectional half-duplex serial bus developed by Intel that facilitates the addition of new types of peripheral devices, the connection and arrangement of peripherals, and the connection of computers to telephones for transferral of data and voice, as well as control. (Daisy chaining is the connection of devices in a series with a signal passing sequentially from one to the next. Half duplex refers to the ability of a connection to pass signals in either direction but only one direction at a time. Full duplex means capable of passing signals in both directions simultaneously.) The USB is the basis for connecting (for example) scanners that also can be used for sending and receiving fax communications. USB is intended to replace the RS-232 standard for modem communications, as RS-232 is not fast enough. USB supports four types of data transfer:

**Interrupt data transfers**, such as transfers from keyboards or mouse movements
**Bulk data transfers**, such as transfers from a scanner or to a printer. These transfers are large and occur as a "burst" (1023 bytes) beyond the capacity of low-speed devices.
**Control transfers** for configuring newly attached devices
**Isochronous data transfers** (streaming real-time transfers) up to 1,023 bytes in length, again beyond the capacity of low-speed devices

A **parallel interface** is a multiline channel that transfers one or more bytes simultaneously. A frequent application is a connection to a printer via a 36-wire parallel interface, which transfers one byte at a time, one bit over each of eight wires. This allows a character to be transmitted as a unit. The remaining wires are used for control signals. Large computer parallel interfaces transfer more than one byte at a time. Because it transfers more than one byte at a time, a parallel interface is faster than a serial interface. A **parallel port** is an I/O connector used to connect a printer or other parallel interface device. A parallel port on a microcomputer is a 25-pin female DB-25 connector.

In a microcomputer, standard communication circuits are built into a small expansion card that plugs into an expansion slot. A standard configuration might include two serial ports, one parallel port, and one game port. In some machines, they are included on a larger **host adapter card** with hard and floppy disk drive control.

A **floppy disk** (or diskette) is a reusable magnetic storage medium. It is a flexible plastic-based disk coated with metal oxide, with both surfaces used for magnetic recording. A modern floppy disk can hold up to 1.44 MB of data. The disk, which is round, is spun inside the drive housing, where a read/write head makes contact with its surface. Floppy disks spin at 300 rpm but are immobile between data transfers. Because of its convenience, standardization, and low cost, the floppy disk has been the usual means of distribution of microcomputer software and of transferring data between users. Magnetic storage media are, however, damaged by exposure to magnetic fields, and they deteriorate gradually over a period of years. Reading and writing to a floppy disk is relatively slow; it takes as long as a second to find a data location on a floppy disk. Speeds must be kept low to minimize wear from the read/write head. At this writing, floppy disks are very cheap, available for 60 cents or less apiece.

Storage on a disk surface is organized according to **tracks** and **sectors.** Tracks are narrow, circular, concentric bands on which data is recorded as discrete points. The thinner the track and the smaller the point (the more bits per inch), the more storage. The capacity of a disk is described in terms of number of bits or tracks per inch of recording surface, or **packing density,** while **bit density** is the number of bits that can be stored within a given physical area. Most disks are organized so that each track holds the same number of bits. As outer tracks are longer, bits are more densely packed in the inner tracks. Sectors are subdivisions of tracks. Sectors hold the least amount of data that can be read or written at one time. To store and retrieve data, one or more sectors are read into memory, changed, and written back to disk, all under the control of the operating system.

The **Zip disk** (Iomega) is a newer technology; a floppy disk variant that is slightly larger in physical dimensions than a conventional 3.5-inch disk, therefore requiring a special Zip drive. Zip disks are available in 100-MB and 250-MB capacities. Zip drives are available for external or internal installation via the SCSI interface or (as an external drive) through the parallel port. The SCSI interfaced drive is quite fast, approaching a hard drive, while the parallel port-connected drive is relatively slow. Zip disks are currently relatively expensive, compared to conventional floppies, currently costing about $11 or $12 each, bought in bulk.

A **hard disk** or hard drive is a storage medium made of a rigid disk with a magnetic recording surface. Hard drive systems are currently offered in one of two types. The IDE (Integrated Drive Electronics) is a hard disk that contains a built-in controller. IDE drives range in capacity, currently up to 6 GB. They are widely used in personal computers. The drive connects via a 40-line flat ribbon cable to an IDE host adapter or IDE controller that occupies an expansion slot. A modern IDE controller can control four drives. The small computer system interface (SCSI, pronounced "scuzzy") is a hardware interface that allows for the connection of several peripheral devices to a single SCSI expansion board (SCSI host adapter or SCSI controller) that plugs into the computer. The advantage of the SCSI is that seven different devices use up only one expansion slot in the computer. SCSI hard disk drives can be installed in a PC that already contains IDE disk drives. The IDE drive is the boot drive, while the SCSI drives provide additional storage.

Minicomputer and mainframe hard disks hold many gigabytes. Hard disks may be fixed in the drive or removable as a cartridge. In contrast to floppy drives, which spin intermittently, hard drives spin continuously at 3,600 rpm or higher and have a fast data transfer rate. Transfer rate is measured in bytes per second and access time in milliseconds. Hard drives are organized in a manner similar to floppy disks.

An **optical disk** is a direct-access disk written and read by laser light. Optical disks have a very large storage capacity, and the laser that reads them can be controlled electronically. Compact disks (CDs) can be used as ROM (CD-ROM), recorded at the time of manufacture. They cannot be erased or reused, although they can be read an indefinite number of times. A variation, the write once, read many times, or WORM, disks can be written to by the user but cannot be erased. A newer technology allows sequential recording on CD, providing a permanent, cumulative data base. Erasable optical disks can be rewritten many times and may eventually replace magnetic disks, as they have much greater storage capacity, have a longer period of data stability ("shelf life"), and are not damaged by magnetic fields. CDs are used increasingly to distribute software and for long-term archiving of data.

The size (capacity) of the hardware required in a computer system for a laboratory application depends on the size of the computational tasks and the organizational philosophy adopted. Small laboratories may be able to develop a system based on microcomputers (personal computers or PCs) while large laboratories may have to use minicomputers or mainframes. A mixed mainframe/PC solution is becoming very common, permitting as it does segregation or distribution of functions and presentation to the user of a "friendly" PC-style interface with the machine.

**RAID** (redundant arrays of inexpensive disks) systems are a form of mass data storage. They enhance the reliability of a computer as well as increase capacity by having it store data on more than one disk. A RAID system consists of several (or many) hard drives with a special controller. Eight levels of RAID system are defined. The simplest, level 1, uses **disk mirroring.** Each disk in the system has a duplicate, holding the same data. Data recording to the pair is simultaneous. If one disk suffers an error, it can be corrected from its twin. A new disk replacing a failed twin can be populated with data from its mirror image. **Disk duplexing** is like mirroring, except that the disk pairs are on different controllers. In RAID level 5, data is stored (with parity bits) across many drives, creating an essentially bullet-proof storage system. Any disk in the system can fail with no loss of data. In a system with **hot swap** capability, a failed disk can be removed and replaced without shutting down operations.

In selecting a computer system, it is very important to distinguish between processing power and storage capacity. Storage requirements for a clinical laboratory system are very great and must not be underestimated. With modern technology data storage can be, for practical purposes, unlimited. Storage at the multigigabyte level is routine even in microcomputers. The ability to use that stored information is another matter. To retrieve particular data from a mass of stored data and to process it into useful information requires processing power, a RAM function, which is, even with modern machines, an expensive limiting factor.

# Operating Systems

To run an application, a computer must respond to its operating system instructions, usually stored on an integral hard drive or on a diskette. Instructions are transferred to RAM. Data is also stored in RAM for processing, then saved in storage memory on disk. All multiuse computers use an operating system, while special-purpose devices controlled by a microprocessor, such as appliances and games, usually do not, as a single program runs all the I/O and processing tasks.

The **operating system** (OS) is the master control program that governs all operations of the computer. It is the first program loaded when the computer is turned on, and its key functional component, the **kernel**, remains in RAM at all times. The OS sets the standards for the application programs that run in it. All programs must work through the operating system, and programs are therefore written to work with specific operating systems. Following are the basic functions of the operating system.

**Job management,** which ranges from loading applications into memory in microcomputers to organizing programs to be run over a period of time in a large computer system.

**Task management,** which controls the concurrent operation of one or more programs. Multitasking is done by running one function while data is coming into or going out of the computer for another. In large computers the operating system governs the simultaneous movement of data in and out through separate channels. Advanced operating systems can prioritize programs, setting the order in which components are run, for example, by assigning high priority to interactive programs that involve an operator and low priority to batch programs that run according to a schedule.

**Data management** The operating system keeps track of data on disk. An application program does not know where its data is stored or how to access it. That function is performed by the operating system's access method or device driver routines. The operating system responds to a message from the application program that it needs data by finding it and delivering it to the program and by transferring output data to the appropriate storage location or display device.

**Device management** The operating system manages all devices, handling all drives and input and output to the display screen and the printer.

**Security** The operating system provides security functions of several types. Through a system of authorization of users and assignment of passwords it can control access to the computer and its functions, especially important in multiuser systems. Depending on the size of the system, it may maintain activity logs and account for use of the system for management purposes. The operating system provides backup and recovery routines for starting over again following a system failure.

# Microcomputer Operating Systems

The operating systems of microcomputers (personal computers) are linked to the historical process of development of the hardware. Currently, most small machines operate on elaborations of the disk operating system (DOS) developed by Microsoft for IBM Corporation in the 1970s. These operating systems are generally known as **IBM compatible.** At the time DOS was developed, the memory capacity of available and foreseeable machines was very limited. It was assumed that data would be retrieved from and stored on magnetic disks; hence the name "disk operating system." This is an important characteristic of the system, as it has been exploited to overcome some of the very serious limitations of DOS. The original Microsoft DOS was written to access memory between 0 and 1 MB. However, the upper 384 KB, variously called upper memory, reserved memory, high memory, and controller memory, was (and is) reserved for system control functions, such as video display. Only the lower 640 K of RAM is available to hold active programs and data. Over the years, the power of machines has increased greatly, and software developers have written increasingly powerful and sophisticated software to use it. However, the DOS operating system, while it has evolved, is still based on the original 640-K memory. This has proven to be a serious limitation, as it assumes an 8-bit system, while machines now function at the 16- and 32-bit levels. Even though the machine may be fully able to process large data files in large application programs, DOS does not recognize and therefore cannot use its capacity. DOS cannot see beyond the basic 640 K called **conventional memory.**

To permit advanced programs to run on DOS machines, strategies to go beyond conventional memory have been devised. They do not change the fundamental nature of DOS but rather exploit its ability to work with disks. In essence, they present the larger memory inherent in the advanced machine to DOS as if it were a disk to be accessed. Normally DOS sends data files to disk for storage. Once there, they are not accessible for processing. Special software is used to present otherwise inaccessible RAM to DOS as if it were just another disk drive. The software products introduced by IBM with its PC DOS 3.0 as VDISK:SYS and by Microsoft with its MS-DOS 3.0 as RAMDRIVE.SYS are device drivers. The presence of the driver makes it appear to DOS that it is in connection with a very fast-responding disk drive. The speed of response is not a confusing factor; in an actual disk drive the rate-limiting factors are mainly in the mechanism of the drive and in finding data in its storage location. This phantom **RAM disk** or **virtual disk drive** may be used to hold data for processing or may run frequently used programs in a location that does not compete for conventional RAM. The drawback is that a RAM disk is still RAM; it is volatile memory that does not survive loss of power.

The 384-K upper memory, between the conventional 640-K and 1-MB, is used for BIOS routines, video and device drivers, and other small programs. While this makes a small amount of RAM in conventional memory available by not competing for it, it is not enough to make much difference. Higher (later) versions of DOS and certain application programs address the limitations of the basic system by finding ways to access memory above 1 MB. These strategies involve the partition of memory into **conventional memory, extended memory,** and **expanded memory.** Extended memory starts at 1 MB; e.g., in a computer able to process using 4 MB memory, 640 KB is in conventional memory, 384 K in upper memory, and 3 MB in extended memory. Special software add-ons, so-called "memory managers," are used to access extended memory not recognizable to DOS. Some of these DOS extended memory applications are able to locate extended RAM and use it. A serious problem occurs when two such programs compete for the same RAM. Third-party memory managers supplied by a program in addition to the operating system and the application delude DOS into allocating upper memory by creating one or more memory-control block (MCB) chains in upper-memory RAM. These upper-memory control blocks (UMBs) contain the programs to be run. The memory manager modifies the lower MCB chain header that signifies the end of the chain into indicating that the chain is extended and points to the upper memory. DOS loads the program there, after which the manager restores the lower MCB chain to its original form. Other managers are able to access extended memory in an analogous fashion. For detailed discussion of these strategies and particular management programs, please see the discussion in Goodman.[1]

## Adding Memory

It is important to keep in mind that a machine may come supplied with less memory than its processors can accommodate. This is often done as a cost-saving measure, as memory chips are relatively expensive. Information inside a RAM chip is organized in a particular way. Most chips hold 1 bit in a particular address location. Some hold 4 bits per address, and others, e.g., PROMs, have 8 bits per address. These chips are called byte-wide chips. Aggregations of RAM chips are organized into "banks" of memory. A memory bank supplies all the data bits addressed by the CPU when one memory address is supplied to the address bus. Since only full banks work, memory is added in sets of full banks. IBM-compatible microcomputers use RAM in banks organized in multiples of 9 bits to include 1 parity bit per byte. Add-on memory is frequently supplied in the form of a single in-line memory module, or **SIMM**. SIMMs are narrow, printed circuit boards about 3 inches long that hold eight or nine memory chips. Each memory chip is rated in terms of its megabit (Mb) capacity. SIMMs plug into sockets on the circuit board. SIMMs are specified by their capacity and configuration. For example, a $1 \times 3$ SIMM has 1-megabyte capacity, organized as 4 megabit chips plus one 1 megabit chip. A $1 \times 9$ SIMM has 1 MB, supplied by nine 1-Mb chips; a 16-MB SIMM has, 16 MB, supplied by nine 16-Mb chips. These are all parity chips. SIMMs with no parity bits would be rated $1 \times 8$, $4 \times 8$, and so on, using eight 1-Mb chips. A number following the chip specification indicates chip speed; e.g., a $1 \times 9$-60 is a 60-nanosecond 1-MB SIMM. SIMMs are installed in multiples of two on microcomputers with a 16-bit data bus and in multiples of four on 32-bit machines.

## Cache

A cache is a reserved section of memory used to improve processing performance. A **disk cache** is a reserved section of normal memory or additional memory on the disk controller board. When the storage disk is read, a large block of data is copied into the cache. This makes the data more readily available than if the slower disk had to be accessed each time the data was needed. Data can be stored in the cache and written to the disk in large blocks. A **memory cache** is a high-speed memory bank placed between memory and the CPU. Blocks of instructions and data are copied into the cache and execution of instructions and updating of data are performed in the higher-speed memory. The larger the disk cache or memory cache, the faster the system performs, as there is a greater chance that the data or instruction required next is already in the cache.

Another disk emulation strategy uses a **flash disk,** a solid state disk made of memory chips used for high-speed data access. While different types of volatile and nonvolatile storage chips are used for solid state disks, a solid state disk looks like a standard disk drive to the operating system. This is in contrast to flash memory cards, which require proprietary software to make them work.

**Windows** is a graphics-based windows environment from Microsoft that integrates with and interacts with DOS. The name derives from a feature in which applications are displayed in resizable, movable regions, or "windows," on screen. The latest versions of Windows contain a built-in DOS extender, allowing it to manage extended memory, beyond DOS's 1-MB memory barrier. Newer Windows applications are 32-bit programs that run on Pentium and Pentium-like CPUs. Windowing allows multiple applications to be kept open while one is being worked on. Windows is a complicated work-around overlay for DOS and retains some complex features that inhibit its usefulness and make it prone to failure.

Windows NT (Windows New Technology) is an advanced 32-bit operating system from Microsoft, introduced in 1993. While it is a self-contained operating system that does not use DOS, it will run DOS and Windows applications as well as 16-bit character based OS/2 applications. Windows NT supports 2 GB of virtual memory for applications and 2 GB for its own use.

In addition to MS-DOS and Windows, minicomputers with the same hardware architecture may use OS/2 from IBM, a single-user multitasking operating system. OS/2 runs not only OS/2 but also DOS and Windows applications, with both a graphical user interface (GUI) as well as a command line interface similar to DOS. Many OS/2 and DOS commands are the same. Version 2.x is written for 32-bit 80386 machines and higher. It provides applications a 512-MB virtual address space. It is generally regarded as a robust operating system. OS/2's graphical user interface, Workplace Shell, is similar to Windows and the Macintosh.

SCO XENIX is a version of UNIX System V for computers using the 80286 processor and more advanced versions. SCO XENIX is a fast multiuser OS that uses less memory than SCO UNIX. For a further description, see the UNIX description in the next section.

**Macintosh** is the name given to a series of 32-bit personal computers from Apple Computer, Inc., using the Motorola 68000 CPU family. Its operating system is based on a metaphorical simulation of a user's desktop on screen. Macintosh introduced a graphics-based user interface that makes use very convenient. The Macintosh family is the largest non-IBM compatible personal computer series in use.

## Minicomputers and Mainframes

Most laboratory computer systems are run on a minicomputer or a mainframe. Much to be desired in the laboratory is an **open system;** one that is vendor-independent and designed to interconnect and work smoothly ("seamlessly") with a variety of products. In an open system, standards are derived by a consensus of interested parties rather than a dominant vendor. A **closed system,** one that uses proprietary elements that cannot be adapted to or joined with products from two or more vendors effectively, ties the user to a single vendor, whose products may be less than excellent or less than flexible and with whom price negotiation becomes difficult.

Several powerful operating systems are available for the large computers encountered in the laboratory. The machines are most often VAX, from Digital Equipment Corporation (DEC), now a component of the Compaq Corporation, or one of a series of machines from IBM.

**UNIX** is a multiuser, multitasking OS developed by AT&T. It is written in C, which can be compiled into many different machine languages, allowing UNIX to run in a wider variety of hardware than any other operating system. Thus UNIX has for many users become almost synonymous with "open system." UNIX has three major components: the **kernel,** which governs fundamental tasks; the **file system,** which is a hierarchical directory for organizing the disk; and the **shell,** the interface that processes user commands. The UNIX vocabulary is very large, containing more than 600 commands used to manipulate data and text. UNIX is set up as a **command line interface** (CLI), with many obscurely designated commands. A CLI requires the user to type in commands when prompted. However, graphical user interfaces have provided a user-friendly look to UNIX users. UNIX is very popular in scientific and academic circles, and commercial versions of UNIX, such XENIX for microcomputers, are available. Indeed, so many UNIX variations were available that AT&T developed several consolidated versions, notably System V. Every major hardware vendor has a version of UNIX, which appears to be becoming the reference standard operating system for processing in a distributed environment. Indeed, most computers that host the World Wide Web are UNIX machines.

The success of UNIX has led to the development of a standard for source code portability between different software and hardware platforms. This is the Portable Operating System Interface (UNIX-like) Open Systems Environment, or POSIX OSE specification.

**LINUX** is a UNIX-like operating system meeting POSIX specification. It is UNIX-like in that superficially it seems to work in a similar fashion, but it is built around a different kernel. It has the unusual virtue of being "free" in the sense of allowing open access to the source code. Indeed, the development of LINUX was and remains a collaborative effort. The LINUX kernel is combined with different sets of utilities and applications to form complete operating systems, also called LINUX, available from various vendors. Since LINUX is developed using an open and distributed model instead of the usual closed model, new versions (often buggy and not completely tested) are frequently available, often over the Internet. Typically, bugs are identified and fixed very quickly. Proprietary versions available through specific vendors are more polished, with useful enhancements.

The strength of LINUX is that it functions very well on a wide variety of mini- and microcomputers from different manufacturers, employing a variety of buses. It is functional on 386/486/Pentium machines, on others using a Motorola 680x0 CPU, on DEC Alpha CPU, on Sun SPARCs, and on PowerPC architecture, including PowerMac, IBM, and Motorola machines. It is an extremely robust and durable system, with records of years of continuous operation without a crash. This makes it very suitable as the operating system for a PC as well as a critical server for high volume, I/O-intense, real-time work demanding flexibility and durability. These qualities lead its partisans to think it will be the dominant operating system on personal computers in the relatively near future.

**MVS** (Multiple Virtual Storage) is the primary operating system used on IBM mainframes. MVS is a batch processing-oriented OS capable of managing large amounts of memory and disk space. MVS/XA (MVS/eXtended Architecture) manages enhancements, including the 2 GB of virtual memory provided with IBM's 370/XA architecture. MVS/ESA (MVS/Enterprise Systems Architecture) manages enhancements like 16 TB (terabyte—1 trillion bytes) of virtual memory, introduced with the ESA/370 architecture. MVS/ESA runs on all models of the System/390 ES/9000 product line.

**VSE** (Disk Operating System/Virtual Storage Extended) is a multiuser, multitasking operating system that runs on IBM's 43xx series. Once called DOS, it is now called VSE to avoid confusion with PC-DOS.

**VMS** (Virtual Memory System) is a multiuser, multitasking, virtual memory operating system for the VAX series developed by Digital Equipment Corporation. VMS applications run on any VAX from the MicroVAX to the largest VAX.

# Distributed vs. Central Processing

In general, computer power can be centralized in a relatively large machine (minicomputer, main frame) or distributed among a smaller central device and one or several interconnected microcomputers. In a fully centralized system the user communicates with the computer using a terminal that has little or no processing power itself, a so-called **dumb terminal** that is merely a conduit to the central computer. A centralized system contrasts with a **distributed system** in which the operator works with a microcomputer that may run its own applications or may communicate with the central computer in an interactive way—a **smart terminal.** The relation between the microcomputers and the central device can be accomplished in two ways, one being the direct connection of each microcomputer to the main computer, the other stringing the microcomputers together on a loop to form a **local area network** or LAN. The main concept is to move tasks off the CPU to the periphery of the system.

The trend seems to be toward distributed processing for several reasons. As computers grow larger, their price increases faster than their computational power. Therefore, a distributed system might be more cost-effective than a large centralized one. If the central unit fails, the entire system is down, and nothing gets done. With distributed processing, the subsidiary instruments can continue to function, at least for a time, often long enough for the main computer to come back up.

Distributed processing allows more efficient exploitation of the devices at any given level. Process data is retained in the peripheral device, and product data is passed along to the next higher level. For example, analytical instruments are now typically task-dedicated microcomputers with the ability to control the analytic process. The programs required to perform the analyses are resident in the machine, as is the ability to perform certain control functions and to hold results in a buffer for a period of time. Only patient results are passed up to the next level. The laboratory system integrates the results from a number of instruments or laboratories into a database, a function that cannot be done at a lower level.

Certain computer functions are slow, do not require much processing power, but occupy significant resources to accomplish. Text editing is a very demanding process and can be done on microcomputers more or less dedicated to the purpose. Only finished (product) text need be passed along to the main computer; all the transactions necessary to develop the document (process) do not compete for resources in the central processor. The microcomputer may be used to develop spreadsheets using any of the commercial programs, and certain personnel records may be kept on removable disks to maintain confidentiality.

Client/server is a software architecture in which interactions with the operator are performed on a local device, e.g., a workstation or a microcomputer (the client), while the underlying data, which is shared by many users, is held

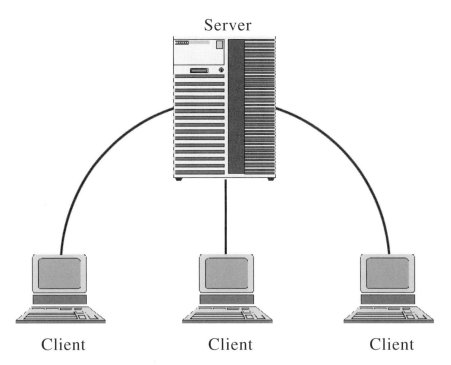

**FIGURE 6-1.** Simple client/server configuration showing thin clients with little computing power .

Server

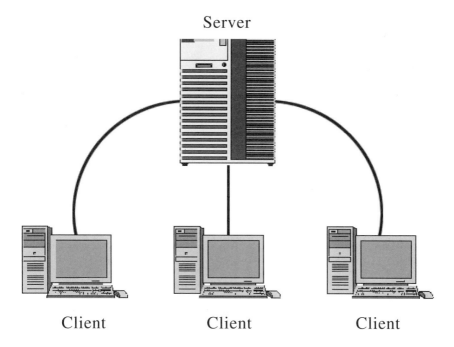

Client            Client            Client

**FIGURE 6-2.** Simple client/server configuration showing fat clients (sometimes called thick clients) with substantial computing power. In this configuration, the server may be a holder of files (a file server).

by a database (server) computer, which can be a LAN **file server,** minicomputer, or mainframe. The client provides the user interface and does much of the application processing. The server keeps the database and receives requests from the client to extract data from or update the database. The client deals with the server, not directly with the database. This adds to the security of the database and introduces substantial efficiency into the process. Clients may be relatively powerful machines with their own applications software ("fat clients") or minimal machines having within themselves not much more than is required for them to interact with the server ("thin clients"). Thin clients are smarter than dumb terminals, but not by much. Figures 6-1, 6-2, and 6-3 illustrate various client/server configurations.

Client/server architecture implies that the server is more to the client than a remote disk drive. The applications used in this architecture are designed for multiple users on a network. There are certain implications in the client/ server setup. For example, two or more users may be using a database at the same time. The server must inform all users of any updates at the same time. In an arrangement where the server is merely a source of files to be downloaded

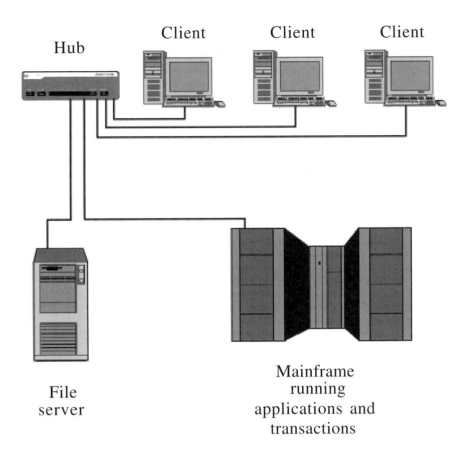

Client    Client    Client

Hub

File
server

Mainframe
running
applications and
transactions

FIGURE 6-3. Complex client/server configuration. A string of fat clients is connected to
a file server and a mainframe running applications and other transactions requiring great
computing power.

to a microcomputer, substantial time is spent simply moving the files. Even if
only a particular file among many is needed, a large number is copied to the
client for the client to sort through. A certain amount of availability of the
network to other traffic, is used up and if the client is logged in remotely via
modem, large data transfers can take hours, very expensive of telephone time.
The client microcomputer is probably considerably less powerful a machine
than the server, so it will take longer to perform the computing tasks needed.
In a true client/server arrangement, the client passes a request for a particular
file to the server, which finds it and sends it to the client. The machine, which
is better able to handle the task of sorting through a large number of files, has
done the job, and the network is spared a lot of traffic.

We can end this discussion by summarizing the components of a computer system and their significance:

**Machine language** determines compatibility with future hardware and software.

**Operating system** determines performance and future hardware/software compatibility.

**Clock speed** is a measure of performance (MIPS rate).

**Number of terminals** determines the number of concurrent users of the system.

**Memory capacity** determines performance of the computer.

**Disk capacity** determines the amount of information available to the computer.

**Communications** capabilities determine access to local and external information,

**Programming languages** determine compatibility with future hardware.

**Fail-safe design** determines reliability of the system.

# Chapter Glossary

**ASCII** (American Standard Code for Information Interchange): Standard code for representing characters as binary numbers, used on most microcomputers, terminals, and printers.

**ASCII file:** Text file on a machine using the ASCII character set.

**application software:** Programs written to fulfill a specific purpose, e.g., text editor, spreadsheet.

**assembly language:** Language in which each statement corresponds to a machine language statement, the statements themselves are written in a symbolic code that is easier for people to read.

**BIPS:** Billions of instructions per second.

**bank:** Arrangement of identical hardware components.

**bit:** Contraction of "binary digit," represented in a computer by a two-stage device (on/off). Microcomputers are rated by the number of bits each register can contain. The early Apples and IBM PCs are 8-bit machines. The 80286 processor is a 16-bit device. The 80486 is a 32-bit device. In general, the more bits, the faster the processor runs.

**bus:** Connection or conduit over which information is passed between computer components.

**byte:** Number of bits that represent a character. A kilobyte (KB) is 1024 bytes. A megabyte (MB) is 1,048,576 bytes = 1024 KB. 20 MB is the equivalent of 10,000 typed pages.

**CD-ROM:** Removable information disk that uses optical recording (laser) technology for storage and reading of data. A CD-ROM has very high storage abilities.

**chip:** Integrated circuit. Chips are squares or rectangles that measure approximately from 1/16 to 5/8 of an inch on a side. They are about 1/30 of an inch thick, although only the top 1/1000 of an inch holds the actual circuits. Chips contain from a few dozen to several million electronic components (transistors, resistors, and so on). The terms "chip," "integrated circuit," and "microelectronic" are synonymous.

**client /server:** Software architecture in which interactions with the operator are performed on a local device, e.g., a workstation or a microcomputer (the client), while the underlying data, which is shared by many users, is held by a database (server) computer, which can be a LAN file server, minicomputer, or mainframe.

**client/server network:** Communications network that uses dedicated servers for all clients in the network.

**clock:** Circuit that generates a series of evenly spaced pulses. All switching activity occurs when the clock is sending out a pulse. The faster the clock rate, the more operations per second can be carried out. Clock speeds are expressed as megahertz (MHz) or millions of cycles per second.

**closed system:** Computer architecture that uses proprietary elements that cannot be adapted or joined with products from two or more vendors. Closed systems are vendor-dependent and designed not to interconnect and work smoothly with a variety of products. See **open system.**

**compatible:** Capable of running the same programs. A matter of degree, since some programs contain hardware-dependent features.

**compiler:** Program that translates a high-level language into machine language. The generated machine language program is called the object program. Compilers translate the entire source program into machine language once before running it.

**computer architecture:** Design of a computer system, based on the expected use of the system for business, science, engineering, or graphics, which in turn determines the type of programs that will be run and how many will be run concurrently.

**computer environment:** Computer configuration that includes the CPU model or variation and all system software. A computer environment sets the standards for the applications that run in it.

**coprocessor:** Separate circuit inside a computer that adds additional features to the CPU or does a specific task while the CPU is doing something else.

**database server:** Fast computer in a local area network used for database storage and retrieval.

**expansion bus:** Series of slots into which expansion boards for peripheral devices (including the monitor) are plugged.

**file server** (network server): Fast computer in a local area network used to store many kinds of programs and data files shared by users on the network. It is used as a remote disk drive.

**firmware chip:** Permanent memory chip that holds its content without power, e.g., ROM, PROM, EPROM, and EEPROM .

**high-level language:** Description of a computer programming language. The closer the language is to natural language the higher it is said to be.

**instruction set:** Aggregate of machine language instructions that directly control a computer.

**integrated circuit:** Electronic device consisting of many miniature transistors and other circuit elements on a single silicon chip. Synonymous with **chip.**

**interpreter:** Device that translates and runs the source program line by line.

**LINUX:** UNIX-like operating system meeting POSIX specification. It works like UNIX but is built around a different kernel. The basic LINUX program is free, and the source code is public. The LINUX kernel is combined with different sets of utilities and applications to form complete operating systems, also called LINUX, available from various vendors.

**logic chip:** Single chip that can perform some or all of the functions of a processor. A microprocessor is an entire processor on a single chip.

**MIPS** (millions of instructions per second): Measure of computational capacity.

**machine language:** "Language" or set of instructions that a machine can execute directly. Machine languages are written in binary code, and each statement corresponds to one machine action.

**memory chip:** Chip that stores information in memory. Random access memory (RAM) chips, the computer's working storage, contain from a few hundred thousand to several million storage cells (bits). Constant power is required to keep the bits charged.

**microcomputer:** Computer in which all parts of the CPU are integrated onto one chip.

**microprocessor:** The ultimate integrated circuit: a single chip containing the complete logic and arithmetic unit of a computer.

**modem** (modulator-demodulator): Device that encodes data for transmission over a particular medium, such as a telephone line, an optical cable, and so on. The standard modem format is designated RS-232. Modem transmission rate is commonly designated in **BAUD.** A transmission range of 120 characters per second is 1200 baud. Modern systems available for PCs run up to 56,000 baud and include facsimile (fax) transmission capabilities (faxmodem).

**motherboard** (system board): Main printed circuit board in a computer system.

**open system:** Computer system architecture for which standards have been derived by a consensus of interested parties. Open systems are vendor-independent and designed to interconnect and work smoothly with a variety of products.

**operating system:** Program that controls a computer and makes it possible for users to operate the machine and run their own programs. Under control of the operating system, the computer recognizes and obeys commands entered by the user. It contains built-in routines that allow the application program to perform operations without having to specify detailed machine instructions. Examples: CP/M, MS-DOS, UNIX, OS2, APPLE DOS.

**programming language:** Language in which a program is actually written by a programmer; It is designed so that people can write programs without having to understand the inner workings of the machine. Examples: BASIC, C, COBOL, ADA, PASCAL, FORTRAN.

**RAM** (random access memory): Memory usable for performing computer functions. Information is maintained in RAM during operations, but it is lost when the machine is turned off. For modern applications, 8 megabytes of RAM is minimal. Much better are 12, 16, or 32 MB.

**ROM** (read-only memory): Portion of the operating system built into a chip that allows the basic functions of the machine to be carried out, including accessing the remainder of the operating system either from a floppy disk or in internal disk memory. During the time the machine is on, the operating system may be held in RAM.

**register:** Small, high-speed computer circuit that holds information about internal operations, such as the address of the instruction being executed and the data being processed.

**SIMM** (single in-line memory module): Narrow, printed circuit board about 3 inches long that holds eight or nine memory chips. Each memory chip is rated in terms of its megabit (Mb) capacity. SIMMs plug into sockets on the circuit board.

**server:** Computer in a network shared by multiple users.

**source program** (source code): Original high-level program before compiling or interpreting.

**UNIX:** Multiuser, multitasking, command line interface, open source operating system developed by AT&T. It is written in C, which can be compiled into many different machine languages, allowing UNIX to run in a wider variety of hardware than any other operating system. UNIX has three major components: the kernel, which governs fundamental tasks; the file system, which is a hierarchical directory for organizing the disk; and the shell, the interface that processes user commands.

**VUP** ( VAX unit of productivity): Productivity unit roughly equivalent to one MIP. (VAX is a proprietary line of equipment made by Digital Equipment Corporation.)

**virtual:** Simulated, conceptual, or extended (environment).

**WORM drive:** Write once, read many times CD device that allows production of laser disks. Data is written to the disk once and can be only read thereafter.

**word:** Computer's internal storage unit. Refers to the amount of data it can hold in its registers and process at one time. A word is often 16 bits, in which case 32 bits is called a double word. Given the same clock rate, a 32-bit computer processes 4 bytes in the same time it takes a 16-bit machine to process 2.

# *References*

1. Goodman JM. Memory Management for All of Us. SAMS Publishing, Division of Prentice Hall Publishing, Carmel, Indiana, 1993

# 7
# Computer Networks

R. ZANE GRAY

The computer's position as one of the indispensable instruments in the laboratory logically leads to the necessity of sharing resources and information through the development of computer networks. Computer networking evolved so that people could share devices, resources, files, messages, knowledge, and information. This discussion is intended to provide a basic understanding of computer networks, from a local network to the Internet. Computer networks can bb e relatively simple or very complicated; our objective is to provide a solid foundation of concepts and terminology on which can be built an understanding of how basic computer networks are established and used.

Computer networking technology has already progressed through several generations of development from local to global. In the 1980s, the first efforts to connect personal computers in a local area to share resources were successful; today's networks can host hundreds of users, and there is nothing local about them. Not only do we use enterprise computing networks, we also use worldwide, global networks, including the Internet, as well as the small office networks where the objective is to share a printer. To build extensive networks, special equipment such as **hubs, bridges, routers,** and **switches** are used to tie computers and peripherals together. Special operating systems and software—**communications protocols**—regulate and enable transactions among them. Systems have grown far beyond the original local area network (LAN) technology, creating a myriad of network acronyms.

**Internet**    Global information system logically linked by unique addresses based on Internet Protocol (IP); able to support communications using the Transmission Control Protocol/Internet Protocol (TCP/IP).

**Intranet**    Internal information system with a single user interface based on Internet technology, using TCP/IP and HTTP communication protocols.

**HTTP**    Hypertext Transfer Protocol. Connection-oriented protocol used to carry World Wide Web traffic between a WWW browser and the WWW server being accessed.

| LAN | Local area network. Network that services a work group within an organization. |
| WAN | Wide-area network. Two or more LANs connected across different areas, such as towns, states, or countries. |
| CAN | Campus area network. Network of two or more LANs that spans several buildings. |
| MAN | Metropolitan area network. Network of two or more LANs connected within a few miles. Usually connected wirelessly. |
| GAN | Global area network. Many LANs around the world connected together. |

LANs of several or many computers and devices sharing resources are less costly than the same number of stand-alone computers and devices. The LAN manager no longer has to install individual software such as spreadsheets, word processors, databases, and presentation creators on individual computers. **File servers** provide the ability to share applications and access information as well as share peripheral hardware components across the network. Support costs are thereby significantly reduced. When upgrades are indicated, a copy installed on one station is available to all.[1-3]

The basic components of a computer network fall into two categories: **hardware** and **software.**

## Hardware

- File server/Web server
- Workstations
- Cabling
- Network interface cards (NIC)
- Hub, or wiring center

## Software

- Network operating system (NOS)
- Workstation operating system
- Network shell

The **file server** stores applications and files for use across the network. A Web server serves up information to requesters. The server is the heart of the network. It usually has more RAM, a larger hard drive, and a faster CPU than the workstations attached. The server manages traffic and provides security for data, but it does not do computations or specific record searches within a database. These are the functions of the client workstations. Larger networks have multiple servers for running applications, searching databases, engineering, and communications. An example of another server would be a **print server** that handles print spooling or storing output from users and managing where and when to send it to different printers attached across the network. A **communications server** handles modem connections and fax modems. A communications server might also be referred to as a **modem pool.**

**Workstations** are typically IBM-compatible microcomputers, Apple Macintosh computers, or high-end engineering workstations. Computations and execution of applications software take place at the workstation. A workstation may also be referred to as a **network node** and is configured according to the job it is expected to do.

**Topology** in a communications network refers to the pattern of interconnection between nodes. It describes not only the physical architecture of the network but also the logical structure. That is, the "logical topology" is the operating systems and communications protocols that allow units to work together.

# Physical Topology

**Linear-bus, token ring,** and **star** are three main schemes to consider for cabling topology. A tree topology may combine elements of the basic three. In a linear-bus system a single cable is installed along a cable path in the ceiling or wall and terminated at each node on the network. Token ring topology lays the cabling in a circle. In star topology an individual wire is run from each workstation to a center location or hub. The star arrangement is easier to manage and administer than linear-bus.

A **linear bus technology** consists of a main or backbone cable with a terminator at each end. All nodes, including workstations, file servers, and peripherals, are connected to the cable. LocalTalk and Ethernet are the logical structures run on a linear bus. Typical linear-bus topology is illustrated in Figure 7-1.

In a **token ring topology,** the main backbone forms a loop with workstations or other elements set along it. Data passes from one node to another around the ring. In the star-wired ring variant the ring loops back to a hub between nodes. A typical ring topology is illustrated in Figure 7-2.

A **star topology** is designed with each node connected directly to a central concentrator or hub. Data moving on a star move through the hub on the way to its destination. The hub manages or controls all network functions. Star topology advantages are ease in configuration and wiring, ease in pinpointing node failure, and ability to add or delete nodes without disturbing the system. Disadvantages include a greater use of cable, added cost of the hub, and failure of the entire system if the hub fails. A typical star topology is illustrated in Figure 7-3.

A **tree** or **branched topology** combines features of linear-bus and star topologies. It consists of small star-configured clusters connected through a linear backbone. The advantage of this architecture is that it readily allows for expansion, with diversification or specialization of nodes in a side branch. Individual segments are wired point-to-point. This topology might be effective in a laboratory in which related functions are grouped in side star clusters. The disadvantages of this topology are relative difficulty in configuration

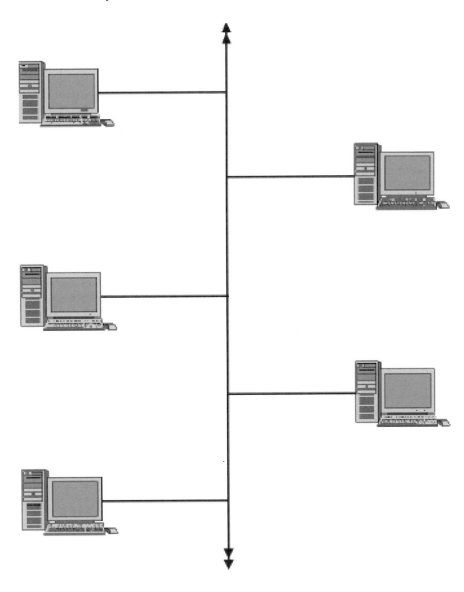

FIGURE 7-1. Linear bus topology.

and wiring, limitation of linear distances by cable type, and failure of the entire system if the backbone cable breaks. A typical tree topology is illustrated in Figure 7-4.

A major consideration in choosing the topology of the computer network is the type of physical cabling system to use. Cable types vary, with each type having physical differences, length requirements, and different impedances.

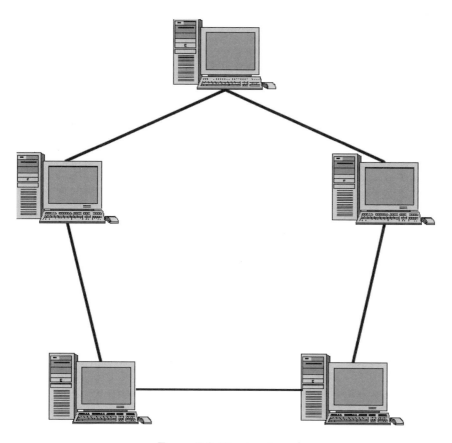

FIGURE 7-2. Ring topology.

Three kinds of cabling are most commonly used: coaxial, twisted-pair, and fiber-optic. Cable types are illustrated in Figure 7-5.

**Coaxial cable** consists of a central conducting copper core surrounded by an insulating material in turn surrounded by a second conducting layer, usually a braided wire mesh. Coaxial cable is used in linear and tree topologies. **Twisted-pair cable,** used in all topologies, comes in several different types. In shielded twisted-pair cable (STP), as in coaxial cable, the main data-conducting wires are protected by a braided wire mesh. Coaxial and STP are the most electromagnetically resistant copper-based cable used in networks. Unshielded twisted-pair (UTP) has two insulated copper wires twisted together with an outside protective jacket. UTP is the most cost-effective and is used in most telephone systems. UTP is gaining popularity with LAN developers because buildings are usually wired for telephone service during construction. The up-and-coming and most expensive wiring solution is

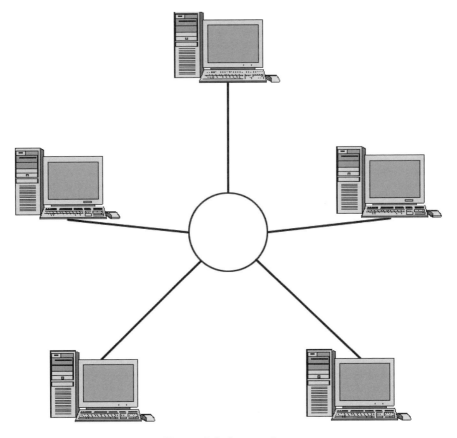

FIGURE 7-3. Star topology.

**fiber-optic cable.** Fiber-optic cable uses pulses of laser light to transmit data over glass cables. It is not subject to outside interference, can handle exceedingly high data rates, and cannot be tapped, making fiber optics an excellent choice for security reasons. Although not a type of cabling system, **wireless** networks are a strong consideration for medical institutions where doctors and nurses use hand-held devices to record patient data instead of being leashed to a data jack.

The important technical considerations in selecting a topology include cost, amount of cable needed, which influences the amount spent on the cable and on the labor of installation, the type of cable needed, and plans for future expansion. Linear bus uses the least amount of cable, and expansion may be easiest on a star; twisted pair cable is the least expensive type of cable.

An institution may decide to install wiring specifically for handling communications needs. The wiring systems are expected to handle the institu-

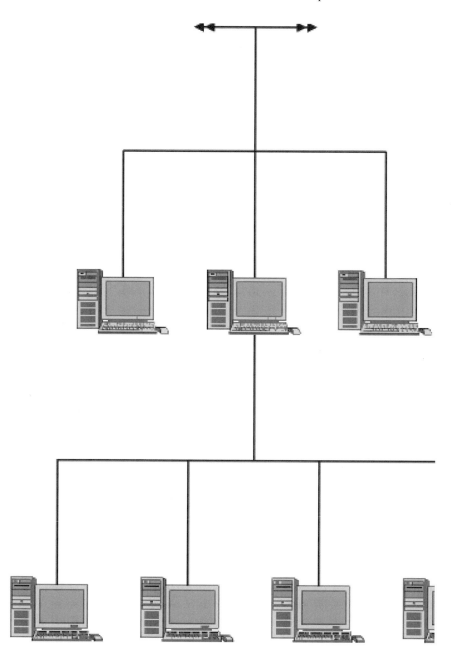

FIGURE 7-4. Tree or branched topology.

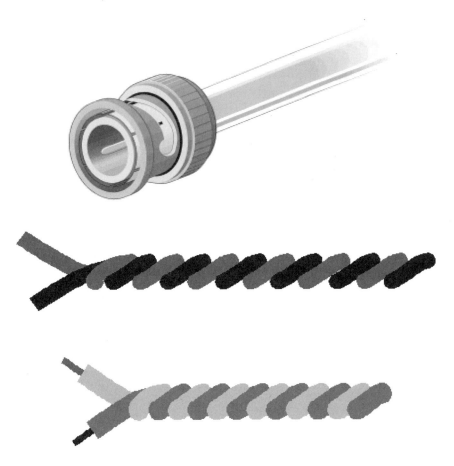

**FIGURE 7-5.** Cabling types. *Top:* Coaxial cable. *Center:* Shielded twisted pair. *Bottom:* Unshielded twisted pair.

tional needs for voice, data, and video communications. Two widely used installations are the IBM cabling system and the DEConnect communication system. The IBM cabling system and DEConnect communication system are installed so that wiring from individual workstations or offices terminates in central wiring closets, creating a star topology.

The next phase of creating a computer network is enabling the passage of data across the new wiring scheme. The network interface card (NIC) must be matched to the topology and cables of the network in order to attach peripherals to the network. NICs can be for a single type of network, or combination cards can be installed to handle a variety of cable types.

# "Logical Topology"—The Communications Protocol

A protocol is a set of rules that governs communications between computers and peripheral devices on a network. Electronic impulses or signals are the carriers of data across the network. The signals carry the protocol or **signaling schemes**. The signaling schemes come in two variations, contention and token passing. **Contention schemes** listen to the network cable and wait for a quiet period before sending out messages. **Token-passing schemes** use a token or specific electronic signal to indicate that a node has permission to transmit a signal. A token is a continuously repeating data frame transmitted onto the network by the controlling computer. When a terminal or the computer is ready to send a message, it waits for an empty token.

Protocols serve as the transport communication schemes for carrying data across a computer network. **Ethernet** is an example of a contention-based protocol. It is a fast and efficient signaling standard and is widely used by the computer networking market. All computers on the network can send data at once. Messages sometimes collide and become garbled before reaching their destination. To compensate, Ethernet networks use a collision detection system called Carrier Sense Multiple Access/ Collision Detection (CSMA/CD). When collisions occur, CSMA/CD detects them and resends the messages. In the token-passing scheme, messages follow a specific order. Messages are held at the local computer workstation until a free token arrives. The free token picks up the message and delivers it to the destination where it is stripped off the token, freeing up the token for the next message. **ARCnet**, **token ring**, and **FDDI** all use token passing signaling schemes. ARCnet (attached resource computer network) was the first LAN system developed; it dates from 1968. It can connect up to 255 nodes in a star topology. FDDI (fiber distributed data interface) is an ANSI standard token-passing network using fiber-optical cabling, capable of transmitting at the rate of 100 Mb/sec over a distance of 2 kilometers. **ATM** (asynchronous transfer mode) is a unique signaling scheme that can simultaneously deliver video and sound across a network. It is used for such applications as cable TV and telemedicine.

The most popular protocol is **TCP/IP** or Transmission Control Protocol/ Internet Protocol. The United States Department of Defense developed TCP/ IP to link computers and maintain connectivity in the event of another world war. TCP/IP functions much the same way as a telephone system. Each computer using TCP/IP must have a unique number to identify it on the network. TCP/IP is routable, flexible, and fault-tolerant, making it *the* protocol for the Internet and institutional intranets. Sequenced Packet Exchange/Internet Packet Exchange (**SPX/IPX**) is a proprietary protocol, owned and developed by Novell. IPX sends data packets to requested destinations and SPX verifies and acknowledges successful packet delivery. Network basic input/output system (**NETBIOS**), on the other hand, enables the use of naming conventions instead of numbering schemes to communicate directly with network hardware without any other network software involved. **NETBEUI** is an extended user interface for NETBIOS protocol. Both NETBEUI and NETBIOS are limited to single LANs because they are nonroutable protocols. To get from one network to another, other hardware must be added.

Hardware that makes a LAN extendible into the WANs, CANs, MANs, and GANs that were discussed earlier comes in various forms, from "dumb" to "intelligent," or programmable. Hubs are the devices most often found in the wiring closet that serve as a central connection point for adding workstations or when longer cable segments are needed. A hub is a box with ports that accept plug-in cables from one area and passes them on to other workstations or servers.

A hub is a common connection point for devices in a network. Hubs are commonly used to connect segments of a LAN. A hub contains multiple ports. When a data packet arrives at a hub it is copied to all other ports so that all segments of the LAN can see all packets. A **passive hub** serves simply as a conduit for data enabling it to go from one device (or segment) to another. So-called intelligent hubs include additional features that enable an administrator to monitor the traffic passing through the hub and to configure each port in the hub. **Intelligent hubs** are also called manageable hubs. A third type of hub, called a **switching hub**, actually reads the destination address of each packet and then forwards the packet to the correct port. Several other terms apply to hubs. A **stackable hub** is a hub designed to be connected and stacked or positioned on top of another hub, forming an expandable stack. Since a hub is basically a concentrator of device connections, a stackable hub is just a bigger concentrator. The stackable approach allows equipment to be easily and economically expanded as it grows in size. Stackable hub features include the ability to mix hubs, routers, and other devices in the same stack; fault tolerance, so that if one hub fails, others can continue to operate; port redundancy, permitting automatic substitution for a failed port; and management of the hubs using hardware and software for the simple network management protocol (SNMP).

Signals tend to lose strength over distance and according to cable size. A physical device known as a **repeater** is designed to tie two long network cable segments together and to boost the signal on to the next connection point. If the next point is on another network, then a **bridge** is introduced to exchange the information, regardless of their specific topologies. **Routers** offer significant capabilities over a bridge, because they don't care about topology or protocol and can address any destination attached to a data packet. The last piece of "other" hardware in the system is the switch. Switches are like hubs, except network management software can be used to program the switches' memory module with information about each node connected to each port. Switches can be programmed to implement contingency plans for disaster recovery. For example, if a portion of the network is blown away in a hurricane, the switch reroutes or turns on another port connected to a specific station that may be designed to back up data. Segments can be turned off through switches during certain periods for security reasons or to squelch damaged segments elsewhere on the computer network.

The hardware components, cabling types, signaling schemes, and cards constitute the physical basis of a network. Software is also an essential element of the computer network. The network operating system (**NOS**) drives the whole basic scheme of planning the network. The NOS runs on the file server and provides the network with the types of services and capabilities specifically associated with the type of network you build. The NOS field is dominated by several major players.

**Novell NetWare** is the number one network operating system used today. The biggest advantage is NetWare Directory Services capabilities, which provides a scheme for arranging an entire organization's network structure, allowing for centralized administration.

**Windows NT** offers the advantage of keeping the entire network operating on Microsoft applications. NT easily interacts with other NOSs. NT provides major growth opportunity, and anyone comfortable using Windows 95 or Windows 98 can easily manage NT in a small environment.

**Banyan Systems VINES** is the third most used network operating system. Banyan VINES supports UNIX, Windows, OS/2, and Macintosh users. It provides basic file and printer services. **VINES StreetTalk** enables every peripheral on the network to be addressed by name. StreetTalk shows whose office each printer is located in, which takes the confusion out of selecting the right peripheral device.

**Macintosh** has been unable to gain a competitive share of the computer networking market. However, Macintosh commands a large and loyal customer base. **Appletalk networks** are fairly simple to set up but are slow compared to the high-speed capabilities of network systems like Ethernet.

**IBM OS/2 Warp Server** was developed by IBM and Microsoft for the purpose of circumventing the 640-KB RAM barrier and to provide dynamic exchange of information between different applications. Few software programs were developed for OS/2 before the Microsoft Windows came to dominate the market.

**Windows 95** deserves special mention, although Windows 95 is not really a network operating system. It runs well on the client side of any of the types of server-based networks we have discussed. It is suited to the peer-to-peer networking concept. Peer-to-peer networking differs form server-based networking in that it does not require a central file server. All workstations are linked together via the cabling system instead of through the server.

# Network Manager

The third essential element in a network, in addition to the physical system and the network software, is the network manager, the person who manages getting the users on board and who must install, maintain, and troubleshoot the network. The network manager must have good people skills, as the people are the customers, not the computers. In addition to the responsibilities already cited, the manager provides technical expertise to network customers and to the key decision makers regarding the technology and use of the network. Therefore, the person designated network manager must have technical, interpersonal, software, and management skills to efficiently care for the network. These requirements can be summarized in three basic categories:

**Operations**

- Application installation
- Management of directories, files, and hardware
- Setting up users and security
- Data backups
- Monitoring performance of the network
- Troubleshooting
- Disaster recovery

**Enhancements**

- Network expansion
- Evaluating/recommending software and hardware products
- Hardware/software upgrades

**Administration**

- Developing policies and procedures
- Validation/documentation
- Training
- Gatekeeping

The network manager must have a comprehensive strategy for managing the network. Several commercial network management applications packages are available. Choice of the one best suited for a particular network strategy involves consideration of current and anticipated future needs. A **management console** is a necessity to provide the ability to collect data about the devices being managed and generating information from the data. Two common **management protocols,** used to communicate with and within a given network are available. **Simple network management protocol** (SNMP) comes with the purchase of hubs and runs regular diagnostic tests to keep up with the status of the management information base. SNMP can locate a problem on the network and allow the LAN manager to quickly access and correct the problem. The other common management protocol is the **common management information protocol** (CMIP), which is more complex than SNMP because it puts network monitoring decisions in the hands of the LAN manager. The manager sets the parameters to be monitored, a task that requires considerable work and maintenance. However, it provides customized control over all components of the LAN. The management protocol should provide some common methods of monitoring and retrieving information about the network. The most common methods follow:

**Protocol analysis** provides information from the physical-layer through the upper-layer protocols. Most network errors are found at the network layer and can usually be handled by the network manager. They consist of such tasks as swapping out a bad network interface card, or reloading a driver.

**Graphical mapping** allows the manager to generate a visual characterization of the network and components using a graphical user interface. Components can be color-coded and the graphical mapping software set to blink when a problem is experienced at that component.

**Polling** periodically queries all devices on the network to determine their status. The manager configures the frequency of polling based on some estimate of functional need, especially on larger networks, as too many polling queries can adversely affect network performance.

**Event logging** is the logging or systematic recording of events. The content of the event messages is captured in a file for statistical analysis and troubleshooting.

**Device configuration** allows the manager to affect the configuration of large numbers of devices from the management console. This is a must in situations where the devices are not physically located near the manager.

Reference was made to **network layers** earlier in the discussion of network management tools. A model called **OSI** (Open System Interconnect) describes a standard for vendors to conform to specifics that would enable most systems to work together. The OSI model has seven functional levels.

**Physical layer** is the connection layer where two or more machines transmit electrical signals across a physical transmission media or cable.

**Data link layer** is responsible for the error-free transmission of frames of data between nodes.

**Network layer** terminates the network connection between two nodes and routes data from one node to another.

**Transport layer** monitors the quality of data transfer between nodes and notifies users when transmission quality deteriorates.

**Session layer** controls when users can send and receive data, concurrently or alternately.

**Presentation layer** ensures that the data is presented to users in a meaningful way.

**Application layer** lets applications exchange information about interconnected systems and the resources they use.

Understanding the network layers in the OSI model enables one to better design and troubleshoot a network. The model works from the bottom to the top and the requirements of each level must be satisfied.

Two other issues the network manager addresses are security and gatekeeping. **Security management** is the process of controlling access to only authorized users of the network. **Gatekeeping,** on the other hand, is the process of controlling applications software being used on the network. Gatekeeping could be grouped into a security category due to the effects uncontrolled applications can have on the network. Users have a tendency to introduce foreign software at the expense of good network usage. Games are probably the biggest issue, next to downloads of all sorts from the Internet. Unauthorized introduction of this foreign software can have deleterious affects on network performance and is a major contributor to the introduction of viruses. Good security practices and user training are the best ways to maintain control of a network. Security is not just passwords; it is viruses, passwords, hardware protection, file access, protecting dial-in access, and rights to the network. Assigning user names and passwords is probably the most common form of security. However, passwords are only as secure as the owner makes them. Instead of running the risk of forgetting their password, some users have a tendency to write their password down or to use one that is too easy to guess. Popular passwords and passwords that are easy to guess are names of children, relatives, pets, or hobbies. Users should understand that it is not a crime to forget a password and that new ones are easily provided for.

Planning of security goals is an important function of the network manager. Security goals must address three issues:

**Confidentiality**—ensuring that data is available only to those who have a need to know and are authorized to see it.

**Integrity**—ensuring that data is reliable by making efforts to prevent and detect deliberate or accidental modifications to data.

**Availability**—ensuring that data, program applications, hardware, and communications links are available to people who need them when they need them.

An effective security policy must be developed and in place to cover these three issues. Data must be backed up regularly and the backups must be protected to the extent that no accidental or deliberate modifications can be made.

Computer hacking does take place. Although the risk of a hacker gaining access to a computer system may seem relatively insignificant, it is still prudent to protect against fraudulent use of resources. It is estimated that at least 75% of computer hacking crimes or destruction of data are inside jobs.

Virus outbreaks, user error, and copyright breaches are the most prevalent logical security breaches. Backup is the best means available to protect against accidental and deliberate loss of data.

The responsibilities for managing a network require technical, administrative, and good people skills. The success of the network manager depends on having good rapport with other network managers, technical support, user training, and a good assistant to ensure continuity and give the primary network manager time to spend on planning and more complicated tasks.

E-mail is a good example of planning uses on the network. It has been estimated that 80% of the amount of traffic on the Internet is generated by electronic mail. So, with all the hype over access to games, news reports, weather summaries, and some not-to-be-mentioned Internet sites, e-mail is proving to be the most useful network application available today. E-mail has many advantages over paper-based communications.

- It reduces postage and writing paper costs.
- It is faster than writing and sending memos or letters and multiple copies are easier to produce.
- Address books are easy to maintain and automatic receipts can be generated to acknowledg messages received.
- It is cheaper than the telephone and no time is wasted on busy signals, idle chitchat, or interruptions.
- Documents such as spreadsheets, graphics, and reports can be attached and forwarded.
- It facilitates communication with the office when traveling.
- Most important, there is an audit trail that can be tracked and traced if necessary.

However, there is no security built into the Internet for e-mail. The Internet was developed for the military with the goal of continued system operation, even if one or more computers within the system ceased to function. By default, a message originating from one system may travel through several other systems before it reaches you or your intended recipient. At any of these system relays, your e-mail can be read. So encryption for confidential information is a must. If your e-mail system does not have built-in encryption, you need to use a stand-alone encryption package on your computer or the network.

Encryption is the scrambling of information in such a way that the information is accessible only to someone who can supply the right authentication keys or crack the code. The network manager should use backup procedures to protect against accidental loss or modifications to data and encryption to provide protection against deliberate abuse of data, whether it is e-mail or other data available through network connections.

Keys or algorithms are the passwords in the encryption world. These may be proprietary or public, public key or private key systems. Consideration must be given to these different keys when choosing an encryption method for the network. Proprietary systems rely on the secrecy of the algorithm itself, which depends on users and managers to maintain. One disgruntled employee can make all information protected by an algorithm vulnerable to unauthorized access. Accordingly, using a product that works on a public algorithm is not weakened by the fact that everyone or someone knows how it works. In fact, the more analysis the algorithm is subjected to, the stronger it gets. For an example of how a public algorithm can remain secure, even when users know the details of the algorithm, consider an algorithm of two numbers multiplied to produce a product such as $12 \times 12 = 144$. It is fairly easy to work out the two prime numbers multiplied to produce 144. However if, a larger number of some 500 digits were produced, then working out its prime factors, would take literally years on even the most powerful computer.

Once you have decided whether to use a proprietary (secret) or public (published) algorithm, the next step is to decide on whether to use a public or private key. Private key is the most widely known key encryption, and it is also the simplest and fastest to implement. Private key encryption is the method of scrambling the data in a way that is relative to the key used. Decryption simply involves feeding the original key back into the program to make the file readable again. Sounds simple enough, but there is one major drawback: how to inform the recipient of the key. If you can find a secure way to do that, then you probably already have a secure means of getting information to your recipient and don't need to encrypt the data at all.

A better way to accomplish secure communications of your data is to use a public key encryption algorithm that places a public and a private key with each user. Public keys can be publicly distributed while your private keys remain private. An example of using a public key would be for you to encrypt a message with your private key and the recipient's public key. You send the message to the recipient; the recipient decrypts the message by using your public key and his private key. The only solution is to have the combination of the two keys. You never need to transmit a private key.

Beware of applications that claim to have built-in encryption and/or password protection on their data files. These applications do not usually scramble the data, so the information is available if the file is examined with a text editor. Some applications whose built-in encryption is easily broken include Microsoft Word, WordPerfect, Paradox, Lotus 1-2-3, Lotus Agenda, and Lotus Organizer. The bottom line is, don't use the built-in encryption in an application unless you are absolutely sure that it uses a secure algorithm. One widely known public key encryption program is called PGP, or Pretty Good Privacy. PGP is available as a DOS program. If you are going to use it with Windows, you can download a front end, which will add a menu-driven interface to the PGP program. PGP has both encryption and authentication features with a facility to display the user's public key in 7-bit ASCII format, which makes it easy to send via e-mail.

All the cables have been pulled, the network equipment installed, an NOS identified, a network management console implemented, and a manager designated; user accounts and a security system have been set up, and a business plan in place. You have a network.

## The Internet

The Internet is a worldwide computer network that has evolved out of a U.S. Department of Defense military research program (Advanced Research Projects

Agency—ARPA) begun in the late 1960s. Its purpose was to develop a geographically large network that would allow communications to be routed through any of many redundant interconnected sites in the event of destruction of particular computers by nuclear attack. From this beginning the network has grown to include scientists, academic and commercial institutions, and individuals around the world. No one "owns" or "controls" the Internet. Each site is responsible for its own maintenance. Certain conventions have come to govern activities on the Internet. The World Wide Web, or simply, the Web, is a part of the Internet, consisting of a vast number of documents stored on computers around the world. A Web page is a document stored on the Web. A Web "document" may consist of text, sounds, still images, or video. Each page has a unique address, or **uniform resource locator** (URL). A collection of Web pages maintained by any agency or individual is called a Web site. A Web server is a computer that stores Web pages and makes them available on the Web. Web pages may contain **hyperlinks** or simply links to other pages on the Web. A link may be highlighted text or an image. Links allow rapid connection to a selected page anywhere in the world. A Web browser is a locally resident program, usually acquired as part of a "productivity suite" including a word processor, spreadsheet, and so on, that allows viewing and exploration of information on the Web. Examples, among several, are Netscape Navigator and Microsoft Internet Explorer. Connection to the Web is accomplished by use of an ordinary telephone line modem, a relatively slow medium operating in the 56-Kbps range or higher; a video cable modem, with speeds up to 3000 Kbps; an integrated services digital network (ISDN), with speeds in the 56–128-Kbps range, and digital subscriber line (DSL) service, with speeds in the 1000–6000-Kbps range.

Actual connection to the Internet is done through a university or company; a commercial online service, such as America Online and Microsoft Network; or through a an Internet service provider (ISP), a company that offers access on a fee-per-time-spent basis.

**Hypertext Markup Language** (HTML) is a computer language used to create Web pages. HTML documents consist of text and embedded special instructions called tags. HTML documents are read using a Web browser, which interprets the tags and displays the document as a Web page, even if the document is on the same computer as the browser. Tags inform the browser about the structure of the document but not specifically how to display it. That is why different browsers may display a single HTML document differently.

# Chapter Glossary

**band:** Range of frequencies used for transmitting a signal. A band is identified by its lower and upper limits. Example: a 10-MHz band in the 110–110 MHz range.

**bandwidth:** Transmission capacity of a computer channel, communications line, or bus. It is expressed in cycles per second (Hertz); the bandwidth is the difference between the lowest and highest frequencies transmitted. The frequency is equal to or greater than the bits per second. Bandwidth is also often stated in bits or bytes or kilobytes per second.

**baseband:** Communications technique in which digital signals are placed on the transmission line without change in modulation. It is usually limited to a few miles and does not require the complex modems used in broadband transmission. Common baseband LAN techniques are token-passing ring (token ring) and CSMA/CD (Ethernet). In baseband, the full bandwidth of the channel is used, and simultaneous transmission of multiple sets of data is accomplished by interleaving pulses using TDM (time division multiplexing). Contrast with **broadband** transmission, which transmits data, voice and video simultaneously by modulating each signal onto a different frequency using FDM (frequency division multiplexing).

**broadband:** Technique for transmitting large amounts of data, voice, and video over long distances. Using high-frequency transmission over coaxial cable or optical fibers, broadband transmission requires modems for connecting terminals and computers to the network. Using the same FDM technique as cable TV, several streams of data can be transmitted simultaneously.

**bridge:** Computer system that connects two similar LANs together.

**browser** (Web browser): Interface to the Web that permits the display of Web pages and other Web services, such as e-mail, discussion groups, and so on.

**bus topology:** Network topology built around a common cable (bus) that connects all devices in the network.

**CAN** (campus area network): Network of two or more LANs that spans several buildings.

**DSL** (digital subscriber line): Internet connection technology with speeds in the 1000–6000-KBps range.

**GAN** (global area network): Many LANs around the world connected together.

**gateway:** Computer subsystem that performs protocol conversion between different types of networks or applications, for example, a personal computer LAN and a mainframe network. An electronic mail or messaging gateway converts messages between two different messaging protocols. See **bridge.**

**HTML** (Hypertext Markup Language): Computer language used to create Web pages. HTML documents consist of text and embedded special instructions called tags. HTML documents are read using a Web browser, which interprets the tags and displays the document as a Web page.

**HTTP** (Hypertext Transfer Protocol): Connection-oriented protocol used to carry World Wide Web traffic between a WWW browser and the WWW server being accessed.

**hub:** Central connecting device for communications lines in a star topology. "Passive hubs" merely pass data through, while "active hubs" regenerate signals and may monitor traffic for network management.

**hyperlink:** Predefined linkage between one object and another.

**ISDN** (integrated digital services network): Internet connection technology with speeds in the 56–128-KBps range.

**ISP** (Internet service provider): Company that offers Internet access on a fee-per-time-spent basis.

**intelligent hub:** Computer that provides network management; may include bridging, routing, and gateway capabilities.

**internet:** Global information system logically linked together by unique addresses based on Internet Protocol (IP); able to support communications using the Transmission Control Protocol/Internet Protocol (TCP/IP).

**intranet:** Internal information system with a single-user interface based on Internet technology, using TCP/IP and HTTP communication protocols.

**LAN** (local area network): Network that services a work group within an organization.

**MAN** (metropolitan area network): Network of two or more LANs connected within a few miles. Usually connected without wires.

**OSI** (Open System Interconnect): Standard to which vendors conform that enables most systems to work together.

**repeater:** Communications device that amplifies or regenerates a data signal to extend the transmission distance.

**ring topology (ring network):** Communications network architecture that connects terminals and computers in a continuous loop.

**router:** Computer subsystem in a network that routes messages between LANs and WANs. Routers deal with network addresses and all the possible paths between them; they read the network address in a transmitted message and send it based on the most expedient route.

**star topology (star network):** Communications network in which all terminals are connected to a central computer or central hub.

**topology:** (1) Pattern of interconnection between nodes in a communications network. See **bus, ring, star** topologies. (2) Interconnection between processors in a parallel processing architecture; bus, grid, or hypercube configuration.

**URL** (uniform resource locator): Unique Web page address.

**WAN** (wide-area network): Two or more LANs connected across different areas, such as towns, states, or countries.

**Web page:** A document stored on the Web.

# *References*

1. Currid CC and Currid AD. Introduction to Networking. Novell Press, San Jose, California, 1997.
2. Martin, J with Kavanagh Chapman, K. Local Area Networks: Architectures and Implementations. Prentice Hall, Englewood Cliffs, New Jersey, 1989.
3. Nunemacher, G. LAN Primer. M&T Books, A Division of MIS: Press, Inc., A Subsidiary of Henry Holt and Company, Inc., New York, 1995.

# 8
# Interfaces

ANTHONY O. OKORODUDU AND DANIEL F. COWAN

A **computer system interface** is a means of communication between a user and a computer system, between two or more computer systems, or between computer systems and other analytical systems. Interfaces not only allow a person to use the machine, they also permit one machine to communicate with another, even one running on an entirely different operating system.

An interface is activated by commands in the programming language. The complexity of the functions and the design of the language determine how hard it is to program. On the human user level, the means of communication are typically the keyboard, the mouse, and the display screen. The keyboard uses a collection of small buttons, each of which is associated with a bit pattern that represent symbols that are then translated into words and commands. The commands of the keyboard are highly specific, requiring rigorously defined sets of actions in a particular sequence that reflects the nature of device that is receiving the message.

A mouse is a small electromechanical device that is pushed across a flat surface and whose movements are translated into cursor movement on the display screen. The display screen has much more flexibility in presentation, recognizing the ability of the viewer to make accommodations for different formats and layouts. Other common devices for human interface with computer systems are joystick, trackball, touch screen, light pen, and voice.

Commands and menus are used for communication between the human user and the computer. A **command line** is the area on screen that accepts typed-in commands. Examples are the command lines in DOS and UNIX, and graphical user interfaces (GUI) of the Macintosh, Microsoft Windows, and other systems. A program that uses command lines is said to be **command-driven.** It is usually harder to learn and more demanding to use, but is more flexible than a menu-driven program. Command-driven programs may be faster to use than menu-driven programs because the user can state a request succinctly.

Every interface has a structure and a defined function. The **structure** provides backbone for the electrical signals which are made up of different voltage levels, frequencies, and duration that pass data from one device or program to another. The electronic signals activate the interface **functions.** Data is read, written, transmitted, received, analyzed for error, and processed for use. The data transferred or transmitted may request functions to be performed, as in the client/server scenario, or may be the subject of the transaction. This data has a precise format, including at a minimum a header, body, and a trailer.

Machine-to-machine interfaces have two components, hardware and software. **Hardware components** are the plugs, sockets, wires, and particular patterns of electrical impulses traveling through them. Examples include the RS-232 interface, Ethernet and token ring network topologies, and the IDE, ESDI, SCSI, ISA, EISA, and Micro Channel interfaces. Electrical timing considerations are very important.

**Software** is the intangible component of the computer that refers to the programs that provide the instructions for the computer hardware. Software communication programs are written in various languages such as assembly, FORTRAN, BASIC, COBOL, C, C++, Visual Basic, and Java. The software makes the hardware function and execute the desired outcome. Software applications run under the DOS, Windows, Macintosh, Unix, and other operating systems. For example, the Simple Mail Transfer Protocol messaging protocol (SMTP) is used in TCP/IP networks for e-mail.

The design of the interaction between the user and the computer is called a **user interface.** The aggregate of rules, formats, and functions for transmitting data between components in a communications system or network is called a **protocol.** More formally, a **communications protocol** is the hardware and software standards that govern transmission between two stations. On personal computers, communication programs include a variety of protocols (Kermit, Xmodem, Zmodem, and so on) that transfer files via modem. On LANs, protocols are part of the Ethernet, token ring, FDDI, and other access methods at the data link level (layer 2 of the OSI model). Mainframe networks incorporate multiple levels of protocols and protocols within protocols.

A data link protocol ensures that a block of data is transferred between two nodes without error. The transaction begins with **handshaking,** the initial transmission of signals back and forth over a communications network that establishes a valid connection between two stations. The "conversation" between the systems may be translated as follows:

*Are you there?* Yes. *Are you ready to receive?* Yes. *Here is the message.* (Message transmission) *Message received?* Yes. *Here is another part of the message.* (Message transmission) *Did you get it?* No. *Here it is again* (Message transmission) *Did you get it?* Yes. *That is all, goodbye.* Goodbye.

The language and message formats between routines within a program or between software components is an **application program interface,** or API. An API is used within a program to activate functions that are either part of that system or external, within another module, program, or system. The specification for an operating system working in a specific machine environment is an **application binary interface,** or ABI. An ABI is specific for a particular hardware platform and operating system.

# Interface Protocols

An interface protocol is a set of rules for communication between two applications allowing them to transmit data in an orderly way. A protocol has four elements:

1. Software programs are used to create or manage the data to be communicated.
2. Data is formatted in an unambiguous way so that it is accurately interpreted by the communicating systems
3. The communicating systems follow conventions (rules) that allow them to respond to each other about their readiness to send or accept data,
4. Communications are structured to assure that delivery is accurate and error free and that erroneous data is not permitted to arrive at all.

# Health Level 7 (HL7)

The HL7 protocol is rapidly becoming the *de facto* standard framework for the development of interface protocol specifications for healthcare applications.[1-4] As a messaging standard it sets the basic communication architecture and provides the vocabulary to accomplish integration. While HL7 provides certain rules, it is not based on highly specific reference architecture. In development of an interface, HL7 might be thought of as providing the foundation for a requirements-based conversation or negotiation between the participants. Only the message definitions for the task are needed and supported in the development of an interface.

The HL7 architecture may be thought of as comprising a set of constituent protocols, each with conceptual differences. It is hierarchical, beginning with high-level groupings and moving toward specific data fields.

**Functional group:** Data areas are grouped according to common application function; for example, broadly used elements such as admission, discharge, and transfer (ADT) information; order entry, result reporting, and billing.

**Message type:** Within the functional groups, one or more message types are implemented to support rules for the various applications. ADT specifies one type of message, while order entry may require many.

**Message definition:** One or more definitions within each message type describe the segments that constitute a properly constructed message. Each message definition includes one or more segments.

**Segment definition:** Segments are logical groupings of data elements. The patient identification segment, for example, includes fields for name, age, sex, and other demographic elements, as well as medical record number, account number, and other administrative elements.

**Field:** Inside segments are groups of fields containing data elements. Each field is defined with a maximum length, which may or may not be used. While length is specified, with some exceptions, internal organization of the field is not necessarily specified. For example, date fields and time fields are specified in format. The HL7 standard recognizes several hundred data elements for communicating patient information, including demographic, clinical, and administrative (such as financial information) elements. Some fields may hold more than one data type.

# Interface Standards

In an attempt to create a standard for the electrical signaling and cable connection characteristics, the Electronic Industry Association adopted Reference Standard RS-232C in 1969.[4] RS-232C defines the way by which data is moved through communication links and it is most commonly used with **ASCII** characters for transmission.

The RS-232C uses a 25-pin or 9-pin D shell connector with a male plug on the data terminal equipment (DTE) end and a female plug on the data communications equipment (DCE). Figure 8-1 is an illustration of a 25-pin RS-232 connector. The names of the signals that correspond to each pin are as follows:

1. Earth ground
2. Transmitted data to DCE
3. Received data to DTE
4. Request to send to DCE
5. Clear to send to DTE
6. Data not ready to DTE
7. Logic ground
8. Carrier detect to DTE
9. Reserved
10. Reserved
11. Unassigned
12. Secondary carrier detect to DTE
13. Secondary clear to send to DTE
14. Secondary transmitted data to DCE
15. Transmit clock to DTE
16. Secondary received clock to DTE
17. Receiver clock to DTE
18. Unassigned

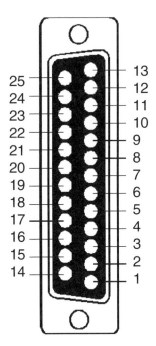

**FIGURE 8-1.** RS-232 25-pin plug. The numbers correlate with various functions, described in the text.

19. Secondary request to send to DCE
20. Data terminal ready to DCE
21. Signal quality; detect to DTE
22. *ning* detect to DTE
23. Data rate select to DCE
24. Transmit clock to DCE
25. Unassigned

Pins 4 and 5 are designated for initiation of the handshaking process that sets and authorizes the transmission.

By the mid-1970s, RS-232C-compliant interfaces were available as options for laboratory instruments (e.g., Beckman ASTRA), and by the mid-1980s, download features were introduced as additional options. The RS-232C has evolved as the most commonly used electrical specification for serial interfacing of laboratory instruments with the information system.

Advances in the 1990s led to the introduction of wireless interfaces that make it possible to connect laboratory instruments to computers by means of electromagnetic waves. The two forms of wireless connections are infrared waves based on a direct-sequence spread spectrum and radio waves using the frequency-hopping spread spectrum (see Chapter 10). This technology has been extended to point of care-testing instruments, e.g., the I-STAT instrument, which uses infrared channels to transmit test results and patient information to the laboratory information system. The use of wireless technology for the interfacing of laboratory instruments with the information system is yet to have widespread acceptance.

## Interfaces in the Diagnostic Laboratory

The laboratory computer may be interfaced to a foreign system such as a hospital system or a reference laboratory. This connection may have several interface components. **Incoming components** bring to the laboratory information system (LIS) admission, discharge, transfer, or ADT information, orders, and queries from the hospital information system (HIS). **Outgoing components** send from the LIS to the HIS ADT information acquired from clinics during HIS downtime; outgoing orders initially received in the laboratory, updating the HIS, such as order entries and cancellations, order status, and results, in response to queries or simply reflecting completion of the test. They also send financial information for a centralized billing service.

Incoming information is received into a file system designed to handle such transactions, which may have to be reformatted to fit the files. These intermediary files are the source of information for LIS functions. The tasks to be accomplished for incoming data are retrieving data from the foreign system; reformatting the data into a form comprehended by the LIS, and writing the data to LIS system files. Outgoing tasks include retrieving data from LIS system files, processing the outgoing records; reformatting the outgoing records into a form comprehended by the foreign system; and sending the data to the foreign system.

Prior to the late 1960s, laboratory instruments were mainly stand-alone and raw data were collected manually for off-line processing. In such instruments, the analyst determines the analyte's concentration from analog data such as the peak height or area of a chromatogram. Examples of such instruments are gas chromatographic and spectrophotometric analyzers. In the late 1960s and early 1970s, laboratory instruments with analog chart capture (e.g., Technicon SMA) and printer capture (Coulter S), respectively, were introduced. The analog data is converted to the digital data by an analog-digital (A-D) converter that resides in either the instrument or the printer. These early connections between the laboratory instrument and analog chart capture devices used parallel interfaces.

## *Parallel Interfaces*

The parallel interface can send several bits (1 to 16 bits, 32 bits or wider) of data across eight parallel wires simultaneously.[3] Figure 8-2 illustrates the parallel interface. The type of handshake used to move the data over the

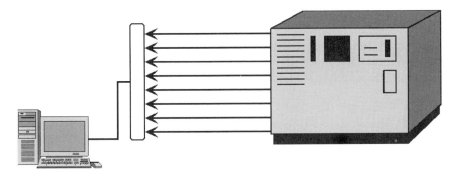

**Figure 8-2.** Parallel interface. Eight signals travel over eight parallel wires from the sender to the receiver.

parallel wires can further classify the parallel interface into four groups. The groups are zero-wire handshake, one-wire handshake, two-wire handshake, and three-wire handshake. This classification is based on how the wires are actually used for the handshake.

The parallel interface has the main advantage of speed; an entire byte can be sent across the wires in a relatively short time. However, it has the major disadvantage of distance, because voltages tend to leak from one wire to another at a rate that is proportional to the length of the wires. Thus, parallel cables are limited to 10 feet to avoid this voltage leakage problem. This limitation made it difficult to use parallel interfaces for instruments and information systems that are far from each other. However, the parallel interface continues to be used for connections between instruments and printers that are in close proximity and where vast amounts of information are being transferred (for example, between the Hewlett Packard 5890 GC and the 3390A printer).

## Serial Interfaces

A solution to the voltage leakage and long-distance problems of the parallel interface was found with the development of the serial interface. The serial interface sends data 1 bit at a time over a single, one-way wire. A serial interface cable contains several wires that have designated tasks: one wire is for sending the data, another wire is for receiving data, and the other wires are used for regulating how the data is sent or received. Based on the mode of data transmission, the serial interface can be divided into one of two types: asynchronous and synchronous.

In **asynchronous transmission**, each character is transmitted without any fixed time between it and the preceding character. As illustrated in Figure 8-3, in the asynchronous systems, each character must have start bit preceding the character and a stop bit after the character. The start bit alerts the receiving device that a

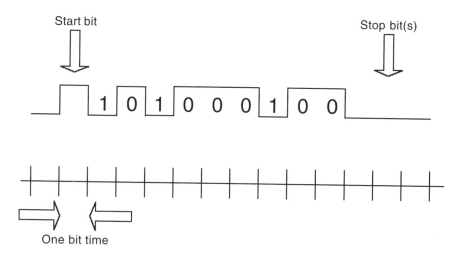

FIGURE 8-3. Asynchronous format for the transmission of the ASCII character E.

character is coming and the stop bit allows the receiver to "rest" before the next character is transmitted. Both the transmitting and receiving devices have internal clocks that are used for synchronizing the transmission.

Unlike asynchronous transmission, **synchronous transmission** sends blocks of characters, which include synchronization (sync) characters in front. The sync character synchronizes the receiver with the transmitter, thus providing a sort of running start for the block. Synchronous transmitters and receivers share a common clock that is sent as a clock bit to the other device. Error detection is critical for synchronous transmission because the characters are sent in block. This need for error check is resolved using one of several error detection techniques, e.g., cyclic redundancy checking. Synchronous transmission can be further divided into **byte-control protocol** (BCP) and **bit-oriented protocol** (BOP). The synchronous BCP primarily transmits bytes of information, and error checking is done at a byte level. The synchronous BOP transmits information as bits, so it is more flexible for transmitting odd-length data (e.g., 17 bits—rarely done).

Laboratory instruments since the 1990s predominantly use serial interfaces for connectivity with the laboratory information system. The serial interface is further classified as simplex, half-duplex, and full-duplex interface.

## Simplex Connection

The communication in the simplex system is unidirectional with one device designated as the sole transmitter and the second device is a receiver. The transmission direction is fixed, e.g., transmission from a laboratory instrument to a printer or a computer system. The simplex interface satisfies the

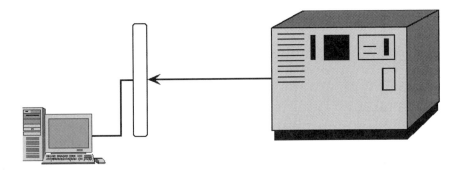

**FIGURE 8-4.** Simplex serial interface. One machine transmits, the other passively receives. The analytical instrument is instructed at its own key pad and sends results to the recipient computer.

needs of a working environment where the second device (e.g., a printer) never needs to transmit or of older instruments, which do not have receiving features (e.g., older blood ABG instruments). This is illustrated in Figure 8-4.

**Half-Duplex Connection**

This bidirectional connectivity supports transmission in only one direction at a time. It is designed for systems that do not have sufficient bandwidth in the communication channels to handle simultaneous bidirectional communications. Half-duplex connectivity (illustrated in Figure 8-5) is used extensively for the interface of laboratory instruments with the laboratory information system.

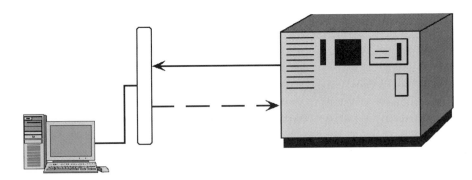

**FIGURE 8-5.** Schematic of a half-duplex serial interface. While one machine transmits, the other passively receives. Conversation alternates. The analytical instrument is instructed by the central computer and sends results to the recipient central computer. These conversations can alternate with great speed.

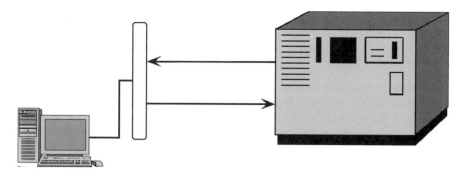

FIGURE **8-6.** Duplex serial interface. Both machines can transmit simultaneously. This is like a telephone conversation in which both parties can talk at the same time. This scheme would not do very well for laboratory analyzers.

### Full-Duplex Connection

The full-duplex, as depicted in Figure 8-6, is a bidirectional system that allows transmission of data or information in both directions between two devices simultaneously. It is used in high-bandwidth channel systems, e.g., cables and radio transmissions.

## Interfaces for Instruments in the 2000s

The laboratories of the twenty first century are characterized by instrument-information systems interfaces, which makes it possible for the interchange of data and/or information between the two entities. The interfaces that most commonly use the RS-232C can be classified as unidirectional or bidirectional. This classification is based on the use of either the simplex serial connection (unidirectional) or the half-duplex serial connection (bidirectional).

### Unidirectional Interface

The unidirectional interface of laboratory instruments to the central information system computer is used in the older models of instruments (Abbott, ADx, Abbott TDx, NOVA STAT Profile, and so on). This interface uses the serial simplex connectivity because the instruments can only transmit data. Thus, to use this unidirectional interface, the order entry is first done on the laboratory information system (LIS). The accession number generated from the order entry is then used to reorder the test at the instrument keyboard or via a bar-code reader. On completion of the testing, the accession number is used by the instrument for transmission of the results to the LIS computer. The unidirectional interface eliminates the need for manual input of test results into the laboratory information system. It eliminates transcription error for test results and may improve the overall turnaround for test results.

### Bidirectional Interface

The bidirectional interface of laboratory instruments to the LIS computer uses a serial half-duplex connectivity. In this interface, the test ordering is done only once at the keyboard of the information system terminal. The order is then available for transmission to the instrument. Based on the mode of transmission, the bidirectional interface is further classified as either broadcast system or host query system.

In the **broadcast system**, the ordered test is announced to the instrument (or instruments, if multiple instruments that can perform the test are interfaced) by the information system, thus allowing the test to be done once the bar-coded test tube is presented to the instrument. On completion of the analysis, the instrument transmits the results to the LIS. Unlike the broadcast system, the **host query system** is characterized by the fact that the instrument first reads the bar code and then asks the information system to download the ordered test information. The LIS computer then transmits the order to the instrument for testing to be performed. On completion of the testing, the results are transmitted to the central laboratory information system.

The bidirectional interface has the additional advantage of allowing the order entry function to be done once (only at the level of the information system) versus the unidirectional interface that requires the order entry to be done at both the information system and the instrument. This feature is important in the reduction of order entry errors. Examples of instruments with bidirectional interface are Sysmex 9500, Axsym, and Vitros 250 and 950.

# Chapter Glossary

**ASCII:** American Standard Code for Information Interchange. It is a character set representation scheme. Each character uses 7 bits, for a total of 128 possible symbols.

**handshakes:** Signals transmitted back and forth over a communications network that establish a valid connection between two stations.

**handshaking:** Process used by two devices to define how they will send and receive data from each other. It defines transfer speed, number of bits that make up a data packet, number of bits that signal the beginning and end of a packet, use of a parity bit for error checking, and mode of operation (e.g., for serial interface: simplex, half-duplex, or full-duplex). If these settings are not acceptable during the handshaking process, communication may fail completely or characters that make no sense may be transmitted.

**interface:** Method by which two independent entities interact with a resultant exchange of data or information.

**joystick:** Small vertical lever mounted on a base that steers the cursor on a computer display screen.

**light pen:** Input device. Selections are made by pressing a penlike device against the computer display screen. Suitable when the user needs to have direct interaction with the content of the screen.

**protocol:** Rules governing transmisson and reception of data.

**RS-232C:** Serial interface that consists of several independent circuits sharing the same cable and connectors. See **Recommended Standard**

**Recommended Standard (RS):** Nomenclature used by the Electronic Industry Association (EIA).

**trackball:** Sphere mounted on a fixed base that steers the cursor on a computer display screen. It is a suitable replacement for the mouse when work space is limited.

**touch screen:** Input strategy in which selections are made by touching the computer display screen. This is suitable in situations where the user works in a dirty environment or has limited dexterity or expertise.

**voice:** Input strategy where spoken words are captured and translated by the computer into text and commands.

**wireless interface:** Transmission media not based on wired connections, including infrared, satellite, and microwave links.

# *References*

1. IEICE Transactions on Communication. 1995; E78B(10): 1365–1371
2. IEEE J. Selected Areas in Communications. 1995; 13(5):839–849
3. White R. How Computers Work. Emeryville, Ziff-Davis Press, 1993
4. Derfler FJ Jr, Freed L. How Networks Work. Emeryville, Ziff-Davis Press, 1996

# 9
# Bar Coding in the Laboratory

Daniel F. Cowan

A bar code is a machine-readable code in the form of stripes, bars, or squares affixed to an object for the purposes of identification.[1] It is a binary system with several elaborations, including one-dimensional, two-dimensional, and matrix codes. The development of bar coding was a response to the need to rapidly identify objects and incorporate information about them into a format that does not depend on the ability of the human eye to interpret subtle variations in the printing or writing of letters and numbers but rather permits machine reading of symbols and relation of the encoded object to a database. It is generally accepted that manual transcription is the most important source of laboratory errors, especially the transcription of numbers. It is estimated that one in 300 keystrokes is an error. A misspelled word may be obvious, but transposition of digits is not. Also, manual transcription is slow and might have to be repeated several times in the progress of a specimen through the laboratory. Speeding data entry and reducing errors may improve overall laboratory productivity.[2]

The first and still very important solution to the transcription problem and to management of large volumes of information about objects was the horizontal one-dimensional bar code, an optically readable automatic identification technology that encodes information into an array of adjacent parallel rectangular bars and spaces of varying width. This format, lacking curves or other subtle variations requiring judgment in interpretation, lends itself to a binary either-or approach suitable for reading by machine, allowing rapid, accurate, and efficient gathering of information necessary to manage large numbers of items. Since the defining characteristic of a one-dimensional bar code system or symbology is the ratio of widths of elements, not absolute size, the codes may be printed in a size and density suitable to a particular application. Density in this context is the number of data characters that can be represented in a linear unit of measurement. On a large item such as a

Based on the chapter, Barcoding in the Laboratory, *in*: Automated Integration of Clinical Laboratories: A Reference. Bissell M, Petersen J, editors. AACC Press, 1997.

shipping container or a railroad box car, the density may be low, while on a label on a small electronic component, density must be very high.

Many different bar code symbologies exist, each designed for a particular purpose. They all are simply methods of representing letters, numbers, and symbols in a highly consistent and stereotypic format; in that sense they are analogous to typefaces or fonts, readily translatable from one display technology to another. The most familiar bar code symbology is the one-dimensional linear array of bars and spaces used to identify nearly everything bought in retail stores, the contents of packages, electronic devices, and so forth. These relatively simple codes are rows of letters or numbers or alphanumeric combinations of bar code characters. These simple codes are references to computer databases in which detailed information about the coded objects is stored. When a labeled object is subjected to many discrete steps in an analytical process, the database must be referenced many times.

Various trade and standards organizations have adopted standards applicable in their particular businesses or areas of responsibility. Among the most familiar of these are the Uniform Code Council, which administers the Universal Product Code (UPC) found on most retailed items; the ANSI standard MH10.8.3 for load and transport packages; the Automotive Industry Action Group (AIAG); and the European Article Numbering (EAN) system, an international standard bar code for retail food packages. The Japanese Standards Association has been active in defining standards for several bar code applications, and recently the Japan Society of Clinical Chemistry has published standards for bar codes used in sample transportation.[3] The American Society for Testing and Materials (ASTM) has issued a standard specification (E-1466) for the use of bar codes on specimen tubes in the clinical laboratory,[4] which extends the Health Industry Business Communications Council (HIBCC) standards generally used in hospitals, laboratories, and other healthcare settings.[5]

# One-Dimensional Codes

A one-dimensional bar code can be defined as an automatic identification technology that encodes information into an array of adjacent varying-width parallel rectangular bars and spaces. A **bar code character** is the smallest component of a bar code symbol that contains data—a single group of bars and spaces that represent a specific number, letter, punctuation mark, or other symbol. In bar code symbology (CIA code 128), the letter A may appear as ▌▌ and the number 5 as ▐▌. In code 39, A is represented by ▌▌, 5 as ▌▌▌. Other codes use other representations. The **aspect ratio**, or ratio of bar height to symbol length, and the absolute height of the characters contain no information and are immaterial in the horizontal codes, except insofar as a certain height is needed to assure that the scanning device or reader can be applied to all the bar elements without the need for precise positioning. The codes read as well from an angle as they do exactly straight across, just so long as the scan includes all the bars.

Horizontal, one-dimensional bar codes are commonly named by reference to the number of wide and narrow elements used to construct a character. The narrow printed element is the reference thickness, or **X dimension**. Thickness is in reference to an internal element, either a narrow line or narrow space. The wide elements are commonly two or three times the width of the narrow elements. Each element may refer to a binary code, i.e., a wide element may represent 1 and a narrow one may represent 0. This is analogous to the keys on a computer keyboard, where each key bears a human-readable cap but when pressed, sends an 8-bit binary encoded message to the central processor. In the **2 of 5 code family**, each character group consists of five elements equally spaced, of which two must be wide. The position of the wide elements in the array determines the coded symbol. In **code 3 of 9**, also called **Code 39**, three of nine elements are wide and six narrow. In the simplest codes, the spaces between the dark elements are merely spaces; in **interleaved codes,** the spaces themselves are wide and narrow data elements, allowing two letters or numbers to be encoded in one array. Thus, in Code 39, an interleaved system commonly used in the health-related industries, the numbers 1–0 appear as

normally printed in a compact group as

The code may include human readable elements:

The code has a certain degree of error correction and error detection. For example, in the Code 39 representation of the number 1 in Figure 9-1, a line crossing the symbol at an angle (A–C) encounters the same sequence of wide and narrow elements as one crossing it horizonitally, and reads it as well as the horizontal scan. However, if a printing defect causes one element to have an irregular border, a scan crossing at that point (A–B) would not encounter the proper ratio of wide to narrow elements required by the code and would not recognize the symbol as a valid representation of anything.

There are more than 50 different one-dimensional bar code symbologies. The examples cited use only two widths of bars and spaces. Certain other symbologies, the **N,K codes**, use three widths of bars and spaces. N refers to the number of modules in a character, and K to the total number of bars and spaces in a character. Standard Code 39 uses 43 characters to represent all

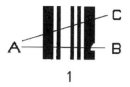

FIGURE 9-1. Although not level, scan A–C produces an accurate reading because line and space proportions are maintained, while scan A–B is rejected because a bar is defective and proportions are not maintained.

capital letters, numbers, and seven symbols, including space , . / + – $ %, using bars and spaces of two widths.

Codes are commonly bracketed by narrow bars that identify the particular code and indicate beginning and end of the data fields, or by some other symbol that serves the same purpose. Typically, a Code 39 symbol begins and ends with * to indicate to the reader (scanner) the specific code symbology. A terminal check digit computed from the coded numbers and added by the printer, provides an error check. If the encoded numbers do not compute to produce the check digit, an error is registered and the scanner does not accept the code.

**Extended Code 39** is a variation that permits use of more characters than can be accommodated by standard Code 39. This is done by using the first 43 characters in the usual way, then representing the remaining characters of the full ASCII set by using two code characters for each ASCII symbol. Extended Code 39 is used mainly when lowercase letters are needed.

The familiar UPC found on retailed items is a 7–2 N,K code, meaning that it is seven modules wide, with each module composed of two bars and two spaces of variable width. The UPC encodes only numbers, which are commonly printed as human-readable text at the bottom of the bar code. Characteristic features of the UPC-A symbology are narrow beginning and ending (left and right) guard bars and the division of the 12-character group into two separately scannable halves by a similar pair of narrow bars. This arrangement allows the manufacturer to be coded in half the symbol and the specific product to be coded in the other half. It also makes the symbol pairs taller than they are long, easier for the simple and inexpensive scanners used in markets to read, and makes positioning of the code in relation to the scanner less critical.

UPC is a relatively simple symbology limited to coding numbers, and it is well suited to simple applications. **Code 128**, another N,K code, is designed to encode the entire 128-character ASCII set, including special codes that enable it to communicate with computers. This symbology is considerably more dense than UPC or Code 39, requiring both check digits and more refined scanners.

At some point, the need to include more and more information requires more of the simple linear bar code format than it can deliver, and a new strategy is needed. This strategy involves stacking one or more linear codes into a two-dimensional array.

# Two-Dimensional Codes

A bar code is defined as any printed code used for recognition by a scanner, including some that do not appear to the human viewer as including "bars." Bar codes can be broadly grouped as one-dimensional or two-dimensional (2D). Traditional one-dimensional bar codes use the width and spacing of bars as the code. Because of practical difficulties in managing linear codes of great length, one-dimensional codes are relatively limited in the amount of information they can contain. Some 2D systems hold well over 1500 characters in an area 2 cm$^2$.

2D symbols store data using two dimensions of a surface, in contrast to the one-dimensional codes, which code data in a linear array. There are two types of 2D symbols. **Stacked symbols** are segments of linear code placed (or stacked) one above another. Their advantage is that they carry much more data than a simple linear array; their disadvantage is that they are relatively bulky. Familiar examples of stacked codes are code 49, code 16K and PDF417. PDF stands for **portable data file**, a reference to the volume of information that can be represented in the code symbol. In contrast to linear codes, which identify the object and refer to a database, a stacked code such as PDF417 contains the data within itself and does not need to frequently refer to an external database. PDF417 can contain 1850 ASCII characters and 2710 numbers. An example of Code 49 and PDF417 are shown in Figure 9-2.

The pattern of vertical lines that border the symbol, most evident in the PDF417 symbology, identifies the particular symbology and orients the reader as to start and stop (left and right) of the code. PDF417 symbology is used to construct portable data files, such as the physical and chemical properties of a material, used in association with material safety data sheets (MSDS). On a reagent label they may include not only information identifying the material but also expiration date, so that the device in which it is to be used may identify a nonusable but otherwise correct reagent. Personal identification cards encoding name, rank, serial number, and various other information are issued as identification cards by the Department of Defense, and several states incorporate PDF417 in automobile driver's licenses.

Stacked codes have the potential for two kinds of error: **erasures**, which are missing, damaged or otherwise undecipherable symbols whose position is known but value is not, and **errors** in which a character is mislocated or

CY 1234CD5678EF901234

Code 49

XY1234CD5678EF901234

PDF417

**FIGURE 9-2.** Representative stacked codes. Each layer is recognizable as a line of bar code.

incorrectly decoded; both position and value of the symbol are unknown. Stacked codes typically include built-in error correction (redundancy) to compensate for damage to the label or some other defect. The information is simply repeated within the label on the assumption that an error will not occur in the same place twice. The amount of redundancy built into the code depends on the application. Redundancy levels are rated 0 to 8. A high level assures high levels of correction, at the upper levels compensating for as much as 50% damage. This capacity requires, however, that the reader be controlled by a computer with substantial processing power.

Finally, complex coding technologies of small size and high data density require considerable precision in production and placement of the label in relation to the reader, since **tilt** becomes an issue. With a simple linear code, tilt is not a problem so long as the scan incorporates all parts of the code (Figure 9-1). With stacked codes, the chance of the scan crossing more than one layer of the code is high. PDF417 manages this problem by employing a separate coding scheme for each of three successive rows. Thus, rows 1, 2, and 3 are distinguishable by the scanner, defining an acceptable level of tilt. The pattern repeats in rows 4, 5, and 6, and so on. Limits placed on the system by acceptable levels of tilt mean that the densely printed label is not suitable for hand application to a specimen; however, it is very effectively used in applications by machine, such as identification of reagents or other supplies used within a closed analytical system.

**Matrix codes** or **matrix symbols** are two-dimensional arrays of squares or cells, each of which carries a bit of binary data. They are much more space-efficient than stacked codes but require more complex imaging devices to read them. Examples of matrix symbols are given in Figure 9-3.

The different symbologies use different strategies for identification of the code and orientation of the symbol for the reader. Most obvious in the examples given are the open top and right side of DataMatrix, the locator bull's eye of Maxicode, and the central bars of Code One.

Because of its ability to pack large amounts of information into a small space, DataMatrix has been adopted as the standard symbology for small-item tracking applications by several trade groups, including the AIAG, the EIA, and Semiconductor Equipment and Materials International (SEMI). Because the matrix can be printed using materials that withstand harsh conditions, such as exposure to heat and caustic solutions, DataMatrix is

Vericode         Data Matrix        Maxicode         Code One

FIGURE **9-3.** Representative matrix codes. Note how orientation elements vary with each code.

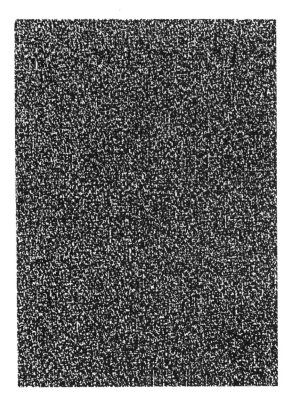

FIGURE 9-4. Intactacode encoding scheme, composed of innumerable minute squares that are uninterpretable without the correct code on the receiving end of a transmission.

used to track electronic component and manufacturing processes. Another advantage of DataMatrix is that it is in the public domain and is highly standardized. A disadvantage of DataMatrix and other matrix codes is the requirement for special readers, which may be several times the cost of conventional scanners.

Other bar code technologies, perhaps better referred to as binary encoding technologies, include the proprietary system IntactaCode, devised by Info*imaging* Technologies, Inc. (Palo Alto, CA). One use of IntactaCode is an application called 3D FAX. In this system each byte of information is represented by a small pattern of black and white dots. A stream of bytes is referred to as a grid. This system may be used to encode information for security when sent over a more or less "public" system such as telefax. Using encoding software on the sending computer, the message is translated into densely packed binary code that may be sent directly from computer to computer or to a printer. The recieving computer contains decoding software to render the message into readable text. A faxed paper message may be fed into a scanner that enters the encoded message into a recieving computer. Variations of this system permit encoding of large volumes of data in a small space. The density depends on the resolving power of the scanner used. The example of encoded text presented as Figure 9-4 contains the text of the first page of this chapter.

# The Bar Code System

A bar code label system consists of defined information to be printed on the label, the software that incorporates the information and controls the printer, the printer, the label stock, the label scanner, the reader, the computer that receives signals from the reader and converts them to usable information, and the database within the computer.

## *Defining Information*

The purpose of the label defines the information that will be encoded on it, such as name and other reference information, whether the label must contain human-readable characters, and so forth. The volume of information required and the circumstances under which the label will be read determine the size of the label and the code symbology selected. With the application defined, the code symbology and other factors determined, a vendor of the code is selected. Prospective vendors may assist in identifying technology options for achieving the desired results.

## *Bar Code Software*

Depending on the complexity of the project, the label may be composed on a computer, using special software. A simple label may be prepared using a word processing program and fonts available with specialty font packages. The first examples of bar code presented in this discussion were printed using fonts that simply substituted for the normal character font. Software may be provided with the printer by a vendor.

## *Labels*

Bar code labels may be printed on any relatively smooth surface, commonly paper, but also cardboard, plastic, metal, or ceramic. In the laboratory, labels are typically plain paper, coated paper, or heat sensitive (thermal) stock. Depending on the application, label adhesives may be water or solvent resistant, peelable, or one-use only. Size of the label is determined by the object on which it is to be placed.

## *Bar Code Printers*

Bar code print quality guidelines are defined under American National Standards Institute (ANSI) standard X3.182-1990.[6] A variety of printing technologies may be used, from a formed-font impact printer such as a typewriter or daisy-wheel printer to a dot matrix impact, laser, or bubble jet printer. Formed-font printers transfer a preformed image of a letter, number, or symbol by striking an inked ribbon against the paper. In dot matrix printing, each character is composed individually by changing the arrangement of a cluster of pins, which strike the paper, or ports that eject minute droplets of ink against the paper. The print technology used is the limiting factor in the clarity, density, and durability of the coded image produced. Scanners tend to have high levels of discrimination but may be defeated by fuzzy, blurred, or run-together printing. This is especially true of high-density linear codes used for tube labels and identification bands and the complex patterns of 2D codes. Depending on the application and the place in which labels are produced, dot matrix impact printers, portable thermal printers, or high-resolution laser printers may be indicated.

Thermal printers are dot matrix devices that use heat instead of impact to transfer images from the print head to the printing stock. **Direct thermal printers** heat the printing pins, which produce small dots on a special heat-sensitive paper. These printers are quiet and relatively cheap; they can be battery powered and light enough to be genuinely portable. The paper's sensitivity to heat and strong light makes it unsuitable for long-term storage, as it deteriorates rather quickly. However, for short-term functions such as specimen tube labeling, direct thermal-printed labels may be a successful solution. **Heat transfer printers** also use heated printing pins, but the heat transfers ink from a ribbon to the label, so heat-sensitive paper is not required. Heat transfer labels are more expensive than direct thermal labels but are more durable and long lasting. Some machines can produce either direct thermal or thermal transfer labels, as needed.

## Laser Printers

Laser printers are flexible and ubiquitous, and they produce symbols of high density and resolution. The product may be stable and durable. The drum-and-toner photocopierlike machines transfer a powder to the paper, where it is fused by light, heat, and pressure to form a clear image. Depending on the toner or other colorant used, the product may be stable and resistant to heat or pressure, although the ink may transfer to plastic objects or sheets that come in contact with it for a time.

## Print Density

Printers capable of 400-DPI (dots per inch) provide high print resolution and therefore permit printing of high-density or complex symbols that can be read by available scanners. This is particularly important with the bulls-eye finder pattern of MaxiCode. Lower-DPI printers produce images with irregular, "fuzzy" edges, more accurately identified by the Data Matrix scanner.

# Bar Code Readers

Three kinds of devices are used to read bar codes. These are the wand or pen, the moving-beam laser scanner, and the fixed-beam scanner. The **wand** is often found in the laboratory, where its flexibility allows it to be used on a variety of objects, such as requisition forms and tube labels. Wands are most effective on small coded labels, where reading is done in one quick pass. They are less effective on codes printed large on items such as shipping containers and reagent bottles. Wands are reliable but require some practice to be used effectively. A common error when scanning with them is to make a quick swipe at the label, missing some of the bars, rather than a smooth and consistent pass across the entire symbol. Wands also require high-quality printing for maximal effectiveness. **Moving-beam laser scanners** are hand-held and passed over the code to be read. They project a thin, red, scan line onto the bar code. They are very fast, performing more than 30 scans per second. Hand-held scanners are most convenient to use on large labels, may be held at a distance of several inches, and are less sensitive to poor quality or fuzzy printing, such as may be found on shipping boxes. **Fixed-beam scanners** require the scanned object to be passed over or under them. The scanners used at super-market checkouts are fixed-beam devices. Smaller versions are appearing in the laboratory, where they are used mainly to read requisition labels, and inside automated analyzers, where labeled tubes are passed by readers.

Code readers are generally attached to computers via RS-232 ports when it is intended that they will be used as the primary data entry device. Sometimes they are connected with a device known as a **keyboard wedge** to allow either the keyboard or the bar code reader to be used as the input device. The same binary signal is presented to the computer whether it is initiated by the keyboard or the scanner.

# Bar Coding in the Laboratory

Bar codes are being used more and more extensively in the laboratory for a variety of functions, including order entry, patient identification, specimen identification, preparation of load lists, efficient real-time bidirectional interfacing of instrumentation, on-line result verification, maintenance of specimen integrity, specimen tracking, data entry, including interpretive phrases, and identification of slide materials.[7] To these individualized processing steps might be added identification of reagents and for inventory control. Bar codes have become ubiquitous in many settings in which highly accurate identification, error-free data entry, and fast throughput are required. A specimen may arrive in the laboratory bearing a bar code label that identifies the patient; it may also identify the test requested. In the blood bank, labels identify bagged blood by ABO type and by other determined antigens. Many automated analyzers use bar coded reagent containers or cartridges, and in some devices, reagent cartridges may be placed in a holder, in any or no special order, to be identified by the analyzer as needed.

The ASTM has designated Code 39, including a standard check digit, as the symbology for printing and reading bar coded labels applied to specimen containers. Code 128 is allowed and is considered by the ASTM as the code symbology of the future, as it contains an integral check digit. A corollary of this designation is that printers and readers used in the laboratory should be able to produce and read both Code 39 and Code 128. The ASTM further specifies that tube labels be no longer than 60 mm and no taller than 10 mm and that tube labels, except for start, check, and stop characters, be human-readable. At a minimum, labels must link the specimen to a patient; they may contain other information, such as patient name and ID number, sample number, date, and priority ( e.g., "routine" or "stat"). Standards for labels used on blood bags are promulgated by the American Blood Commission[8]

Bar coding imposes certain requirements on the laboratory computer system. The LIS must be able to print specimen labels with a bar coded accession number, download patient information and orders to the appropriate instruments in real-time, read bar codes to prepare load lists for instruments that cannot accept a real-time interface, read bar codes for on-line verification of patient information and to track specimens through the testing process, and ideally, to support hand-held instruments for phlebotomist use when identifying patients and identifying samples.[7]

Before undertaking a bar coding project, objectives should be clearly defined. The tasks that lend themselves to bar coding are identification of patients and specimens, tracking specimens, identification of reagents, and maintenance of a reagent and supplies inventory, all of which can be done without bar coding. A benefits analysis should focus on reduction of handling costs, reduction of the number of lost specimens, and reduction of transcription errors. Some of these benefits may be quantifiable as dollars saved, while others are matters of judgment, such as convenience, error reduction, and shortened turnaround time, reflected mainly in client satisfaction, a notoriously subjective parameter.

Vendors specialize in different aspects of bar coding. Some supply preprinted labels to the user's specification; others provide on-demand printers and software to drive the printers. Some vendors can promise integration of a bar code printer and reader into an existing computer system, while others cannot. The buyer should be cautious of proprietary systems that may effectively lock the buyer into a single source of supply of bar code supplies or bar coded reagents.

The more automated a laboratory becomes, the more it will rely on a sophisticated system of specimen identification. In a fully automated laboratory, the entry of a test request into the laboratory information system can result in the production of bar coded labels that include not only the name of the patient, but also the test or tests requested on a sample. In some laboratories, the labels may be taken by the phlebotomist on rounds. In a laboratory with a wireless communication system linking phlebotomists to the laboratory, a request received in the LIS is immediately relayed to the phlebotomist, who receives it via radio device. The device incorporates both a bar code reader and a portable lightweight thermal printer. The phlebotomist, directed to the patient by information displayed on the hand-held device, uses the reader on the patient's bar coded wristband (both hand-held and wristband positively identify the patient) to open a transaction with the laboratory. Blood is drawn and information entered into the hand-held, which prints labels with the patient identifier and the requested test. The labels are affixed to the tubes, and the phlebotomist then indicates that the transaction is complete, either by scanning the wristband again or by entering a command into the hand-held. The device communicates the collection to the LIS, which acknowledges the status of the specimen as "collected," noting date, time, place, and collector. Since the specimen is now accessioned into the laboratory, on return the phlebotomist puts the labeled tubes into the automated processing line, which, guided by the information on the labels and governed by computer program, passes them along the appropriate processing sequence. For some specimens, processing might include sample division with production and application of bar coded labels to aliquot tubes or, in a different testing sequence, to blood smears, which are then directed along the line for machine sorting. Eventually, specimen tubes are stored still bearing the original bar coded label, pending further need. None of this random-entry automated processing is possible without the reliable, discrete identification and control system provided by bar coding.

## Chapter Glossary

The following list includes terms that are often encountered in relation to bar coding.

**AIM:** Automatic Identification Manufacturers Inc., a trade association.

**alphanumeric:** Character set that contains the letters A–Z and numerals 0–9.

**ASCII character set:** 128 characters including both control and printing characters.

**aspect ratio:** Expressed as X:Y; when referring to 2D codes, the ratio of either module height to module width or the height to the width of the entire symbol.

**background:** Spaces, quiet zones, and area surrounding a printed symbol.

**bar:** Darker element of a printed bar code symbol.

**bar code:** Automatic identification technology that encodes information into an array of adjacent varying-width parallel rectangular bars and spaces.

**bar code character:** Single group of bars and spaces that represents a specific number (often one) of numbers, letters, punctuation marks or other symbols. This is the smallest subset of a bar code symbol that contains data.

**check character:** Character within a symbol whose value is used to perform a mathematical check to ensure that the symbol has been decoded correctly.

**code word:** Symbol character value.

**element:** Single bar or space.

**element width:** Thickness of an element measured from the edge closest to the symbol start character to the trailing edge of the same element.

**error correction** (also referred to as data redundancy): Symbol characters reserved for error correction and/or error detection. These characters are calculated mathematically from the other symbol characters.

**error detection** (also referred to as data security): System that prevents a symbol from being decoded as erroneous data. Error correction characters can be reserved for error detection. These characters then function as check characters.

**Finder pattern** (also called recognition pattern): Pattern used to help find the symbol, determine the symbol version, and determine the symbol's tilt and orientation, as well as providing additional reference points to calculate the data square positions and to account for surface curvature.

**matrix code:** Arrangement of regular polygon-shaped cells where the center-to-center distance of adjacent elements is uniform. The arrangement of the elements represents data and/or symbology functions. Matrix symbols may include recognition patterns that do not follow the same rule as the other elements within the symbol.

**module:** Narrowest nominal width unit of measure in a symbol. One or more modules are used to construct an element.

**numeric:** Character set including only numerals 1–9.

**overhead:** Fixed number of characters required for start, stop, and checking in a given symbol. For example, a symbol requiring a start/stop and two check characters contains four characters of overhead. Thus, to encode three characters, seven characters are required to be printed.

**quiet zone (clear area):** Spaces preceding the start character of a symbol and following a stop character.

**stacked code:** Long multirow symbol broken into sections and stacked one on another similar to sentences in a paragraph.

**symbol character:** Unique bar and/or space pattern defined for a particular symbology. Depending on the symbology, symbol characters may have a unique associated symbol value.

# *References*

1. Sharp KR. A short, basic course in bar code. ID Systems 1990; Nov:74–80
2. Dito WR, McIntire, LJ. Bar codes and the clinical laboratory: Adaptation perspectives. Clin Lab Man Rev 1992; Jan–Feb:72–85
3. Japan Society of Clinical Chemistry, Committee Report. Jpn J Clin Chem 1996; 25:122–125
4. American Society for Testing and Materials, Standard Specification for Use of Bar Codes on Specimen Tubes in the Clinical Laboratory. (E-1466) Annual Book of ASTM Standards. Philadelphia
5. Provider Applications Standard, Health Industry Business Communication Council, Phoenix
6. American National Standards Institute, Bar Code Print Quality Guidelines X3.182-1990. New York
7. Haas DJ, Murphy L. Bar codes in the laboratory Lab Comput Autom 1989; 6:49–55
8. Guideline for the Uniform Labeling of Blood and Blood Components. American Blood Commission, Arlington, Virginia

# 10
# Wireless Communication Networks in the Laboratory

Daniel F. Cowan

As the settings in which medical and other health services change, the need for mobility, flexibility, and efficiency in communication increases.[1] Wireless medical technology is in use in diverse settings, including aircraft,[2] ships,[3] and ambulances,[4] as well as the hospital and medical office environments.[5] The replacement of paper records by electronic records changes the way information is collected, stored, and transmitted, requiring changes in procedures that formerly depended on manual data entry and the accumulation and filing of pieces of paper. Wireless communications technology permits an unprecedented degree of mobility of people and transportability of equipment, while retaining functional connection to a central laboratory information system, which may itself be integrated into a larger information structure.[6]

Wireless technology may also replace cable connections in stationary installations, such as from one building to another, when for cost or convenience issues laying of cable is not deemed desirable. The costs of antennae and other connections at each site are calculated to be less than the cost associated with leasing telephone lines or paying cable, installation, and support fees or when electrical interference with cable transmission degrades signal quality to unacceptable levels.

Available wireless technology can support national, regional, and local networks. Wireless local area networks (LANs) are most applicable in the laboratory. Wireless LAN technology allows wireless communication between components of an electronic information system. Wireless systems allow continual contact with laboratory personnel moving freely or **roaming** around a

This discussion was prepared using information provided by Aironet Wireless Communications, Inc., Fairlawn, OH, a subsidiary of Telxon Corporation, Akron, OH; Spectrix Corporation, Deerfield, IL; Cerner Corporation, Kansas City, MO; and Proxim Inc., Mountain View, CA. Parts were previously published as the chapter Specimen Procurement: Wireless Networks, *in*: Automated integration of clinical laboratories: A reference. Bissell M, Petersen J, editors. AACC Press, 1997.

facility and permit either relatively settled or mobile instruments to interface directly with the central computer system, without the laying of complex, extensive, and expensive cable systems. Wireless LAN technology is in use in a variety of industries, and the technology in general has been well established and verified as reliable.

## Conventional LAN

In a conventional wired LAN, all components are connected by a set of wires, interface devices, and communications protocols. In such a system, among the problems to be solved are routing of messages to an appropriate recipient and preventing traffic collisions that could result in the corruption or loss of data. **Token ring systems** pass messages in one direction from node to node in sequence. Messages are passed in the form of "tokens," repeating frames (packets of data transmitted as a single entity) that are transmitted along the network by the controlling computer. When a station on the net wants to send a message, it waits for an empty token, into which it puts the address of the destination and the message. Every computer station on the net monitors every token it passes to see if it is the addressee. If it is, it "grabs" the message and passes the empty frame (free token) along. A nonaddressed node simply passes the message along. In this system, each segment in the system is a separate link. Since messages are sent in sequence in one direction only, there is no possibility of collision. Token ring networks are capable of transmission rates that vary with the carrier—4 megabits per second (Mbps) with a shielded pair of twisted wires, 16 Mbps with unshielded twisted pairs, and 100 Mbps over optical fiber. A typical maximum usage rate is 60%–70% of capacity. Large frames of data may be transmitted. The strength of the token ring network is its ability to uniformly support heavy traffic. However, token rings are not cheap, with an average connection running from $200-$300.

In **Ethernet systems,** up to 1024 nodes are connected by electric wire or optical cable. Ethernet broadcasts messages over its wires. All stations can "hear" all traffic and must sort out messages by specific address. The system must therefore contend with the possibility of collision of messages; it does so using **collision detection protocols.** A standard Ethernet LAN has a transmission rate of about 10 Mbps. The frame size is a little more than one third a token ring frame. While Ethernet costs are relatively low, about $65-$100 per connection, an Ethernet LAN can support only about 40% network use. Loads above that level are associated with a deterioration in performance. The attraction of Ethernet LANs are low installation cost, reliability, and a broad base of vendor support.

In wired systems, distance between nodes is generally not a problem, as the system is powered by house current or incorporates signal boosters. Power levels (signal strength) are therefore relatively constant throughout the system. Security of access depends mainly on controlling access through terminals, using passwords, and similar contrivances. Someone not on the network has no possibility if intercepting messages, and sources of interference are relatively few. Because the power levels in the network are low, the wired LAN is not a source of interference with other devices. Transmission error rates in the controlled cable are low and predictable. The obvious drawback to wired systems is that the user is always tethered by wire to a specific location, and adding or relocating a terminal may mean stringing new wire or cable, which requires time and money and intrusion into work spaces.

# Wireless LAN

In the wireless LAN, some part or all of the cable of the conventional system is replaced by broadcast energy, either radio waves or infrared light. In such systems, several problems must be addressed. The first is that the message is literally thrown into the air, effectively negating conventional measures for collision avoidance or detection. Anyone within range with an appropriate receiver has the possibility of intercepting the message. Range is limited, as electromagnetic energy falls off with the square of the distance from the source. This means that a wireless system must contend with signals of varying strength. An interfering or colliding transmission may be stronger than the message, negating several approaches to collision detection. Interference from similar energy sources must be controlled or eliminated.[7,8] Finally, roving units of wireless systems are battery dependent, and management of battery power is a major issue.

Two major types of local wireless communications technologies are in use, **radio frequency** (RF) and **diffuse infrared** (DIR). Each seems to have an application, with certain advantages and disadvantages. What may be a disadvantage in one setting may be a strong plus in another.

Wireless local area networks are built around a structure or "backbone" of access points (**hubs, repeaters,** or **routers**) placed according to a plan in the facility to be covered. Depending on the plan, which will vary according to the size of the facility, the routers may relay through a series of radio devices directly to a host computer or may be connected to it by a wired LAN, using Ethernet or token ring technology. The object terminal device—a handheld unit, a personal computer, or a stationary instrument—is called an **end node.** Routers receive, buffer, and transmit messages to and from the end nodes. With RF, the distance over which the router can communicate with an end node is influenced by the structure (composition) of the building, the contents of the building, and the type of antenna used. Workable distances range up to 3000 feet. With proper antennas, wireless RF communications can take place over up to 2 miles, line of sight, with no obstructions. With DIR, distances are much shorter, within the range of 50 to 100 feet.

## Wireless Technology

Wireless technology depends on the transmission and receipt of signals from a remote device to a host device or between host devices, without the use of physical connections. Certain functions are implied. Each node and each router have a specific identity. Each node and router must maintain contact even though no message is being sent. Routers must buffer (hold) messages until they can be delivered. Each node and router must acknowledge receipt of each message. For the operator to be able to move about, the end node must be taken into the territory of new routers, which must be able to recognize it in its new location. This is done by the end node frequently checking with or **polling** the system to determine whether it has moved out of the territory of the original router and needs to locate a new one. It seeks the best point of access to the system, using criteria such as signal strength, the message traffic being carried by the routers, and the distance of the router from the host computer.

## Applicability of Wireless LAN Technology

In the laboratory and in the hospital or clinic setting, wireless networks are applicable in any circumstance in which there is an advantage to not having system components linked by wire and in which information will ultimately be entered into a computerized information system.[9] A few examples[6] may be given.

1. A phlebotomist carrying a hand-held receiver is dispatched to a patient room or clinic. The receiver contains a work list that is continuously updated by the central laboratory computer and perhaps a device for reading bar coded patient-identifying wristbands. The receiver can read the bar code and identify the patient, display the tests ordered, and on completion of specimen collection, confirm collection to the laboratory computer. It can also cause bar code labels to be printed by a similarly portable printer at the point of collection. The specimen arrives in the laboratory already accessioned and labeled, ready to enter the analytical path. In the event that an order is changed or an order for a different patient is received in the laboratory, the roving phlebotomist's work list is updated and he or she is dispatched to the new patient without having to return to the laboratory to receive the new assignment.

2. A point-of-care instrument with an appropriate send/receive device is linked to the central computer. The test result is subjected to the same quality control procedures as a hardwired instrument in the laboratory; the test result is displayed locally and also entered into the laboratory record. Billing information is collected automatically. Appropriate log-on procedures allow identification of the operator and collect workload information. Operator performance is monitored, perhaps by comparing

specific operator results to reference standards and to all operator results. A satellite laboratory may be established quickly in a new location, or a cart carrying diagnostic instruments may be rolled from a central location to a point of service.

3. In a paper-based medical record system, typically a paper chart is carried or a cartload of charts pushed from examining room to examining room or bed to bed. In a hospital with an electronic medical record, it may be necessary to have a computer terminal at every bed and in every examination and consultation room—a great expense in terminals, terminal servers, wiring, and maintenance. A wireless system allows a notebook computer to travel with the physician or a battery-operated microcomputer on a cart to substitute for the chart cart. Unlike paper records, which may be sequestered or in use by someone else, the electronic record is always available on line. The record displayed on the remote device is as current as the moment a test result is verified in the laboratory. Further, laboratory (and other) orders may be entered at the bedside by the physician without having to make a trip to the nursing station.

The common feature in these three examples is an increase in efficiency, promptness, and accuracy and a reduction in paperwork that together increase productivity and quality of services.

An additional example might be the need to integrate operations of newly consolidated laboratories in buildings some distance apart. Use of focused RF antennas obviates the need to string cable or to lease a telephone line between buildings.

## Connecting the Node

A node may be a hand-held unit, a computer, or an instrument. **Hand-held** or **walk-around units** typically contain the RF or DIR transceiver, its antenna, and a battery. For laboratory as well as for other applications, they also have a graphical user interface (GUI) screen for display and a keyboard or touch-screen input system or both. These devices can also include an infrared bar code label scanner for positive patient identification and a computer connection, such as a serial RS-232 port into which a portable bar code printer is plugged. This allows on-site printing of labels for collected specimens. The hand-held device seems most applicable in specimen collection.

**Note pad, notebook,** *or* **laptop computers** commonly incorporate a socket into which a function card is placed. These cards, which conform to the Personal Computer Memory Card International Association (PCMCIA) standard, are removable specialized modules that can hold memory, fax/modems, radio receivers, network adapters, and so on. Vendors of wireless systems can provide an IR receiver or a spread spectrum radio that plugs into the PCMCIA slot, allowing the computer to communicate as a terminal with the central information system. The advantage of this kind of system is that it allows users such as physicians to take it into the clinic or on rounds using it to access the most current laboratory studies and to place orders. The limitations of such a system are mostly related to battery life and quality of the display.

A **desktop computer** may be incorporated into a wireless network as a stationary but relocatable terminal. Radio cards may be plugged into an internal socket or via a communications port.

In theory, **stationary instruments** may be connected through a wireless LAN. There appear to be no major technical issues involved. At this writing we are not aware of any sites in which large stationary analyzers have been connected with the LIS through a wireless LAN.

## Diffuse Infrared Systems

DIR systems use infrared frequency band ranges from 3 micrometers ($3 \times 10^{-6}$ meters) to 750 nanometers ($7.5 \times 10^{-7}$ meters), just beyond the visible light range. For practical purposes, infrared in this range behaves exactly as does visible light, with the exception that it is not detected by the eye. In this application infrared radiation is produced by fast-switching light-emitting diodes (LED), which produce only incoherent, non-self-reinforcing light. The light is deliberately not focused or directed, as diffuse lighting is the essence of the system.

In contrast to directed IR transmissions, such as keyboard-to-computer and remote controller-to-television, which require the devices to be pointed directly at each other, DIR signals are bounced off walls, floor, and ceiling, allowing the communicating devices to be oriented randomly. Since infrared radiation does not pass through opaque surfaces and energy falls off rather quickly with distance, for practical purposes a receiver is needed for every room in which the technology is used, and the rooms should not be more than 25 feet on a side. Under ideal circumstances, in an open space without obstructions, transmission may be effective up to 100 feet. For large open spaces, several antennas linked to a base station may be used to provide coverage. Individual handheld units are identified by the assignment of specific Ethernet addresses to each. The central controller awaits indication that a particular unit has data to send or receive. On request, the controller assigns the unit a specific time slot in which to send and receive, thus avoiding interference and collisions.

With DIR technology, error rates are calculated at a set distance between transmitter and receiver. One standard used is 50 feet. At this range an expected error rate may be in the range of $10^{-6}$. In an ideal environment the rate may be as low as $10^{-7}$. In a poor one, errors may garble the data.

An important disadvantage to DIR is interference from certain types of light, and this may be a determining consideration in choice of technology. DIR can handle transmission of large amounts of data. Transmission rates in the neighborhood of 4 Mbps are achieved. Transmission rates are limited by the switching rate of the LED. Advances in LED technology promise rates of up to 10 Mbps or higher, without much change in cost. The short range and inability of DIR to penetrate opaque surfaces may be an advantage if security is an important issue. DIR may be preferred to RF transmission in environments with a great deal of radio interference, in which metal structural components or large machines interfere with radio transmission, or in which radio frequencies might interfere with a manufacturing process. DIR may also offer advantages in network management, allowing more simultaneous users than might RF systems. With all these considerations, DIR may offer an effective and relatively low cost wireless LAN.

## Radio Frequency Systems

Radio-based telemetry systems are now widely used in medical applications and increasingly are regulated by both the Food and Drug Administration (FDA) and the Federal Communications Commission (FCC). The Wireless Medical Telemetry Service (WMTS) of the FCC reserves the frequencies of 608–614 MHz (megahertz), 1395–1400 MHz, and 1429–1432 MHz for primary or coprimary use by eligible wireless medical telemetry users.[10] This action was taken to protect the frequencies used in medical telemetry from in-band interference. The FCC now defines medical telemetry as "the measurement and recording of physiological parameters and other patient-related information via radiated bi- or unidirectional electromagnetic signals."[10] "Eligible WMTS users" include licensed physicians, healthcare facilities, and certain trained and supervised technicians. Eligible healthcare facilities are those offering services for use beyond 24 hours, including hospitals and other medical providers but not ambulances or other moving vehicles.[10]

WMTS rules include limitations on transmitter output power, out-of-band emissions, and protection of other services. Interestingly, users of the WMTS are coprimary with the radio astronomy service operating in the 608–614-MHz band and devices operating within 80 km of certain radio astronomy facilities, and 32 km of certain other radio astronomy facilities must have special permission from the WMTS.[10] "Primary users" of a frequency band have priority of use and may not be subject to interference by "secondary users," who may however, have to accept interference from primary users. Primary users tend to include commercial broadcasters and the military. Coprimary users have equal priority that must be resolved by means such as distance and power limitations. Most medical telemetry users operate as secondary users in select commercial broadcast bands—channels 7–13 (174–216 MHz) and channels 14–46 (450–470 MHz)—and in the private land mobile radio service (PLMRS) 450–470 MHz band. The medical telemetry application must accept interference from these primary sources. Also, the FCC has allocated previously vacant television channels in the range of 7–46 for digital television (DTV). Some telemetry equipment may also operate on a shared basis in industrial, scientific, and medical (ISM) bands. In addition, the FCC began accepting applications for high-power land mobile applications for the 450–460-MHz band on January 21, 2001.[10] The message in all this is that demand for and use of the limited number of broadcast-usable radio frequencies is great and increasing. Attention was vividly drawn to this issue in 1998, when DTV transmissions from a local TV station in Dallas interfered with medical telemetry systems in two hospitals.[11,12]

Radio frequency transmissions consist of a basic **carrier frequency** to which data can be added by **modulation** of the carrier frequency. Modulation of the carrier frequency produces sidebands that carry the data. Receivers contain **demodulators** that extract information from the sidebands and delete the carrier frequency. In order for RF transmissions to be received, the operator must know the transmission frequency so that the receiver may be tuned to it and must use the appropriate corresponding method of demodulation. Different uses of portable radio require transmitters of differing power output. Typically the transmitter power of portable two-way radios (walkie-talkies) is 2.0–5.0 W, of cellular telephones 0.6 W, and of transmitters of the type discussed here 0.1 W. Walkie-talkies typically broadcast at a bandwidth of 12.5 kHz (kilohertz) and telephones at 25 kHz. RF wireless devices broadcast at much higher frequencies.

RF transmissions in the narrow band 450–470 MHz range are fast but penetrate solid objects poorly, and they require a Federal Communications Commission (FCC) site license. The FCC has assigned particular bandwidths for nonlicensed use—the ISM band. The most widely used wireless applications in healthcare operations employ the non-FCC licensed **spread spectrum technology** in the frequency bands 902–928 MHz and 2.4–2.484 GHz (gigahertz). The 902–928 MHz band is best used in an area that requires a broad zone of coverage, while the 2.4–2.484 GHz band is more efficient in handling large volumes of data. Spread spectrum transmission involves continuous change in carrier frequency across the spectrum according to a unique pattern recognized by both sending and receiving devices. It is used for security and allows multiple wireless transmissions in the same space.

Two technologies are used, **direct sequencing** and **frequency hopping**. Direct sequencing, or direct sequence coding, is simultaneous broadcasting over many radio frequencies. Direct sequence spread spectrum (DSSS) radios broaden bandwidth transmission by increasing the data bit rate. Each bit is divided into subbits. The subbits are called **chips** and the process **chipping**. DSSS radio transmitters use unique spread codes. For a receiver to interpret the transmission and extract information from it, it must use the same spread code. The receiver matches the spread code to the spread signal, removes the effect of chipping, collapses the spread signal to the data sidebands, and demodulates the signal to extract the data. The process of dechipping and collapsing the spread signal also includes filtering at a narrow bandwidth to remove interference from other radio sources. Further, the use of large numbers of chips (over 10), signal spreading, and collapsing results in significant

**processing gain;** an increase in the signal-to-noise ratio. These are design features and can be specified for the application.

Frequency hopping spread spectrum (FHSS) is the transmission of signals over frequencies that shift every few milliseconds according to a defined sequence. To an observer, the sequence appears to be random, but in reality it is not: the transmitter and receiver must both know the pattern. The FCC allows FHSS systems to define their own channel spacing, permitting a maximum of 500-kHz bandwidth in the 900-MHz band and 1-MHz bandwidth in the 2.4-GHz band. To keep spectrum use uniform and random, 50 channels are used. While the transmission pattern is definable, it is not permitted to use specific channels selectively or to broadcast for a long time on a single channel. These constraints allow for a full use of the spectrum and reduce the likelihood of collision between transmitters. Only receivers that know the transmitter's hopping sequence can receive the message. Transmissions using other sequences cannot be received. Communications protocols govern those instances when two different transmitters attempt to use a particular frequency simultaneously.

DSSS and FHSS each have advantages and disadvantages. Direct sequencing is the more commonly used of the two and is faster than frequency hopping, while frequency hopping broadcasts at lower transmission rates and requires more computer processing overhead. Transmission rates of equipment supplied by various vendors for DSSS technology are in the range of 240 Kbps (kilobits per second) to 2 Mbps and for FHSS 38.4 Kbps to 1.6 Mbps. DSSS has a decided advantage in battery power management.

## Installing Wireless Technology

Wireless technology is actually a hybrid system. Network cabling over token ring or Ethernet lines terminates in one or more access points. These access points are combined receivers and transmitters (transceivers) with antennas sited at points selected after a technical survey to determine actual transmission of signals through the proposed facility. The site survey is extremely important, as it determines the number and placement of transceivers as well as sources of interference and places where the signal is received poorly if at all—"dead spots".

Each antenna can service a number of mobile transceivers and is therefore in a way analogous to a terminal server. In a typical large installation, antennas are placed close enough to allow operational fields to overlap. In RF installations, this overlap occurs along the length of a floor and with antenna fields in the floor above and below. The effect is much like a cellular telephone antenna array, with the mobile unit moving from one cell to another, never outside the range of the field as a whole. Should one antenna unit fail, its lost function is assumed by antennas overlapping its field. Figure 10-1 illustrates a typical multifloor layout of antennas for an RF wireless system.

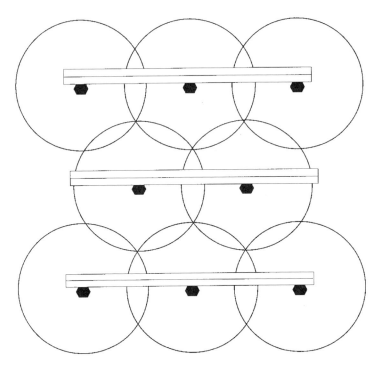

**Figure 10-1.** Layout of antennas (transceivers) in a multistory building. Note that the antennas are sited in staggered rows to eliminate "dead" areas. All radio cells overlap to provide continuous coverage.

## Security

The security of wireless systems has several aspects: unauthorized reception, interference with the broadcast signal, and interference by the broadcast signal with other systems.

### Unauthorized Reception

Unauthorized reception of the transmitted signal is prevented in several ways. In the case of DIR, the signal is contained within a room or closed space. It is picked up only by an authorized device in the local area. As light does not pass through opaque surfaces, a receiver outside the room cannot pick up or introduce signals. RF presents security issues and solutions of a different sort. Spread band radio was developed by the military with the specific intention of providing secure message transmissions. To receive a transmission, a radio listener must be tuned to the proper frequency. This process is familiar to any user of a commercial radio receiver. With spread band transmission, the message is broadcast over an array of frequencies whose bandwidth must be known.

Interception of a specific frequency does not produce a readable message. Using DSSS, with proper equipment transmissions are easily mapped back to the original data. All that is required is capturing the signal and translating it back. Translation is easily done with a well-defined algorithm. Whether the gain is worth the effort depends on the kind of information being transmitted. It is unlikely that laboratory results would justify the effort and expense. To intercept an FHSS transmission, the listener must know the transmission frequency sequence. This is much harder to crack, even with sophisticated equipment, and FHSS is therefore substantially more secure than DSSS. Further security is inherent in the fact that spread band transmission using the frequencies commonly employed has a very short range, typically in the range of a few hundred feet. A receiver must be in the building to receive. If necessary, security can be enhanced using supplemental encryption devices, with reduced performance at increased cost.

### Interference with the Broadcast Signal

Evaluation of interference with broadcast signals is an important component of the precontract site evaluation. Controllability of light sources and site architecture are important issues with DIR. Building construction (presence or absence of steel members), shielding, room contents, and the like determine distances RF will travel. Radio sources must be evaluated.[8,13,14]

DSSS, using set frequencies, is more susceptible to outside interference, while FHSS, spending only milliseconds at a given frequency, is essentially immune to outside interference. **Multipath interference** is a form of interference caused by the broadcast frequency bouncing off surfaces, such as walls and doors. DSSS cannot avoid causing this kind of interference with its own signals without manipulating antennas, while FHSS is able to evade it by constantly shifting away from it as it moves to new transmission frequencies. This is an important consideration in large DSSS networks, in which users receive signals from multiple access points. While overlapping fields of transmission guarantee that a user will receive a signal from multiple access points, overlap causes interference and degrades performance.

### Interference by the Broadcast Signal

A major source of concern is the possible effect of RF transmission on medical monitoring (telemetering) equipment.[8,13] Two approaches to avoiding this potential problem are used. One is to use RF bandwidths at a distance from those used by the monitoring devices. Another is to keep the broadcast power level low. Currently no industry standard exists regarding the susceptibility of monitoring equipment to RF and how much electromagnetic force an RF device may emit, although such standards are under development in both North America and Europe. RF can potentially interfere with analytical instruments, but this is not generally a problem at the power levels used. The effect on any new instrument must be evaluated.[8]

## Battery Power Management

While fixed components of a wireless LAN, such as the antenna units and stationary instruments, may use building current, walk-around or hand-held units must rely on battery power. These units impose what appear to be incompatible demands on a battery. A unit must be light and small, yet it must remain charged to a functional level for a useful period of time—say, a work shift of eight hours or longer—without recharging. Few batteries are up to this task. In general, DSSS amplifiers are less efficient and use more power than FHSS amplifiers and require heavier batteries and more frequent recharging. The problem is addressed by managing the use of battery power. Two strategies are used to conserve battery power. One simply turns the device off for the period of time when it is not actually relaying data; the other keeps it on continuously but at a greatly reduced level of power consumption—the "sleep" mode between data transfers. Each has its particular application.

An on/off cycle (**polling rate**) may be incorporated into the operation of the mobile device. This cycle is configured to the particular application of the device. Typical cycle times may be in the range of one per second to 15 per second. During the off or down period, messages accumulate in a buffer in the backbone LAN. During the on period, the device signals the LAN that it is ready to transfer data. On signal, transmission occurs. Though very short, this scheme of power management is able to usefully extend the power reserve between charges.

The on/off cycle applies with DSSS RF, but it will not work with FHSS, as the unit must be continuously live for synchronization to be maintained. Frequency-hopping devices use the sleep mode for power conservation, although it is less effective than on/off cycling.

## Safety Considerations

The only theoretical problem caused by DIR is injury to the retina. The protective mechanisms of the eye respond to visible light but not to invisible IR, so retinal injury by heat transfer is possible. However, retinal injury is not thought to be a problem with DIR wireless LANs, as the energy levels produced by the LED are well below the level known to produce eye injury. While a safety standard has been developed by the American National Standards Institute for eye exposure to infrared lasers (ANSI Z136.1-1993), there is none from this agency for incoherent, LED-produced IR. One approach taken has been to keep LED emissions well below the stringent levels prescribed for laser emissions. Vendors should certify the emissions levels of their devices.

Radio waves are a form of radiation and may raise a concern about possible biological effects on persons chronically exposed to RF.[15] Radiation is especially a concern as higher and higher frequencies are used, as it is the high frequencies that produce the short wavelengths with the greatest potential to penetrate and, as ionizing radiation, interact with tissues. However, this is not a practical concern to users of RF, as the intensity level of radio emissions in

RF systems is well below the level at which ionization occurs. To assure that safe levels are used in any given system, vendors should certify that they comply with ANSI standard C95.1-1982, which specifies that a hand-held RF device operate at a power level less than 0.7 watts.

# Chapter Glossary

**band:** Range of frequencies used for transmitting a signal, identified by its lower and upper limits; for example, a 10-MHz band in the 100—110-MHz range.

**DIR** (diffuse infrared system): Communication system using the infrared frequency band ranging from 3 micrometers ($3 \times 10^{-6}$ meters) to 750 nanometers ($7.5 \times 10^{-7}$ meters), just beyond the visible light range.

**direct sequence coding:** Simultaneous broadcasting over many radio frequencies, using unique spread codes known only to the transmitter and the intended receiver.

**end node:** In a network, the object terminal device: a hand-held unit, a computer, or a stationary instrument.

**Ethernet system:** Network topology consisting of up to 1024 nodes connected by electric wire or optical cable (bus topology). Ethernet broadcasts messages over its wires. All stations can "hear" all traffic and must sort out messages by specific address.

**frequency hopping spread spectrum** (FHSS): Transmission of radio signals over frequencies that shift every few milliseconds according to a defined sequence known only to the transmitter and the intended receiver.

**hand-held unit (walk-around unit):** Device designed to carry out certain functions without direct connection to a computer; typically contains an RF or DIR transceiver, its antenna and a battery; may have a graphical user interface (GUI) screen for display and a keyboard or a touch-screen input system or both.

**multipath interference:** Form of radio interference caused by the broadcast frequency bouncing off surfaces, such as walls and doors.

**PCMCIA** (Personal Computer Memory Card International Association): Nonprofit trade association founded to standardize the PC card or PCMCIA card.

**PC card (PCMCIA card):** Removable module that can hold memory, modems, fax modems, radio transceivers, network adapters, solid state disks, or hard disks. All are 85.6 mm long by 54 mm wide (3.37 inch $\times$ 2.126 inch) and use a 68-pin connector. Thickness varies with the application.

**polling:** Network communications technique that determines when a terminal is ready to send or receive data. The computer continually interrogates its connected terminals in sequence. If a terminal has data to send or is ready to receive, it sends back an acknowledgment and the transmission begins.

**processing gain:** In broadcasting, an increase in signal-to-noise ratio—an improvement in the clarity of the signal.

**RF:** Radio frequency system broadcasting over a variety of wavelengths.

**sideband:** In communications, the upper or lower half of a wave. Since both sidebands are normally mirror images of each other, one of the halves can be used for a second channel to increase the data-carrying capacity of the line or for diagnostic or control purposes.

**spread spectrum transmission:** Radio frequency transmission that continuously changes carrier frequency across the spectrum according to a unique pattern recognized by both sending and receiving devices.

**token ring network:** Communications network that uses the token-passing technology in a sequential manner. Each station in the network passes the token on to the station next to it. Messages are passed in the form of "tokens," repeating frames (packets of data transmitted as a single entity) that are transmitted along the network by the controlling computer.

**wireless LAN:** Network in which some part or all of the cable of the conventional system is replaced by broadcast energy, either radio waves or infrared light.

# *References*

1. Grimm CB. Wireless communications: Taking healthcare by storm. Healthcare Informatics 1995; 12:52–59
2. Gandsas A, Montgomery K, McIntire K, Altrudi R. Wireless vital sign telemetry to hand-held computers. Stud Health Technol Inform 2001; 81:153–157
3. Allen A. From early wireless to Everest. Telemed Today 1998; 6:16–18
4. Curry GR, Harrop N. The Lancashire telemedicine ambulance. J Telemed Telecare 1998; 4:231–238
5. Lovell NH, Celler BG. Implementation of a clinical workstation for general practice. Medinfo 1005; 8:777–779
6. Cowan DF, Martin M. Specimen Procurement: Wireless Networks In: Bissell M, Petersen J, editors. Automated Integration of Clinical Laboratories: A Reference. Washington, DC, AACC Press, 1997
7. FDA Public Health Advisory. Risk of Electromagnetic Interference with Medical Telemetry Systems. July 10, 2000. fda.gov/cdrh/safety/emimts.html
8. Paperman WD, David Y, McKee KA. Electromagnetic interference: Causes and concerns in the health care environment. Healthc Facil Manag Serv 1994; Aug:1–15
9. Bunschoten B, Deming B. Hardware issues in the movement to computer-based patient records. Health Data Manag 1995; 3:45–48, 50, 54
10. Federal Communications Commission, Wireless Medical Telemetry Service. fcc.gov/Bureaus/Engineering_Technology/Orders/2000/fcc00211.doc
11. Food and Drug Administration, Center for Devices and Radiologic Health Advisory. Interference Between Digital TV Transmissions and Medical Telemetry Systems. March 20, 1998. fda.gov/cdrh/dtvalert.html
12. Joint Statement of the Federal Communications Commission and the Food and Drug Administration Regarding Avoidance of Interference Between Digital Television and Medical Telemetry Devices. March 25, 1998. fcc.gov/Bureaus/Engineering_Technology/News_Releases/1998/nret8003.html
13. Tan KS, Hinberg I. Effects of a wireless local area network (LAN) system, a telemetry system, and electrosurgical devices on medical devices in a hospital environment. Biomed Instrum Technol 2000; 34:115–118
14. Schlegel RE, Grant FH, Raman S, Reynolds D. Electromagnetic compatibility of the in-vitro interaction of wireless phones with cardiac pacemakers. Biomed Instrum Technol 1998; 32:645–655
15. Carlo GL, Jenro RS. Scientific progress—wireless phones and brain cancer: Current state of the science. Med Gen Med 2000; 11:E40

# 11
## Essential Software
### Databases, Spreadsheets, Word Processing, and Presentation Software

SUE SCHNEIDER

One objective of this essay is to provide an understanding of the widely used categories of software as well as how one might select software for one's own use. The most commonly used categories and considerations for software selection and use are discussed, with an emphasis on databases and database software.

Another objective is to highlight the many usages of the term "database." Under the name "database," one can buy a container of sets of related data, a software development product, or an application or system. It is up to the consumer to understand how the seller is using terminology.

In today's workplace most companies purchase a **suite** of software products. The minimal suite contains word processing, spreadsheet, presentation, and database software. Most personal computers purchased by individuals come with a suite of software products already installed; more than 85% of the time it is a Microsoft suite of products targeting personal or business use.

## Software Categories

**Word processing software** facilitates the creation, editing, storage, and publication of documents. Word processing software stores the material one types, plus various hidden codes for formatting the document, in a specialized file in a format unique and proprietary to the vendor of the software. Besides text paragraphs, sections, chapters, and so on, documents can contain embedded tables as well as other objects such as images, spreadsheets, and graphs. When word processing software starts up, it is ready for you to start typing your research paper, letter, report, essay, or book. As we moved through our formal education we had many opportunities to learn to express ourselves with the written word. Word processing software helps us store and publish our written communications.

**Spreadsheet software** facilitates the creation, storage, and publication of worksheets. Worksheets are specialized files, composed of rows and cells, used to process numbers via formulas and functions, create graphs and charts from the numbers, and create financial, statistical, and other mathematical reports. Spreadsheets deliver the ability to perform complex mathematical functions, analyze statistics, and graph results quickly and easily. Spreadsheet software stores the worksheets in specialized files with a format unique and proprietary to the vendor of the software. If our education or experience has led us into bookkeeping or accounting or analysis of numerical information, we had to learn about some form of ledger sheets. Worksheets are an automated form of ledger sheets.

**Presentation software** facilitates the creation, storage, editing, previewing, and showing of slide shows. Presentation software helps one build a slide show presentation, enables one to insert images, text, spreadsheet cells, graphs, and so on into the slides, provides a place to store presentation notes, and prints handouts. Presentation software stores the slides to be used in the presentation in a specialized file with a format unique and proprietary to the vendor of the software.

**Database software** is used to build databases and user interfaces to those databases. "Database" is a widely used and imprecise term. In this discussion, a **database** is a facility where data is collected and stored for the purpose of generating information and knowledge needed to solve problems. The actual set of procedures and displays used by that facility is called a "User Interface". Databases are organized, accessible, structured, and secured to varying degrees. Below are some descriptions of databases.

**Example 1.** A generic office file—a filing cabinet of paper files—is a database. It is organized by the files' tab contents, by topic or alphabetically. Access and security are handled by physical control devices, such as locations and drawer locks. Its structure is the physical folders. The folder content may or may not have a specific sequence, structure, or standard format. This database is updated by adding, deleting or changing folder contents by whoever has access and motivation. The user interface is called "filing."

**Example 2.** The campus telephone directory, a soft-cover book, is a database. It is organized by person or entity name. There are few access or security restrictions. It has a simple name/number structure presented in a standard format. This database is updated only by a single entity, the publisher, but it can be read by all (a read-only database). In addition to looking up a number in the book, another user interface to the databases, called the operator or directory assistance, is available via the telephone.

**Example 3.** The Laboratory Information System (LIS) provided by Our Vendor is referred to as a database, as are various components of the LIS. Technically, it is more accurate to refer to this item as an "application" or system; i.e., OurVendor Corporation's proprietary software tools and programming languages are applied to the significant task of supporting the processes of operating and administering clinical and anatomic laboratories. It has both a physical and a logical structure. Both structures are highly complex, sensitive to change, and require specialized resources to maintain.

This application's database contains hundreds of files organized by numerous keys, such as patient identification number, encounter number, accession number, and so on. It is accessible via a personal computer, secured with passwords, and requires training to access the information sought. The complex user interface is composed of various menus, screens, and reports whereby patients are registered, orders are placed, tests are resulted, and charts are printed. There is also a user interface especially for administering the system itself as well as to help administer the department workload.

The user interface provided by this version of OurVendor's LIS is an example of a style of interface—a DOS-based interface versus the GUI (graphical user interface) used with Windows or Macintosh operating systems. The user interface provided on a newer version of OurVendor's LIS is a graphical user interface.

**Example 4.** The Pathology Department's budget spreadsheet is a database. It is organized by worksheet name; its accessibility and security are performed via access to the Pathology network; and its structure determined by the author of the spreadsheet.

**Database software products are *not* databases. Database software products are tools or tool kits used to build databases and/or entire applications.** Use of a database software product enables one to do the following:

- Design the organization, accesses, and structure for data to be collected and retrieved.
- Define data security measures and their implementation.
- Enforce data integrity within its files.
- Design and develop interfaces for people to interact with the database to enter data, to perform a function, to generate information, to develop knowledge.

Various vendors, such as Microsoft, Oracle, IBM, Sun, Apple, et al., market multiple lines of software products as databases. There are many technical and proprietary differences among these vendors that are beyond the scope of this discussion. However, a database that will be updated by several people concurrently may have to be deployed under a more robust database than what is delivered by Microsoft Access to most desktops or home computers. In this situation what is wanted is a database that is highly reliable and provides security or locking at the record level (when someone is updating a record, the record is not available for another to update).

These more robust or enterprise-level software products cost significantly more to acquire and require qualified technical assistance to develop and administer. Three of the more popular products are Microsoft's SQL Server, IBM's DB2, and Oracle's product line. Different products have different features and trade-offs, such as power versus ease of use. A product may initially be selected for ease of use which over time is found to be criteria of lesser value than the criteria of power and scalability.

**Other Useful Software**

**Graphics packages** can be a helpful addition to suites of products. They make it possible to capture or edit photographs or other scanned images and graphics, as well as "screen shots" that can be embedded in training materials, reports, or presentations. When the standard graphics program is insufficient for particular tasks, an add-on advanced program may be used. Some vendors also offer multimedia products. Most scanners and digital cameras arrive with graphics software; however, one may be working with images captured by another party.

Advanced graphics programs directly support many different file formats and can read other file formats if the appropriate external import filters and drivers are installed along with associated scanner or digital camera hardware.

**Project management software** interacts with an individual planning or coordinating the effort needed to accomplish a change in the status quo. The individual identifies the tasks to be done, the time and resources needed for each task, task dependencies, and available resources. The software calculates the critical path of the project and, when effort expended and project completions are input, calculates the status of the project. Timelines and Gantt charts can be printed, providing a framework for effective communication among all concerned parties.

Formal project management is not consistently performed in many healthcare organizations. The level of project management followed is usually relative to the project stakeholders' perception of the magnitude of the project and/or appreciation of the consequences of its success or failure and/or the experience of the project leader. Real project management is usually applied to large-budget projects with accountability such as mandated or contracted target dates.

**Personal information manager** programs help schedule time, manage contacts, track appointments and to-do lists, and record journal notes—replacing the paper-based organizer.

# Selecting Software Products

The first step in choosing a software product is to determine if a standard suite of software and standard hardware setup are in use at the company for which you work. If so, get that software and use it until such time as you determine that you have special requirements that cannot be met by that software. Using a standard setup does not preclude you from obtaining another vendor's software for a specialty or niche need. Acquisition and support of specialized hardware and software is often a financial and a resource issue. Availability and experience of support staff may be a determining factor. Databases developed for and used in research tend to require more memory and a larger hard drive than the "standard" personal computer. Also having the same setup on a home computer as at the office facilitates working from either location.

If your employer or primary network of associates does not have a standard software suite and you must make a selection yourself, then the first step is to identify your requirements—what you expect the software to do—in a list of questions. The more detailed the list, the more rigorous the selection process and the more time it will take, and the more likely you are to make a satisfactory choice. Next, prioritize and rank the importance of the items in the list. Then ascertain by vendor or product how well they meet your requirements.

Some key questions to ask:

- "What do I want to do with this software?"
- "What does it cost?"
- "How well does this vendor's software meet all my requirements or considerations?"
- "What kind of hardware do I have?" (IBM compatible PC, Apple, other)
- "What is the operating system installed on my hardware? And what version?" DOS, Windows 3.x, Windows9x or NT or 2000, Unix, Linux, and so on)
- "How will this software facilitate my working with others in my area as well as in my professional network?" This is a very important requirement. "Can I easily exchange work products such as spreadsheets, documents, images, and reports with the majority of people with whom I work?" Every vendor's file format is unique and proprietary. Many vendors provide "drivers" so that other vendors can read or translate that vendor's file format. Vendors frequently change file formats with each new version of their software. The new version will read older version formats but may write only the latest format. If you are the only one with the newest version of the software, no one else can open files you create.
- "When it breaks or when I'm learning to use it, where do I get help?" Most vendors provide a variety of help resources, from self-study and tutorial materials embedded in their software to onsite or telephone support representatives, as well as by e-mail and a knowledge base on the Internet. When running the software and needing help there are many potential sources: Look for the word "Help," try the F1 key to find software documentation, position the cursor on a menu item and see if a Help tag appears, position the cursor on a menu item and right-click with the mouse to see if any options appear or see if you have a "Getting Started"manual.

Arrange to have a hands-on, demonstration of the software you expect to use the most. Try it out. Buyer beware: Not all "databases" are ready to use right out of the box.

# Matching the Product to the Task At Hand

Suppose you want to create a *table*. You should determine which software is best suited to your task: word processing, spreadsheet, or database software. All three can create and automatically format the table for you.

- For a table that includes complex formatting such as bulleted lists, custom tabs, numbering, or hanging indentations, use word processing software. But if the table will be enhanced or need some specialized business rules applied to it, use database software.
- For a table that includes complex calculations, statistical analysis, or charts, use spreadsheet software. However, if your table entries will exceed 255 characters in length, do not use spreadsheet software; instead, use word processing or database software.
- For powerful sorting and searching capabilities, use either database or spreadsheet software.
- If you need to store and update more than 10,000 records or the data elements may expand, create the table in database software.
- For a table that can easily be included in a presentation, use word processing software.

In an integrated suite, the database software can publish or export a report or query for processing by the word processing or spreadsheet software.

When starting up word processing software, you expect to create a document and the software begins ready to accept typing, to create a document. Word processing software replaces the typewriter. Spreadsheet and presentation software similarly replace specialized office equipment, and what they do is implied in their names.

What office equipment does database software replace? Database software takes on a function performed by a highly trained, technical staff in a data processing or information services department and puts the components of that function onto the desktop in the business area. It is not automatically ready to accept data.

Database software is different from word processing and spreadsheet and presentation software. It requires instruction. To use database software, one must be ready to design a database using a technique called **Relational Database Design** and to design and develop a user interface with which to interact with the database.

Unless you've been specially trained or have specific experience, you may not be ready to design and develop a database and its user interface. Let's review some of the techniques used to design a database.

**1. Spreadsheet Design–**This is a very common way for those accustomed to spreadsheets to design tables. The resulting tables typically have lots of redundant data and duplicate fields. Redundant data and duplicate fields cause problems when one tries to get data out of the database (do a query).

**2. Old Software-Driven Design**–The "old" database system, Paradox or dBase or FoxPro or OurVendor, dictates how the tables are structured because the tables are imported/copied into the new database. (Vendor advertising assures us that their products will convert these old databases, **but** the user interface is not automatically converted.) By doing an import or automatic conversion, the design limitations of the old databases come with them. Often redundant data was built into these tables so that it could appear on a single screen/form; modern database software does not have that limitation. Redundant data can cause problems in getting data out of the database or in updating it. The problem with redundant data is that it usually means redundant data entry and a lack of data consistency and integrity within the database.

**3. Flat File Design, or "Let's Keep It All in One Table"**–The problems with this type of structure are numerous: duplication, wasted space, no unique index, difficult or impossible to retrieve the data, and so on. Flat-file design is like creating a mansion from a two-bedroom ranch house, with extra floors and rooms and portable buildings added on without the use of an architect or building inspector. Databases with this type of structure are also called "flat files" because there is no built-in hierarchy or relationship between the records. Figure 11-1 is an example of a flat file redesigned into a database table.

**4. Multi-Valued Fields Derivative**–Putting Address, City, State, and Zipcode—four pieces of data—all in one field becomes a problem when you want to sort by State or find out who lives in Texas City (see Figure 11-1).

**5. Relational Database Design.** Before starting to use a database software product, do the following:

- **Step 1.** Determine the purpose of the database and write it down on paper.
- **Step 2.** Review current methods of collecting and presenting the data (forms and reports) to be stored in the database. This is the current process's user interface.
- **Step 3.** Identify the tables needed. Develop a list of data elements on paper, and group the data elements logically, as the data is in the real world. This identifies database objects (data elements and tables). You might have a table for Patients, which would contain data elements for each patient's First Name, Last Name, Patient Identification Number, and so on. In addition to numeric and alphanumeric data types, you may have a data element that is an image data type or a memo data type (equivalent to 8 pages of text).
- **Step 4.** Finetune the tables by "normalizing the data." Database design theory includes data design standards called **normal forms.** The process of making your data and tables meet these standards is called **normalizing data,** or **normalization. Normalization** is the process of putting things right. The Latin word, *norma,* identifies a carpenter's tool for assuring a right angle. In geometry, a line at right angles to another is said to be "normal" to another. In relational database design, normalization has a specific mathematical meaning having to do with separating elements of

| NAME | EMP# | PHONES | ADDRESS |
|---|---|---|---|
| John James | 1 | w-643-2127,h-281-777-1232 | Rt 0440, Texas City, TX |
| Sallyy Rider | 2 | w-74339, h-935-5129,pg-641-8237 | 301 Univ Blvd |
| Celma Stevens | 3 | 771-0712 | POBox 123 |
| Phil Beaxon | 4 | W1-281-330-8779,w2-72834,pg-641-6668,cell-281-409-7889, fax-935-6678 | |

2

| First NAME | Lst Name | EMP # | PHONES | ADDRESS |
|---|---|---|---|---|
| John | James | 1 | w-643-2127,h-281-777-1232 | Rt 0440, Texas City, TX |
| Sallyy | Rider | 2 | w-74339, h-935-5129,pg-641-8237 | 301 Univ Blvd |
| Celma | Stevens | 3 | 771-0712 | POBox 123 |
| Phil | Beaxon | 4 | W1-281-330-8779,w2-72834,pg-641-6668,cell-281-409-7889, fax-935-6678 | |

3

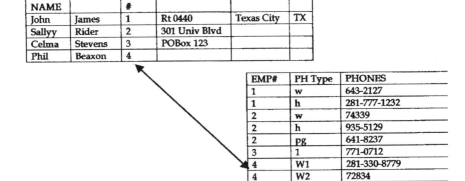

| First NAME | Lst Name | EMP # | ADDRESS | CITY | ST |
|---|---|---|---|---|---|
| John | James | 1 | Rt 0440 | Texas City | TX |
| Sallyy | Rider | 2 | 301 Univ Blvd | | |
| Celma | Stevens | 3 | POBox 123 | | |
| Phil | Beaxon | 4 | | | |

| EMP# | PH Type | PHONES |
|---|---|---|
| 1 | w | 643-2127 |
| 1 | h | 281-777-1232 |
| 2 | w | 74339 |
| 2 | h | 935-5129 |
| 2 | pg | 641-8237 |
| 3 | 1 | 771-0712 |
| 4 | W1 | 281-330-8779 |
| 4 | W2 | 72834 |
| 4 | Pg | 641-6668 |
| 4 | Cell | 281-409-7889 |
| 4 | fax | 935-6678 |

FIGURE 11-1. "Flat file" to third normal form.

data (such as Patient Identification Number, First Name, Last Name, Date Of Birth, Doctor Identifier Code, and Ordered Test) into affinity groups (tables) and defining the normal, or right, relationships between the groups.

Redundant information is eliminated and tables are organized (by you) to make managing data and future changes in table structure easier. *If the tables are normalized, then each data element/table attribute will be a fact about the key, the whole key, and nothing but the key.*

The key is analogous to an index or a label. Keys are used by filing systems to access individual records. In the example Patient Table, Patient Identifier Number could be a key, as could the combination of First Name and Last Name. The Patient Identifier Number is the better candidate for a primary key, as it will be unique.

In normalizing data, tables are divided into smaller, easier-to-maintain tables. Then relationships between the tables are defined so that the database software knows how to join tables in the queries, forms, and reports that you also develop. Tables are represented as joined together by drawing lines between them, such as between Patients and Orders, and a way is found to annotate that relationship as a one-to-many relationship.

To establish a relationship, the two tables must have a field in common. This field must be the primary key in one table and may be a foreign key in another table. A primary key uniquely identifies each record in the table and is present for each record in the table. The University of Texas Medical Branch's patient-identifying Unit History (UH) Number is an example of a primary key for a Patient table, whereas Accession Number and Ordered Test might be the primary key for the Orders table. The Orders table could contain the UH number as a foreign key to relate the order to the patient.

Having identified specific tables (things about which you want to store data) and the relationships between them, you now have a logical model of your database on paper. It will be checked out and tuned when you work through the next step.

- **Step 5.** Using imagination, intuition, industry standards, and knowledge of current methods of collecting and presenting data, think through the planned use of the database.
- **Step 6.** Design and build the user interface, menus, navigation paths, queries, forms, reports, and security that will be needed. There are articles, books, and courses on graphical user interface design as well.
- **Step 7.** Finally, go to the computer, turn on the database software and translate the logical model on paper to a physical implementation.

Traditionally, creating databases with a hierarchical or relational structure has been the purview of central data processing departments. Marketing of database software products, corporate administrators' continuing belief in silver bullets and other magical solutions, a department's need for responsive tactical information services, and market advances have moved the tools of relational database design from the central data processing department to individual desktops. However, planning for training in these tools is usually absent, resulting in a potential user who may or may not have a desire to be a database programmer being assigned to do database design and programming, to develop a database in Microsoft Access, and to install the database on a network. It could happen to you.

# Additional Commentary on Medical Informatics

Expanding on the term *"engineering"* used in an earlier chapter, when you design and develop a database and its associated forms and reports (the user interface), you are using database software to build an application or tool or database for a specific need. You will be more successful following a development life cycle, a "methodology," to develop an application. Find a methodology that has proven successful in a situation similar to yours.

The methodology could include developing a prototype or full working model as well as concurrently or serially developing a more robust, fully tested and documented production system ready for deployment. A tool suitable for quickly building a prototype or even a full working model may not be the tool that is suitable for building the more robust production version. Quite often they are different. On the other hand, when a production database appears to be too expensive or difficult to sell, a lower-cost prototype can be developed to provide "proof of concept" to obtain the funding to build the production version.

When you get into the "deployment" activity mentioned in an earlier chapter, was the end product a prototype or a production model? It may be that the database needs to be ported (converted) to a more robust database product such as Oracle, SQL Server, or DB2 because it now has to support more concurrent user update or a higher volume, or it requires more security. These database products can require more knowledgeable resources to use them effectively. It is possible to be redeveloping your database within the deployment phase.

Two other unique activities that arise during deployment are data conversion and loading as well as additional exception research and reporting. Familiarizing yourself with the content of a methodology that has proven successful will help you be proactive in your engineering and deployment activities.

# Summary

This discussion has briefly touched on some of the software most frequently used in business. As technology and ways of doing business are changing faster than ever, parts of this discussion referring to specific products and specific vendors could be out of date in less than two years. After all, the latest trend is to put yourself and your work "on the Web," the Internet. Many software products assist you in doing that. The newer releases of UTMB's standard software suite have the ability to publish a document, image, report, or graph in a form acceptable to a Web browser with a click of your mouse. Developing technology using mobile devices with built-in cellular chips will allow you to access your database away from the office.

A major point to be emphasized is that buying a database software product does not get you as close to having an effective database as buying word processing software gets you to having an effective document. As we move through our formal education we have many opportunities to learn to express ourselves with the written word. Word processing software helps us store and publish our written communications.

This same formal education may introduce us to computers and to a programming language in the same manner as we are introduced to a foreign language. Courses to develop the skills needed to design and organize an application or a database are not usually part of the curriculum. Database design and user interface design are areas where you will need to either get more education or buy some experience, depending on your available time and resources.

## Chapter Glossary

**database:** Any storage facility where data is collected for the purpose of generating information.

**data normalization:** Process of making data and tables match database design standards. The objective of these standards is to eliminate redundant information to make managing data and future changes in table structure easier. If the tables are normalized, each data element/table attribute will be a fact about the key, the whole key, and nothing but the key.

**presentation software:** Software that interacts with an individual developing, editing, and arranging slides for presentations.

**integrated software suite:** Term used when all the components of the suite can exchange information with each other, requiring minimal effort for the individual using the software.

**project management software:** Software that interacts with an individual planning or coordinating the effort needed to accomplish a change in the status quo. The individual identifies the tasks to be done, the time and resources needed for each, task dependencies, and available resources. The software calculates the critical path of the project and, when effort expended and project completions are input, calculates the status of the project.

**spreadsheet software:** Software that interacts with an individual processing numbers, creating graphs and charts from the numbers, and creating financial, statistical, and other mathematical reports.

**user interface:** Methods and techniques used to interact with a computer and the software running on the computer at the behest of the user. There are two major types of interface: character and graphical. A character interface utilizes the keyboard as its input provider and happens character by character, line by line. A graphical interface is visual and utilizes a mouse or other pointing device in addition to keyboard input and mouse events. Everyone's graphical interface may be different in appearance whereas all character interfaces resemble one another. Windows and applications written for it present a graphical user interface.

**word processing software:** Software that interacts with an individual typing, changing, formatting, spellchecking, and printing textual documents.

# 12
# Clinical and Anatomic Pathology Database Design

SUE SCHNEIDER

This chapter will provide a more detailed look at clinical and anatomic database design for the following reasons.

- Personal computer software vendors' marketing of database software appeals to nontechnical, computer-friendly professionals and desperate (and/or disparate) clinicians.
- Health care lags behind other industries in utilization of information technology.
- Financial executives often fail to understand the laboratorian's or the clinician's or the scientist's need for information technology beyond billing for services.
- Financial executives generally control the information technology available to the laboratorian or the clinician or the scientist unless they build their own technology.
- Clinically meaningful information patterns that exist in the electronic laboratory record are obscured by current data management and presentation approaches.

Most of the software on your PC facilitates an activity that you already knew learned how to do—write a paper, analyze numeric data, create a poster presentation. Database software facilitates an activity that you may not have been trained to do—design and develop databases and applications.

Creating databases has traditionally been the purview of central data processing departments. Many factors have shifted database design from the central data processing/information services department to individual desktops. However, planning for and training in database design and implementation is usually absent in departments outside of information services. This frequently results in an individual who may or may not have a desire to be a database designer/programmer being assigned to develop a database.

Today, clinical and laboratory databases engender common complaints:

- Expected flexibility is not achieved.
- Requests for information take too long and consume a high proportion of resources.

194

- On-line response for decision support or research does not exist or takes too long.
- They are difficult to understand, hard to use, "too clicky."
- Requests for change due to business changes take too long and cost too much.
- They don't contain the specific data requested.

The source of these problems is inherent in the database design process itself and in the several definitions and uses of the term "database" (as stated in Chapter 11, people use the term to mean container of sets of related data, software product or application or system). A remedy is often determined to be a move from the current database support service provider to another provider with its own set of problems. The new provider is either a vendor of one of many products in the marketplace or you initiating the development yourself with your resources or your organization's information services department initiating the development as part of your organization's strategic plan.

Embedded within each vendor product is a database engine on which these products are designed to run. The database engines are typically developed and supported by yet another vendor. The database engine serves as the physical file system manager, the infrastructure for database system being used. There is a strong tendency for vendors to promote their database products as "all that's needed." If there were such a thing out there, we'd all be signing up for it.

In the case of LIS systems vendors, some support their product's operation on multiple database engines while others support their product's operation on their own proprietary database engine, promising interfaces to everything.

## Designing a Database

For purposes of this discussion, let's assume that we have various databases in place that support daily patient care, but options for laboratory management decision support, utilization review, and outcomes research are difficult to use, consume significant resources, are inflexible, and/or take too long. Let us outline and review the activities needed to design a database to address these functions–a Medical Informatics Database For Research and Decision Support. The scope of work for the database is an integrated view of patient data for research, outcomes research, and utilization review.

Database design is similar to a juggling act, with the database designer having to consider a wide range of factors that may all have a crucial effect on the final database. The activities may be grouped into three stages: (1) Data Analysis and Logical Design, of which data normalization is a part, (2) Physical Design, and (3) Optimization. In each stage, there are specific rules to be followed. A major portion of the process is easy to understand and execute by personnel who may not have extensive knowledge of generic database or any specific vendor's database engine. However, the optimization stage is highly dependent on the brand of database software and the brand of the hardware operating system and is outside the scope of this chapter.

## *Data Analysis and Logical Design*

First, there is the data itself. The database designer must understand or investigate the meaning of each data element, eliminate ambiguity and semantic issues, reduce redundancy, accurately identify data interdependencies, and catalogue the data. An *analogy* might be recycling bins: paper, glass, metal, plastic. Each bin contains a separate type of entity with certain attributes or properties—And Metal, for example, subdivides into aluminum cans, aerosol cans, all other cans, and all other metal, depending on how the bins will be handled later.

With clinical data, there are factors to consider revolving around the organization itself: the purpose and perspective of the database. For example, a laboratory test has a result. The result may be a simple format such as a number, reference ranges, and unit of expression. Or it may be a surgical pathology case report that includes images. Now apply purpose and perspective: Is the organization a hospital or a laboratory or both or more? Is the perspective that of care provider, researcher, administrator, laboratory medical technologist, pathologist, all of the above? If a care provider, the result reference range is needed with each result. If a laboratory technologist, a chronological history of all the reference ranges used for each test is also required.

Analyzing the data itself, its purpose and use, is of tremendous value because that activity is key to creation of a database structure that reflects the needs of today and a structure that is generically correct enough so that future, unanticipated requirements can be quickly and easily addressed.

After Data Analysis is complete and the logical structure is defined, emphasis must shift to fitting the structure to the specific vendor database engine being used to implement it. Each vendor's database engine has its own set of facilities—things that can be done—and its own set of constraints—things that must not be done. The exact details of facilities and constraints still vary from vendor to vendor. And the final design must operate within acceptable performance criteria. The more database engines with which the database designer has experience, the more flexible and portable the final design. This is important when you need to upgrade hardware or migrate/convert to a new vendor's database engine.

To summarize the outcomes of Data Analysis:

- Data interdependencies are identified.
- Ambiguities are resolved.
- Data can be grouped into related sets.
- Relationships are identified.
- A basis of shared data is provided.
- Data becomes closely defined.
- Data is easy to maintain.
- Data redundancy is eliminated at a logical level.
- The organization allows flexibility.
- A Logical Model is defined.

By performing data analysis, the database designer creates an unambiguous set of relations among all the data elements. The relationships are, in fact, the first view of the record types that will eventually make up the physical database. Following are some of the benefits of performing data analysis:

- The analysis is data-oriented, not process-oriented, and less subject to impact by business/procedural changes.
- Logical and physical considerations are separated.
- Rules are relatively easy to apply.
- Techniques are sound and mathematically proven.
- The analysis operates at a real level, with currently used forms, reports, and documents, existing files, planned outputs, and currently used computer screen shots.

Tasks to be performed are collection of samples of available input, file, and output documents and layouts; carrying out data normalization steps; optimization of normal forms; and cataloging the results in a database directory. Little attention is paid at this point to the business processes.

Next, the Logical Model is reviewed and the business processes identified in the scope of work. The natural data relationships that exist within an organization are mapped into the Logical Model to ensure that business needs are met and to provide for the necessary future flexibility. Sometimes the model is referred to as an Entity Model or a Business Model. The most significant aspect of logical design is that it deals only with an organization's environment, its data and processing needs; while the logical design is being created, the database designer is not also juggling with the problems of the database engine's facilities and constraints and performance standards. When the logical design is completed, the result is a portable database design that meets the clinician and laboratorian's needs.

Two key factors that influence any logical design are data relationships and required access paths between related data elements. It is possible to develop the Logical Model and the Business Model concurrently and then integrate them to a single logical design. A desirable offshoot of this activity is a collection of data about data, a data dictionary or metadata, that defines what the data is, where it originated, where it is stored, how frequently is it updated, and so on.

Outcomes of logical design are:

- A logical database design that is portable and flexible, regardless of the hardware or the database engine to be used. The logical design enables the database designer to create a physical structure that will meet the organization's requirements.
- If the organization has not yet selected a database engine, the logical design depicting the interrelations and dependencies of data provides an easy-to-understand tool to use in evaluating vendors.
- One of the downsides of database design being directed by an entity outside clinical management control is that the physical aspects are too often dominant in the design process. Experience shows that software developers are more comfortable beginning the design by considering how the database software will handle the system rather than the data

relationships and structures needed to meet clinical/research/decision support requirements.

The final design stage is taking the database design through a series of iterative steps that ensure that the final design meets performance objectives in terms of information, response and run times, security, recovery, and storage utilization within the particular database engine's facilities and constraints.

# Practice Example

So let's create our database. We'll use the outline of steps from Chapter 11 as our starting point and flesh it out with actual data elements and mock work products.

**Step 1.** The scope of work for the database is to be an integrated view of patient data for research, outcomes research, and utilization review—a medical informatics database for research and decision support.

**Step 2.** Review current methods of collecting and presenting the data (forms and reports) to be stored in the database. These are the user interfaces of the current processes.

- Patient Chart produced by OurVendor's LIS
- Patient Chart and Notes produced by care providers and their staff
- Treatment protocols
- Patient Billing System data storage
- Various procedure coding schemes: ICD9, SNOMED, DRG, and so on
- Forms used/reports produced by existing systems and processes that contain data pertinent to the database's purpose

**Step 3.** Identify the sets or categories of data about which you intend to store facts—i.e., the tables you will need. Tables are today's equivalent of files. From the forms and reports reviewed in Step 2, develop a list of data elements, on paper, and group the data elements logically, as they are in the real world. This identifies basic database objects, data elements and tables. Figure 12-1 lists some the data elements we might see in some of the pieces of the patient record we are analyzing. Figure 12-2 lists some of the tables we might derive from the list of data elements.

From this list of elements and an understanding of their definitions, sources, and usage, we define a table for patients containing data elements for the patient's First Name, Last Name, Patient's Identifying Unit History (UH) Number, and so on. We may define a table of Patient Encounters to chronicle patient interaction with the organization, a table of Ordered Procedures, a table of Procedure/Test Results, and Lookup Tables, such as a Doctor Table with Doctor Code (ordering and attending), Doctor Name, Specialty, and other pertinent data you plan to store for each doctor.

In addition to numeric and alphanumeric data types, there are many other data types: an image data type, a memo data type (equivalent to eight pages

| | | |
|---|---|---|
| U H Number | S S N | Verified Time |
| Encounter ID | Height | Result |
| Patient Name | Weight | Result Units |
| Date of Birth | Home Telephone | Normal Low |
| Address | Work Telephone | Normal High |
| City | Test Ordered | Abnormal Flag |
| State | Order Date . | Corrected |
| Zipcode | Drawn Date | Case Nbr |
| Sex | Drawn Time | Location Code |
| Race | Result Mnemonic | Date Vitals |
| Blood Type | Verified Date | Checked |
| Weight | Lenth of Stay | |
| Temp | Discharge Date | |
| Systolic | Admitting DRG | |
| Dystolic | Discharge ICD9 | |
| Respiration | Order ICD9 | |
| Pulse | Accession Number | |
| Lab | Procedure Ordered | |
| Attending Physician | Diagnosis | |
| Ordering Doctor | Clinical Summary | |
| Order Location | Gross Description | |
| Admit Date | | |

FIGURE 12-1. Data element list.

of text), a "blob" data type that is virtually unlimited in size, or a multimedia data type for a video clip.

Many of UTMB's current systems were built before technology allowed such a variety of data types, so our pathology case reports are physically stored in small segments that work for the current system but are difficult to use to input data and harder to browse horizontally across many cases. These physical segments in OurVendor's LIS even contain various special characters embedded within the text for formatting by that system. These create special challenges when converting a stored case report (old technology) to newer technology database storage with more diverse data types.

**Step 4.** Refine the table design by "normalizing the data". Review the groupings of data and the normal, or right, relationships between the groups. The next section will provide a more detailed example of clinical data normalization.

Redundant information is eliminated and tables are organized to make managing data and future changes in table structure easier. *If the tables are*

| | | |
|---|---|---|
| Patient Encounters | Orders | Inpatient Stays |
| Doctors | Results | ICD9 Codes |
| Locations | Procedures | SnoMed Codes |

FIGURE 12-2. Table list.

*normalized, then each data element/table attribute will be a fact about the key, the whole key, and nothing but the key.*

The key is analogous to an index or a label. Filing systems use keys to directly access individual records. In the example Patient table, UH Number could be a key, as could the combination of First Name and Last Name. The UH number is the better candidate for a primary key as it is unique.

In normalizing data, tables are divided into smaller, easier-to-maintain tables. Then relationships between the tables are defined so that the database software knows how to join tables in the queries, forms, and reports you develop. These relationships resemble trails left by those browsing the database, say from Patient to Test Results or from Client to Test Order to Test Result. Relationships are represented by drawing lines between tables and a consistent method to annotate the relationship as one-to-one, one-to-many, or many-to-many. Having identified your tables (things about which you want to store data) and the relationships between them, you now have a logical model of your database on paper. Figure 12-3 shows partial detail of a logical model, showing the relationship between the Patient Encounter and the Order.

In Figure 12-3, two of the tables of our logical design are shown. The annotation used is a single asterisk for each field that is a Foreign Key, two asterisks and PK for each field that is part of the Primary Key of the table, and an arrow whose direction indicates the relationship. The figure shows that each encounter can have one or more orders associated with it, and the Encounter Number is the field that links them together.

**Step 5.** Test and tune the logical model. Using your imagination, intuition, industry standards, and knowledge of current methods of collecting and presenting data, walk through the planned usage of the database. Add foreign keys and relationships as needed.

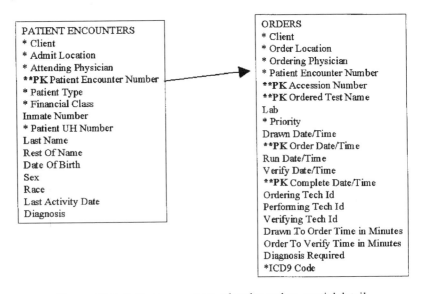

FIGURE 12-3. Patient encounters related to orders, partial detail.

**Step 6.** Still on paper, validate the logical model: design a "mock-up" of the user interface, menus, navigation paths, queries, forms, reports, security, and so on that will be needed.

**Step 7.** Finally, we are ready to go to the computer, turn on the database software and translate the logical model on paper to a physical model. After we validate its operation, we are ready to load it with data.

## Physical Design

Loading the database with data does not make it ready to use unless you know how to use whatever toolkit comes with the database engine. Most of us prefer a user interface to the database, an application designed and programmed to support how we do our work. The interface may have been developed concurrent with the database design or it may start now. Or you may buy a software package that promises to become the user interface to your database. It depends on the resources you have and the methodology you are following.

How ready to use is our database? The answer is quite subjective. Let's say we are hungry and are going to have a sandwich. How do we get a sandwich? One scenario is to go to the store, wander around the grocery store (which may be organized for the convenience of the stockers rather than the sandwich shopper), find and retrieve all the ingredients, and then make a sandwich. Another scenario is to go to the nearby deli and pick up a sandwich made to our order. We get our sandwich quicker, and behind the scenes someone else found and retrieved and stored the sandwich ingredients. Or we let our personal valet know of our sandwich request. Our valet brings us the perfect sandwich quickly. In this scenario, we have the least involvement in obtaining the sandwich, although we paid for all that was involved in bringing it to us.

Again, how do we get that sandwich? How hungry are we? Will any sandwich satisfy or do we have a particular craving? How much time and money are we willing to spend? The point is that even in the grocery store we do not obtain our ingredients directly from the producer; the sandwich ingredients have to be obtained and stored by others in a healthful manner involving various food industry and department of health standards. Similarly, interfacing data into a database and its logical and physical design must be carefully done using technical methods and skills that are not usually found in the clinical or financial areas.

Figure 12-4 is a partial view of our logical database design, identifying some of the tables and some of the relationships. At this level, neither the contents of the tables nor the properties of the relationships are listed.

Figure 12-5 shows the key to it all. We have the data in appropriate tables and we are able to start at any table and move to the related data in any other table. We have our database designed, physically implemented, and loaded with data. What is hidden from view are the database engine specific objects that were implemented to meet business and performance criteria: logical views, indices, cross-reference tables to enable many-to-many relationships, and so on. What is still needed is a user interface with a data directory to shield us from having to remember what data is in the database and in which table.

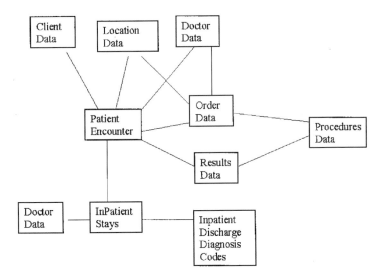

**FIGURE 12-4.** Logical database design, partial view.

Let's use our imagination with Figure 12-5 and extract some data for our analysis and management decision support.

- We need to gather some information about observation patients' laboratory turnaround times. How would we do that? We would find all the patient encounters whose patient type implied "observation" then, using the encounter identification number, we would pull all the related orders within any specific time period. Was the physician ordering tests that we send out? What was our turnaround time on each, on average? Is the laboratory service level standard still appropriate?
- How about gathering some order volumes and turnaround times for client BigWheel for the past six months? Pull all the orders for that client where the order date is within the six-month range, counting the accessions and averaging the order-to-verify time. Now you have the data to respond to BigWheel.
- How about reviewing the cholesterol levels found in the general population? Pull all the cholesterol test results and using the encounter numbers relate the results the patient data to obtain sex, race, and data of birth, and using the patient UH, relate the results to any inpatient stays the patients might have experienced.

These are the tip of the possibilities iceberg.

From the Doctor Data, we can extract all the orders for any given doctor. Conversely, we can recap all the orders by doctor or by doctor by order month. We can extract all the results of a particular test and then identify who had it or who ordered it or the average result. We can define a set of patients and then extract all their test results.

So, even without a user interface that is programmed just for you, today's tools are easier to learn than programming languages. All you need is a good database design.

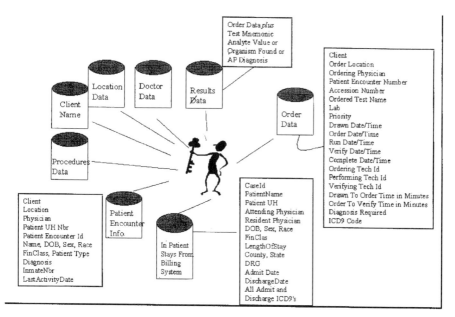

FIGURE 12-5. A medical informatics database.

# Data Normalization Applied to Clinical and Laboratory Informatics

This section will take a small subset of our medical informatics data and step through the data normalization process. It is easier to do than it is to read about. Five rules will be presented in their normal, technical lexicon, enabling you to recognize them if or when a database administrator or software developer tosses "data normalization" into a conversation with you. Data normalization is only one part of database design protocol. Less experienced software developers tend to stop at third normal form or claim that normalization is useless. And it is a key facilitator and integral part of a flexible database design with proven data integrity, as well as a design that is easy to change.

A semantic note: In data normalization, the actual activity that occurs is **data elimination.** The goal is to eliminate data from each table until there is no longer anything to take away and each remaining data point is a fact about the table's primary key, the whole primary key, and nothing but the primary key.

## Rule 1: Eliminate Repeating Groups

*Make a separate table for each set of related attributes, and assign each table a primary key.*

Figure 12-6 presents an unnormalized list of data. In the original, unnormalized list of data, each patient description is followed by the laboratory test results received on that patient. Some might have 10 test results, others might have hundreds of results, and some might have no test results. To answer a question such as "What is Dan's current cholesterol level?" we need to first find Dan's

| UNNORMALIZED LIST |
|---|
| Patient Number |
| Patient Name |
| Lab Code |
| Lab Location |
| Lab Name |
| Accession Id 1 |
| Procedure Id 1 |
| Procedure Name 1 |
| Test Result 1 |
| Procedure Order Date 1 |
| Procedure Ref Range 1 |
| Procedure Chart Date 1 |
| Accession Id 2 |
| Procedure Id 2 |
| Procedure Name 2 |
| Test Result 2 |
| Procedure Order Date 2 |
| Procedure Ref Range 2 |
| Procedure Chart Date 2 |
| Clinic Code |
| Clinic Location |
| Clinic Name |

FIGURE 12-6. Unnormalized list to data.

patient record, then scan the tests associated with the records. This is awkward, inefficient, inaccurate, and extremely untidy. And there is the possibility that Dan may have more than one patient record, a data integrity issue.

Applying Rule 1, moving the test results into a separate table helps considerably. Separating the repeating groups of test results from the patient information results in First Normal Form. The Test Results table will contain one record for each test result for each patient. The Patient Number in the Test Results table matches the primary key in the Patient table, providing a foreign key for relating the two tables. Now we can answer our original question with a direct retrieval by finding all records in the Test Results table where Dan's Patient Number and the test identification number for cholesterol appear together. Figure 12-7 presents the First Normal Form.

## Rule 2: Eliminate Redundant Data

*If an attribute depends on only part of a multivalued key, remove it to a separate table.*

In the test results table, the primary key is made up of the Patient Number, the Accession Identification Number, the Procedure Identification Number, and the Order Date. This makes sense for the test result, because it will be different for every combination of patient, accession, procedure, and order date. But the Procedure Name depends only on the Procedure Identification Number. The same name will appear redundantly every time its associated identification number appears in the Test Results table.

Suppose you want change the procedure name and make it more meaningful. The change has to be made for every patient who has had that procedure.

| PATIENT TABLE 1st Normal Form | TEST RESULTS TABLE 1st Normal Form |
|---|---|
| Patient Number | Patient Number |
| Patient Name | Accession Id 1 |
| Clinic Code | Procedure Id 1 |
| Clinic Location | Procedure Name 1 |
| Clinic Name | Test Result 1 |
| | Procedure Order Date 1 |
| | Procedure Ref Range 1 |
| | Procedure Chart Date 1 |
| | Lab Code |
| | Lab Location |
| | Lab Name |

FIGURE 12-7. First Normal Form.

If you miss some you'll have several patients with the same procedure charted with different names. This is known as an "update anomaly," another data integrity issue.

Or suppose that the last patient who had that procedure is removed from the database. The procedure is not stored anywhere! This is a "delete anomaly," another data integrity issue.

To avoid these problems we need Second Normal Form. Separate the attributes depending on multiple parts of the key from those depending on a single part of the key. This results in one more table: Procedures, which gives the name of each procedure. And depending on our situation, we might also store Laboratory Code in the Procedures table, if we order the same procedure from different laboratories that use different names and numbers for the same test.

Now we can change the charted spelling of a procedure name with one change to one table. The improved name will be available throughout the application. Figure 12-8 displays the Second Normal Form.

The attribute, reference range, is left in the Test Results table because it applies to the entire key. Where should it be stored? That depends on who I am. Am I the laboratory or the care provider? When performing the procedure, the reference range is stored in the Procedures table and passed on to the chart as part of the result. In fact, the laboratory must keep a chronological record of the reference range variances. When caring for patients, the reference range is stored in the Tests table. For purposes of this example, we'll be care providers and store the reference range in the Test Results table.

## Rule 3: Eliminate Columns Not Dependent on Key

*If attributes do not contribute to a description of the key, remove them to a separate table.*

The Patients table satisfies First Normal Form, as it contains no repeating groups. It satisfies Second Normal Form, since it does not have a multivalued key. But the key is Patient Number, and the Clinic Name and Clinic Location

**PATIENT TABLE**
**2nd Normal Form**

Patient Number
Patient Name
Clinic Code

**CLINIC TABLE**

Clinic Code
Clinic Location
Clinic Name

**TEST RESULTS TABLE**

Patient Number
Accession Id
Procedure Name
Test Result
Procedure Order Date
Procedure Ref Range
Procedure Chart Date
Lab Code
Lab Location
Lab Name

**PROCEDURE
TABLE**

Procedure Id
Procedure Name

FIGURE 12-8. Second Normal Form.

describe only a clinic, not a patient. To achieve Third Normal Form, clinic attributes must be moved into a separate table. Since they describe clinics, Clinic Code becomes the key of the new table.

The Test Results table also satisfies First Normal Form. However, Laboratory Code, Laboratory Name, and Laboratory Location describe the laboratory that performed the procedure. Laboratory Name and Location must be moved into a separate table.

The motivation for this change is the same as in Rule 2. We choose to avoid update and delete anomalies. For example, suppose no tests from TheBigLabCorp were currently stored in the database. With the previous design, there would be no record of TheBigLabCorp in our database. Figure 12-9 displays Third Normal Form.

## Rule 4: Isolate Independent Multiple Relationships

*No table may contain two or more 1:n (one-to-many) or n:m (many-to-many) relationships that are not directly related.*

Actually, third normal form looked pretty good, and it is sufficient for most situations. However, we are dealing with clinical and anatomic data in our database. And this rule is especially applicable to designs where there are many data relationships. An example of a 1:n relationship is that one patient can have many laboratory tests. An example of an n:m relationship is that a patient can have many laboratory tests and many patients can have the same laboratory test. Or a patient can have many tests performed by different laboratories and be seen at different clinics.

Suppose we want to add a new attribute to the Patient table, Maternity Flag Date. This will enable us to look for patients who are/were pregnant and who have had their blood sugar checked. Rule 4, Fourth Normal Form, dictates against

| PATIENT TABLE | CLINIC TABLE |
|---|---|
| Patient Number | Clinic Code |
| Patient Name | Clinic Location |
| Clinic Code | Clinic Name |

**TEST RESULTS TABLE**

| Patient Number |
|---|
| Accession Id |
| Procedure Name |
| Test Result |
| Procedure Order Date |
| Procedure Ref Range |
| Procedure Chart Date |
| Lab Code |

**PROCEDURE TABLE**

| Procedure Id |
|---|
| Procedure Name |

**LAB TABLE**

| Lab Code |
|---|
| Lab Location |
| Lab Name |

FIGURE 12-9. Third Normal Form.

using the Test Results table because Maternity Flag Date is not directly related to the Test Result Table. The Patient table is also a poor choice because multiple pregnancies can occur over time, a violation of Rule 1, First Normal Form.

The solution is to create a new table, Maternal Cross Reference, containing the Patient Number and the Maternity Flag Date; the two fields would also comprise the primary key of this new table. Figure 12-10 shows the maternity flag table.

## Rule 5: Isolate Semantically Related Multiple Relationships

*There may be practical constraints on information that justify separating logically related, many-to-many relationships.*

Suppose our organization is changing and our patients can now be seen at more than one of our clinics. Or suppose we require more precision relating patient visits to laboratory tests. We create a new Patient Organizer table containing the Patient Number, an Encounter Identification number, a Clinic Code; we add the Encounter Identification Number to the Test Results table; we remove the Clinic Code from the Patient table. With this new table, we would be able to relate all of a patient's laboratory test results regardless of the clinic at which the patient was seen. We could further refine it so that we could ensure that a patient has only one patient record no matter how many patient identifiers the patient may have. Inpatient stays could also be integrated into this database in a similar manner for a comprehensive patient view as well as population view. Figure 12-11 displays final table designs resulting from the original unnormalized list.

**MATERNAL XREF**

| Patient Number |
|---|
| Maternity Flag Date |
| Est Fetal Age |

FIGURE 12-10. New table—Fourth Normal Form.

| PATIENT TABLE | TEST RESULTS TABLE | PATIENT ORGANIZER |
|---|---|---|
| Patient Nbr | Patient Number | Patient Nbr |
| Patient Name | Accession Id | Encounter Id |
| Encounter Id | Procedure Name | Clinic Code |
| Date of Birth | Test Result | |
| Race | Procedure Order Date | |
| Sex | Procedure Ref Range | |
| | Procedure Chart Date | |
| | Lab Code | |
| | Encounter Id | |

| CLINIC TABLE | LAB TABLE |
|---|---|
| Clinic Code | Lab Code |
| Clinic Location | Lab Location |
| Clinic Name | Lab Name |

| MATERNAL XREF | PROCEDURE TABLE |
|---|---|
| Patient Number | Procedure Id |
| Maternity Flag Date | Procedure Name |
| Est Fetal Age | Lab Code |

FIGURE 12-11. Final table designs.

# Summary

This chapter outlines a necessary and complex protocol for designing a database. We start with current system screens, files, reports, and other documents and go through Data Analysis, including Data Normalization, to create a logical model and business requirements analysis to create a business or entity model. The logical model and the entity model are integrated for the logical design. The logical design is then transformed into a physical design by the application of database-engine-vendor-specific facilities and constraints along with performance requirements. In database design, designing tables is the heart of the matter. In the design process, you are concerned with going from an external view of the data as it exists real world today (data model) to a physical view implemented in a proprietary vendor database technology, then back to an external view (user interface) through which you interact with the database to accomplish your job.

One nugget worth remembering is that designing a database appears to be easy to the Microsoft Access Power User or to an untrained eye. And it is easy, if you really know the data and the technology involved and the scope of work and the design techniques discussed herein. Database design is like the children's toy, a wooden egg painted to look like a person in ethnic costume. As you play with the egg, you figure out that the egg opens and contains another egg painted to look like a person in a different costume. And there is a third egg inside the second, and so forth. There is more to database design than meets the eye. There is more—or less—to that vendor database system than meets the ear.

# Chapter Glossary

**database:** Collection of information related to a particular subject or purpose; an information storage and retrieval facility where data is collected for the purpose of generating information and discovering patterns. It does not have to be stored on a computer. It may have a user interface or not; it may be relational or not.

**database engine:** Internal, highly technical file management system into which a logical database design is physically implemented. Some database engines are Microsoft Jet, Microsoft SQL Server, IBM DB2, and Oracle.

**database application (database system):** Collection of forms, screen, tables, queries, and reports utilizing a Database managed by a Database Engine. For example, OurVendor's LIS is a database application.

**database management system:** Collection of utility and administrative functions supporting the database engine. Its level of sophistication directly affects the robustness of any Database System. It provides security and file management practices additional to those delivered with the computer/network on which it runs. This level varies from vendor to vendor. For example, Oracle is a complete database management system; DBase, FoxPro, and Access are not.

**data integrity:** Desirable condition of data frequently taken for granted by clients. It means, for example, that there are no duplicate records in the database, that there are no "orphan" records (a test result without a patient) in the database, and that steps have been taken to ensure that the integrity remains over time and use of the database.

**data normalization:** Process of making data and tables match database design standards. The objective of these standards is to eliminate redundant information to make managing data and future changes in table structure easier. If the tables are normalized, each data element/table attribute will be a fact about the key, the whole key, and nothing but the key.
Rule 1. Make a separate table for each set of related attributes and give each table a primary key. Each field contains the smallest meaningful value and repeating groups are eliminated.
Rule 2. Make a separate table for each set of related attributes and give each table a primary key. Applies only to tables with a multiple field, primary key. If an attribute depends on only part of the key, remove it to a separate table. Each non-key field should relate to the ENTIRE key.
Rule 3. If attributes do not contribute to a description of the key, remove them to a separate table.
Rule 4. No table may contain two or more 1:n or n:m relationships that are not directly related.
Rule 5. Make a separate table for each recurring attribute and give each table a primary key.

**foreign key:** Field or set of fields within a table that equal the Primary Key of another table. Foreign keys are how we relate one table to another. For example, the Patient table contains a field called Location Code, which is also the Primary Key of the Location Table. This is used by the relational database system to be able to find the Location Name whenever it needs it with the Patient while storing only the Location Code with the Patient record. So when the Location changes its name, we only have to change it once in the Location table and have the change appear in all subsequent uses of that Location Code.

**logical model:** Visual representation of how the database components relate one to another. There are multiple levels in the logical model, the highest being the topics within the database, the lowest being all the data elements about all the topics and all of their relationships.

**metadata:** Collection of data about data; a data dictionary that defines what the data is, where it originated, where it is stored, how frequently is it updated, and so on.

**physical model:** Representation of how the database is physically stored in the computer's file system.

**primary key:** Field or set of fields that uniquely identify each record stored in the table. The power of a relational database system comes from its ability to quickly find and bring together information stored in separate tables using queries. In order to do this, each table should include a primary key to ensure the uniqueness of each record. A primary key may be one or multiple fields within the record.

**query:** Means of retrieving data from the database using specified criteria and displaying it in the order specified. Queries create a logical view of a subset of the data in the database and do not permanently occupy physical storage.

**record:** Technical term for a row of data in a relational database. Table records contain facts or attributes or data elements or columns.

**relationships:** Definitions of how pieces of data relate to one another. A one-to-one relationship exists when one record in the primary table corresponds to one record in the related table. A one-to-many relationship exists when one record in the primary table corresponds to multiple records in the related table. Many-to-many relationships exist in the real world and are implemented in databases via two, one-to-many relationships through a cross-reference table.

**referential integrity:** Something database engines do as a result of the relationships established in a database design. Integrity ensures that data necessary for the relationship is not accidentally deleted, and it cascades updates and deletes throughout the relationship per the designer's specs. Referential integrity means that a patient record must exist in the Patient Table prior to adding a Patient Test Result record to the Test Results table. If it is turned off, a test result can be added to the table without its corresponding patient. Referential integrity is a feature that comes with relational database engines and does not require any programming to be available.

**table:** Technical term for a file in a relational database, a collection of data about a single, specific topic such as a patient or a clinic or a test result. Tables contain records or rows of data, one record per patient or clinic or test result. Using a separate table for each topic means you store that data only once which increases your efficiency and reduces data entry errors. Tables organize data into columns (called fields) and rows (called records). Table records contain facts or attributes or data elements. For example, in a patient table we might expect to find a single record with facts about the patient, i.e. the patient's data of birth, sex, race, social security number. A database table is similar to a spreadsheet in appearance only.

**user interface:** The methods and techniques used to interact with a computer and the software running on the computer at the behest of the user. There are two major types of interface: character and graphical. A character interface utilizes the keyboard as its input provider and happens character by character and line by line. The individual is restricted to following a set course of actions every time an activity is worked through completion.

A graphical interface is visual and utilizes the mouse and 'images' and events as its input provider. Everyone's graphical interface may be different in appearance whereas all character interfaces look pretty much the same. Did you know that the operating system on your PC is called the Disk Operating System (DOS) and that Windows is the user interface to DOS? Windows and applications written for it offer a graphical interface, a GUI. With the Internet, we have text-only user interfaces or graphical ones, dynamic ones and static ones.

# 13
# Process Modeling
## Using Computer Simulation
## in Laboratory Management

AMIN A. MOHAMMAD, JOHN R. PETERSEN, GBO YOUH

Simulation is defined as a means of seeing how a model of a real system will respond to changes in its structure, environment, or underlying assumptions.[1] The value of a model simulation is that it allows exploration of proposed changes in a real, operating system without having to bear the risk and costs of change until the optimal system has been identified and tested. For the purpose of this chapter a system is defined as a combination of elements that interact to accomplish a specific objective. The two types of systems are **manufacturing systems** such as large production facilities, small jobs shops, machining cells, assembly lines, and so on and **service systems** such as healthcare facilities, amusement parks, restaurants, and banks.

A clinical laboratory is a service system usually found within a larger, more complex entity, e.g., a hospital or clinic. To carry out tasks, the clinical laboratory uses a variety of resources such as analyzers, medical technologists, technicians, and sample processors. The task might be the processing and analysis of clinical samples, whole blood, serum, plasma, urine, or cerebrospinal fluid. The human and machine resources perform multiple yet well-defined and repetitive activities on the samples. The various activities performed by these resources are interrelated and must work cooperatively to produce prompt and accurate test results to help in the diagnosis and treatment of diseases. The steps used by the laboratory resources to handle, analyze, and report results on a sample often result in complex interactions that can be very difficult to analyze via human intuition. The economist Herbert Simon called this ability of the human mind to grasp real-world complexity "the principle of bounded rationality".[1] This principle states that "the capacity of the human mind for formulating and solving complex problems is very small compared with the size of the problem whose solution is required for objectively rational behavior in the real world, or even for a reasonable approximation to such objective rationality." From this perspective it is no wonder that just the sheer number of clinical samples and the various tasks performed on each sample are enough to stagger the imagination. However, when the interaction of the various elements that make up the clinical laboratory is taken into account, the system is even more difficult to analyze.

211

The operational complexities of a clinical laboratory are mainly due to two factors; interdependencies between elements and variability in overall behavior of the different elements that make up the system. The interdependencies can be easily understood by realizing that one sample generally has more than one test ordered on it. Thus, in many instances the sample must be tested using different resources, such as different analyzers and more than one technologist. Lack of availability of either medical technologist or analyzer will cause delays in reporting test results. Variability in this system occurs due to variability in sample arrival patterns, analyzer speed, processing for the various sample types, number of tests ordered on each sample, and so on.

## What Is Simulation?

Simulation is the use of a computer to construct a model that is designed to imitate and capture the dynamic behavior of a system in order to evaluate the different ways of improving its efficiency. By using simulation, insights into the complex dynamics of a system can be gained that cannot be obtained by using other techniques. Since simulation accounts for interdependencies and variation, it is one of the best ways to analyze a complex system like a clinical laboratory. No one knows when the first model of a clinical laboratory or even when the first simulation model was built. However, testing an idea or a concept via live or mathematical models is not a new concept and can be linked to basic physical concepts developed by Aristotle and Archimedes. Models today are used to understand and evaluate known phenomena and then to perform experiments to predict the behavior of a real system. Some of the better-known models include the prediction of weather, positions of planets with respect to the Sun during certain time intervals, variations in the stock market, and forecasting election outcomes.

Clinical sciences have used animal models in attempting to understand and find cures for various diseases. The clinical observation of a disease, searching for a hypothetical etiology, and finally confirmation by recreating the disease state in an animal can be considered modeling. Studying the effect of various drugs on the animal model can be thought of as testing the model. The knowledge gained using this animal model is then used to experiment on human beings and finally develop a cure. In simulation the experimentation is done on a computer by building a model of the scenario in question. Numerous software programs are commercially available. Most will simulate and collect performance statistics, such as turnaround times for samples and resource and analyzer utilization, and provide a summary for further analysis. Some of the programs also provide a realistic graphical animation of the processes being modeled, in addition to allowing a user to interact with the model and optimize the system.

Simulation can be separated into two basic techniques, those directed at discrete events and those directed at continuous events. A discrete event is an action that occurs at a unique point in time. Examples of discrete events are a sample arriving in the laboratory, a sample being loaded into a centrifuge rack, the centrifuge rack being loaded into centrifuge, and the process of centrifugation. The underlying principle of these events is that each has been a change in the system state. When modeling discrete events, the computer maintains a timing device known as a simulation clock, which advances with each discrete event taking place at a fixed point in time. If the event represents an initiation of an activity that will conclude in the future, the simulation adds the completion time to a list of future events and advances the clock to the next time at which the event is due. Discrete event simulation also employs statistical methods for generating random behavior and to estimate the model's performance. This is sometimes referred to as the Monte Carlo method because of the similarity to the probabilistic outcomes found in games of chance.

A continuous event is an action that continues without stopping and involves a change in a physical or chemical property over time. These types of events are often represented by differential equations. Examples of continuous events are biochemical reactions, temperature logs, and the flow of water in a river. Changing model variables that are tied to the simulation clock at a well-defined rate best simulates continuous events.

# Why Use Computer Simulation for Laboratory Management?

A clinical laboratory is a dynamic system where various processes, which although well defined and repetitive, are applied to a very large number of samples. Managers must make operational decisions in order to provide the best turnaround times (TAT) for test results and to deal with the variability of the different events, such as arrival of stat samples, and the variety of tests ordered. Finally the outcome, i.e., the test result, is highly dependent on the ability of different people to interact with each other and with the available instrumentation. Thus management of a clinical laboratory is a very complex task, because every section of the laboratory must work in unison to provide the fast and high-quality results required to help manage patients.

Other major challenges facing the clinical laboratory are containing cost and increasing productivity while at the same time improving customer satisfaction. Although the patient is the ultimate customer of the clinical laboratory, it is the physicians, nurses, and other healthcare providers who make the decision of which laboratory to use. Their satisfaction usually depends on the TAT. While not the best indicator of laboratory quality, it is usually perceived that the faster a laboratory is able to turn out a test result, the happier the customer. Test turnaround time depends on numerous factors such as arrival patterns of routine and stat samples, test ordering pattern on each sample, human resources, type of analyzers, and degree of automation. Out of these five variables, sample arrival patterns and test ordering patterns have the greatest degree of variability and change over time, requiring continuous process optimization in order to adapt to them. Of the remaining three variables, human resources constitute 60% of total laboratory cost, imposing a constant need to find the minimum number of medical technologists to meet the laboratory goals of quality results, fast TAT, and minimized cost.

The final two variables, the type of analyzer and degree of automation, constitute fixed costs. Once an analyzer is purchased, leased, or rented, it is not changed for 3 to 5 years. Deciding on an appropriate instrument is a difficult task due to the often large capital investment involved and the availability of a wide range of analyzers having different specifications, strengths, and weaknesses. Additionally, decision making is complicated by the manufacturers of these analyzers who may be unwilling to release information that will not show their instruments in the best light. Almost all clinical laboratories make acquisition decisions based on experience, intuition, and limited experimentation.

However, with the current emphasis shifting toward "getting it right the first time" to save money, the trial-and-error approach is not only expensive but time consuming and disruptive to laboratory operations. If computer simulation, which provides a powerful planning and decision-making tool, is used, it can capture system interdependencies, account for the variability in the system, model any analyzer desired, show changes of behavior over time, provide information on multiple performance measures, and force attention to detail in the design of the evaluation; finally, it is less costly. A good simulation model gives laboratory management unlimited freedom to try out different ideas, instruments, routines and staff assignments risk free—with virtually no cost, no waste of time, and most important, no disruption of the current system. In addition, the exercise of developing a model itself is highly beneficial, since it forces one to work through the operational details of the process, sometimes enough to understand and solve a problem.

## How Is Simulation Done?

Simulation by itself is not a solution to a problem but rather is a tool to evaluate the problem. Simulation is a computer model of an existing system that has been created for the purpose of conducting experiments to help identify the best solutions to a specific problem. Therefore, development of a simulation model follows the standard scientific protocol, which involves formulating a hypothesis, setting up an experiment, testing the hypothesis through experimentation, and drawing conclusions about the validity of the hypothesis. The first step in developing a hypothesis is actually asking the right question. The most common questions that are asked by laboratory management are as follows:

* Can the existing process deliver the desired TAT all the time?
* How many full-time equivalents (FTE) or medical technologists are needed to ensure that the desired TAT is met on a regular basis?

- Is it more appropriate to perform chemistry and immunoassay testing on different platform or on the same platform?
- How many more FTEs will be needed to accommodate a specific increase in test volume?
- What is the best instrument combination for meeting the laboratories TAT goals?
- How will a change in process impact overall laboratory efficiency?
- How much buffer capacity (i.e., ability to maintain the desired TAT during labor shortage due to sick leave, vacation, and so on) does a laboratory have?
- What is most appropriate for laboratory: modular or total laboratory automation?
- What real savings can be expected after implementing a process change?
- What impact will an imaging technology, such as MICRO 21, have on the hands-on utilization by a medical technologist working in a hematology laboratory?
- What impact will front-end automation have on test TAT and labor utilization of FTEs working in the receiving and processing area of the laboratory?
- Will total laboratory automation work without the capability for centrifugation and sample aliquotting?

After formulating the hypothesis, the next step is gathering operational details. Simulation models will work with inaccurate data but will not work with incomplete operational information. The formulation of the hypothesis is an extremely important step since there are times when this process by itself will present solutions, leading to the development of various "what if" scenarios. After an understanding of the operational details has been gained, the pertinent data for each process is collected. The model is then built and run for a period of time, which may be a simulated day, week, or year. The model generates performance statistics, such as turnaround times, resource utilization, instrument utilization, and so on. The simulated turnaround times are then compared with the actual turnaround time to validate and calculate the standard error in the model. The model is then optimized to minimize the standard error and used to perform "what if" analysis.

# Simulating the Receiving and Processing Area of a Laboratory

Computer simulation can be used in many areas of a clinical laboratory. Its application can be best explained by describing the process required to simulate the receiving and processing area of the laboratory. The receiving and processing area of any clinical laboratory is its Achilles heel. Not only are the processes occurring in this section diverse, but they are also manual. Figures

13-1 and 13-2 show the operations typically occurring in the order entry and processing areas. They display the actual operations of the receiving and processing areas of the clinical laboratory at the University of Texas Medical Branch. Any sample tested in a laboratory has to go through these or similar processes. Any errors introduced in receiving and processing adversely affect all subsequent laboratory processes.

To evaluate changes in this portion of the laboratory, a simulation model can be built. The simulation can be used to answer any of the following questions:

- Can the existing process deliver a stipulated TAT of 15 minutes for stat samples and 60 minutes for routine samples?
- What will be the impact on TAT of routine and stat samples when two or three processors call in sick or go on a vacation?
- What are the minimum FTEs needed to provide stipulated TAT all the time?
- Evaluate the inefficiency introduced by continuous arrival of stat samples.
- How much additional work can be handled by the system?
- Evaluate the optimal number of computer terminals, centrifuges, and refrigerators, and study the impact of centrifuge downtime on test TAT.
- Quantify the labor savings by the introduction of process changes such as physician order entry.
- Evaluate and quantify the impact of front-end automation on test turnaround time and labor utilization.

Most of the events occurring in the receiving and processing area of a clinical laboratory are discrete processes, and therefore discrete event simulation is the technique of choice. As discussed previously, when using discrete event simulation, the changes in the state of the physical system are represented by a series of events that occur at discrete, time-limited intervals. Figure 13-3 shows the logic diagram of how discrete event simulation works for the receiving and processing area of a laboratory.

At the onset the model creates a simulation database and programs scheduled events such as sample arrivals. The arrival of a sample is event 1. Since the arrival pattern has already been scheduled at the onset of simulation, it is also called a scheduled event. However, event 2, capturing a medical technologist for a specified time period, is conditional on the availability of the medical technologist. Hence, event 2 is called a conditional event. If a medical technologist is not available, the sample is routed to a waiting queue and will stay there until a medical technologist becomes available. Assuming the time taken by a medical technologist to complete event 2 is described by a normally distributed random variable having a mean of 120 seconds and a standard deviation of 30 seconds, the start of event 2 can be assigned using a random number generator based on the mean and standard deviation for (for

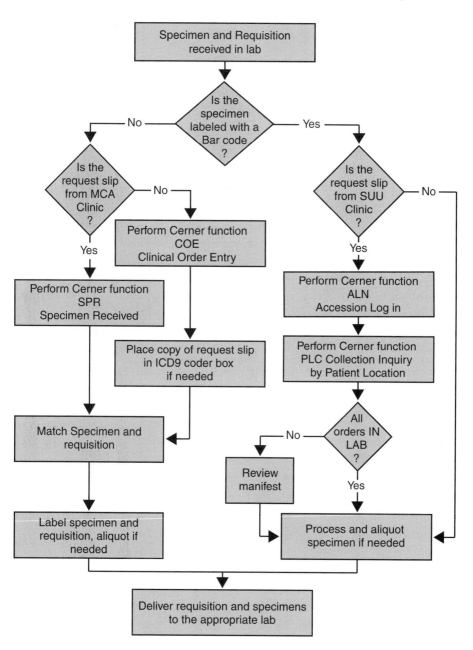

FIGURE 13-1. Work flow in the specimen-receiving area of the clinical laboratory. MCA = medical clinic A; SUU = surgical clinic, urology; Cerner = vendor of the laboratory information system.

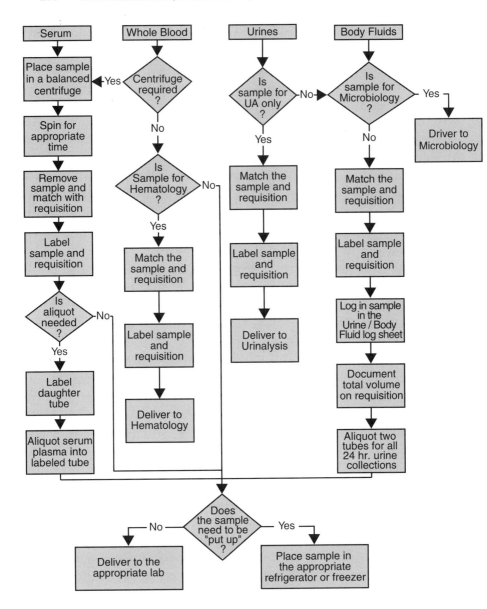

**FIGURE 13-2.** Work flow of various sample types within the laboratory.

example) 90 seconds. This allows the model to schedule the completion of event 2 in the future. In this case the time will be the sample arrival time plus 90 seconds. The logic associated with event 2, "Use medical technologist for 90 seconds," is then executed. The simulation clock is advanced to the sched-

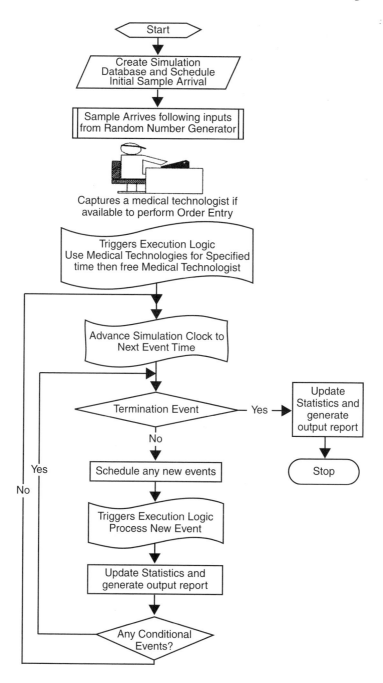

FIGURE 13-3. Logic diagram for the development of a simulation exercise in specimen receiving. and processing.

uled completion time, i.e., sample arrival time plus 90 seconds. Event 2 then terminates, and the medical technologist is made available for the next sample.

The model then refers to the set of instructions to determine whether the process terminates here or moves on to next step, event 3. If the specimen is a hematology sample and it doesn't need any further processing, then the sample exits the receiving and processing area. The model updates the statistics such as exit time and logs TAT as the difference between the exit and sample arrival time. However, if a chemistry sample that needs further processing is scheduled, the model moves on and schedules event 3, which may be "Put the sample into a centrifuge." If there is a wait time associated with event 3, the model schedules the completion of event 3 by adding a specified wait time to the existing value on the simulation clock. The simulation clock is then advanced to the completion of event 3 and any resulting statistics are updated. Depending on the logic used to develop the model, the sample is advanced to the next event or the process terminated by exiting the model.

Thus, the process that a sample has to navigate through in a laboratory is broken up into numerous single discrete events. The end of one event is the beginning of the next event, and so on. The model unites the individual events into a continuum by repeating the following sequence: (1) identify the event scheduled to occur next; (2) set the simulation clock variable to the time equal to the time of the next event; (3) update statistical inputs wherever required; (4) compute the actions associated with the most current event; (5) schedule the occurrence of the next event; and (6) move the simulation clock to the time of occurrence of next event. This general logic is applied in the simulating the various steps illustrated in Figures 13-1 and 13-2.

The building of a model of the receiving and processing functions requires specific information to be gathered:

- Arrival pattern of the different sample types. This includes information such as number of routine, stat, hematology, coagulation samples hourly
- Test ordering pattern on different sample types. The pattern will be an indication of the number of samples requiring aliquots or needing to be tested at more than one station or instrument
- Number of computer terminals available for test accessioning
- Number of available centrifuges
- Shift assignments for different technicians working in the receiving and processing area
- Time and motion analysis for various processes occurring in the section. A minimum of 40 readings must be taken for each process occurring in the laboratory also enabling understanding of how different resources handle a process.
- Layout of existing laboratory

The simulation is typically run for 24 hours and the statistics, such as TAT of different samples, hands-on utilization of medical technologists, and utilization of different computer terminals and centrifuges, are recorded and displayed at the end of running the model. The number of simulation runs is determined by the confidence level and tolerated error in overall analysis. It can be easily calculated by using the following equation:

$$N = [(Z_{\propto/2}) \times S / e]^2$$

where $\propto$ = significance level = $1 - 0.95 = 0.05$ at 95% confidence level
   $e$ = tolerated error in overall analysis
   $S$ = standard deviation of sample population
   $Z$ = derived from standard normal distribution table for 95% confidence level $Z = 1.96$

Typically, 10 replicates will be able to assert with 95% confidence that the simulated TAT is off by ± 10% from the real TAT collected during the data collection phase.

# Case Study

A quality assurance report from a clinical laboratory in a major academic center revealed a 20% failure rate in meeting the stat TAT for chemistry samples. Since most of the stat samples come from critical care sites such as the emergency room, intensive cardiac care unit, and pediatric intensive care unit, it was necessary to determine the cause of the failure and institute a process change. Consequently, a continuous process improvement (CPI) committee was formed, which examined the various processes that occurred in the laboratory for one month using traditional procedures and came up with the following recommendations:

- Add two additional processors on the day and evening shifts.
- Institute a dedicated stat station that is staffed at all times and is responsible only for handling stat samples.
- Add three centrifuges and two computer terminals to speed up test order entry.
- Acquire a front-end automation system that will automate centrifugation, aliquotting, and sample routing to the different areas of the laboratory.
- Develop standard operating procedures for handling the various processes in the laboratory.
- Batch routine samples and handle stat samples as they arrive.

A cost analysis showed that it would cost the institution around $1 million to implement these changes; more important, there were no guarantees that the changes would improve the TAT. Figure 13-4 shows the arrival pattern for stat and routine samples for this laboratory. On a typical day the laboratory processes around 2,400 samples. Figure 13-5 shows the flow of the various processes and the time it takes to finish each process.

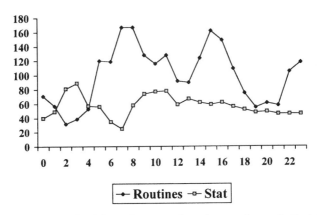

FIGURE 13-4. Arrival times for stat and routine specimens in the laboratory.

A simulation model was built by taking into consideration the various resources and their respective shifts and the number of centrifuges and order entry stations. The number of personnel, centrifuges, and order entry stations available before the process change is shown in Table 13-1. The physical layout of the receiving processing area of the laboratory is shown in Figure 13-6. Drawing the layout to match the laboratory's actual layout is important, as it allows estimating the amount of time a resource will spend in moving from one workstation to another.

The model was validated by visual inspection of the various processes occurring in the laboratory. Fifteen replications of the model were run and performance statistics such as labor utilization, sample TAT, and so on were collected and averaged. Figures 13-7 and 13-8 show the comparison between the actual and simulated TAT. According to computer simulations using resources theoretically available, all stat samples should be processed within 30 minutes; however, in the real laboratory only 80% of samples were processed in that time (Figure 13-7). A similar discrepancy was noticed for routine samples (Figure 13-8).

Detailed analysis of the collected data revealed that approximately 60% of the time the laboratory was short by two technologists. This shortage was due mainly to employees calling in sick, and 95% of call-ins occur during the day shift. By reducing the day shift staff by two in the model, TATs compared very favorably with the actual laboratory TATs (standard error < 8%). The stipulated TAT for stat samples for this laboratory was 30 minutes, and based on computer simulations, this TAT could be achieved if the laboratory were fully staffed. Thus, by simulation, the ability of the laboratory's process to deliver the stipulated TAT could be verified. That is, the process was not the problem; staffing was, contrary to the analysis performed by the CPI team.

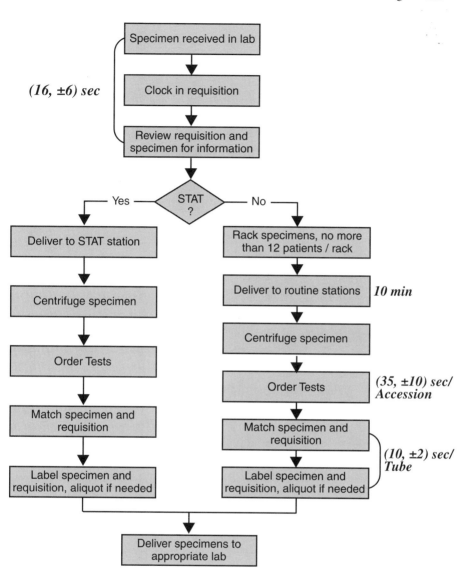

**FIGURE 13-5.** Flow diagram with time intervals.

**TABLE 13-1.** Resources.

| Shifts | No. Resources | No. Centrifuges | No. Order Entry Stations |
|--------|---------------|-----------------|--------------------------|
| Day | 5 | 5 | 5 |
| Evening | 6 | 7 | 7 |
| Night | 5 | 7 | 7 |

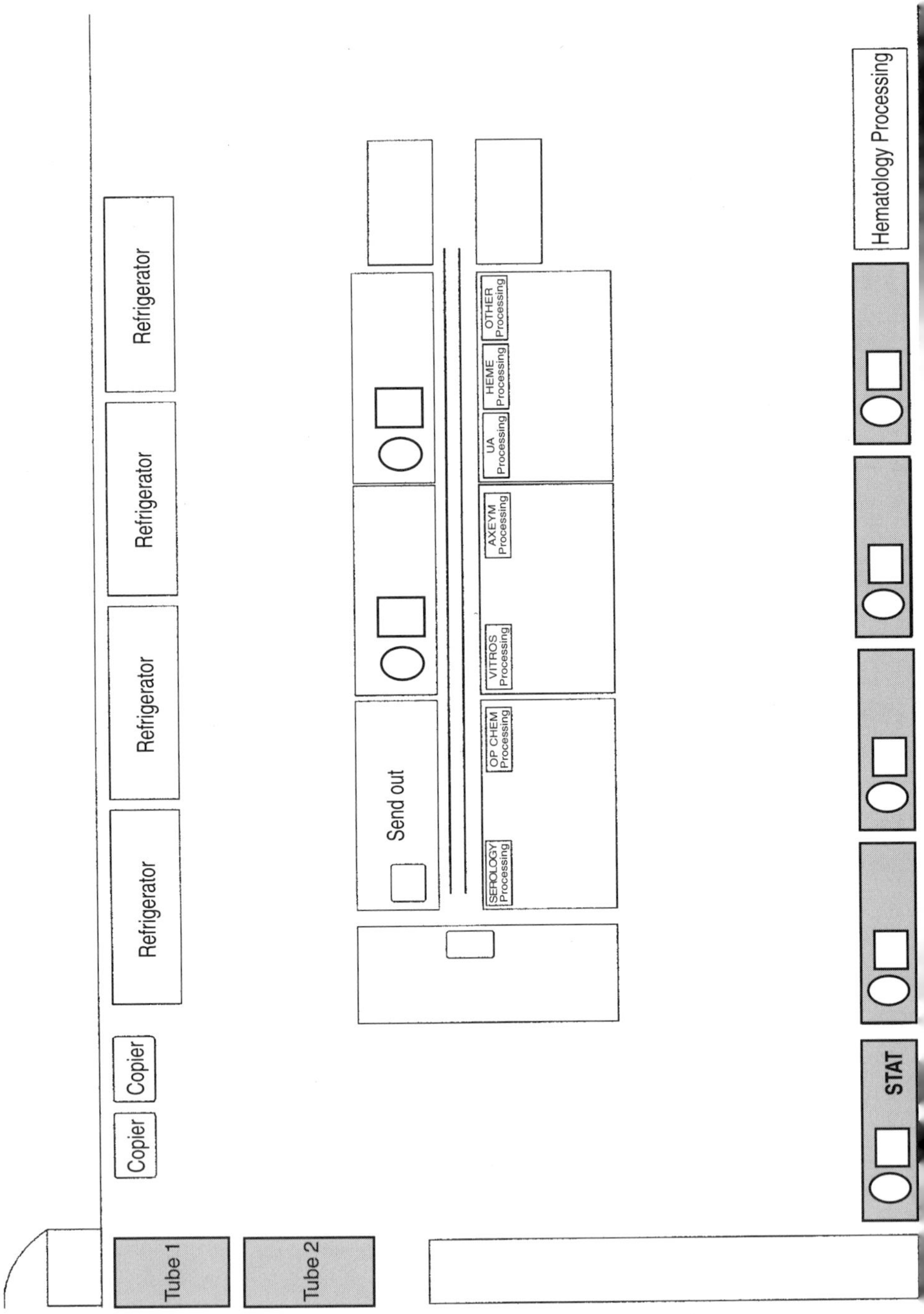
Refrigerator
Refrigerator
Refrigerator
Refrigerator
Copier
Copier
Tube 1
Tube 2
Send out
SEROLOGY Processing
OP CHEM Processing
VITROS Processing
AXEYM Processing
UA Processing
HEME Processing
OTHER Processing
STAT
Hematology Processing

Figure 13-9 shows the predicted utilization of the different people working during day, evening, and night shifts. With the exception of the two people on the day shift, most of the staff was less than 70% utilized. It has been our experience that expecting utilization greater than 70–75% on a regular basis causes employee burnout and hence absenteeism and a high turnover rate of personnel. We consider utilization between 65% and 70% to be optimal for human resources. From close inspection of Figure 13-9 it is also apparent that day and evening shifts have very little buffer capacity in terms of available labor. This was estimated by simulating the reduction of a staff position sequentially on a per shift basis and studying the impact on the overall TAT of all samples. The study showed no significant deterioration in TAT of stat samples when one position was eliminated on either the day or evening shifts. However, the utilization of all other personnel increased by approximately 15%, thus causing their utilization to go over the optimum utilization rate of 70–75%, potentially causing burnout. A significant increase in TAT for the night shift, however, was observed only when two of its positions were eliminated.

The simulation model of the existing laboratory was then modified to include front-end automation. A simulation model of the FE 500, a front-end processor manufactured by TECAN (TECAN AG) for Abbott Diagnostics, was built and validated. This submodel was then inserted into the existing model, and its impact on TAT was studied. Interestingly, the simulation showed a significant increase in the TAT for both the stat and routine samples. Examination of the model before front-end automation revealed that this increase in TAT was due to change in two processes, order entry and centrifugation, that had been occurring simultaneously. The introduction of front-end automation caused the two processes to occur sequentially rather than simultaneously, causing an increase in TAT.

Using simulation to identify and quantitate the effect of changes on the receiving and processing processes resulted in the recommendations that physician order entry should be the first process change. In this context, physician order entry involves the test order being placed and transmitted electronically from the care unit to the laboratory, with samples labeled on the unit with labels printed and applied on site. This would ensure that samples arriving in the laboratory would be bar coded, reducing if not eliminating the need to manually enter the patient demographics and test orders into the laboratory computer system. Once this is done, introduction of front-end automation can occur. This stepwise process of changes, although intuitive, would not have occurred because of two conflicting schools of thought, the first stating that the time gained in automating the aliquotting process would more than offset the order entry time and thus lead to an overall reduction in TAT. The second belief was that the sample order entry process was causing

FIGURE 13-6. Layout of the receiving and processing area.

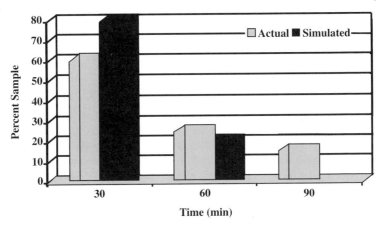

FIGURE 13-7. Comparison of actual and simulated turnaround times for routine samples.

the bottleneck and that front-end automation would increase the TAT. Furthermore the savings estimated before simulating the process were overly high, causing the estimated return on investment to be off by approximately two years.

Another important scenario evaluated using simulation was that of assigning one station dedicated to the ordering and processing of only stat samples. The simulation model showed that this would not expedite the processing of stat samples but would instead cause a delay of approximately 50 to 60 minutes in TAT because of other changes that would flow from that change. Therefore, because of this discovery through simulation, all technicians were told to process samples in following order: (1) stat samples; (2) in-hospital routines; (3) in-hospital clinics; and (4) outreach samples. Simulation also indicated that additional order entry terminals and centrifuges would not result in an improved TAT. Rather it was determined that the number of routine samples

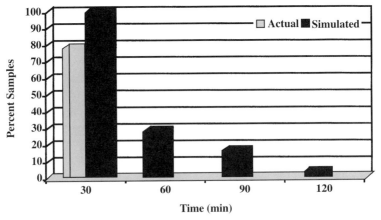

FIGURE 13-8. Comparison of actual and simulated turnaround times for stat samples.

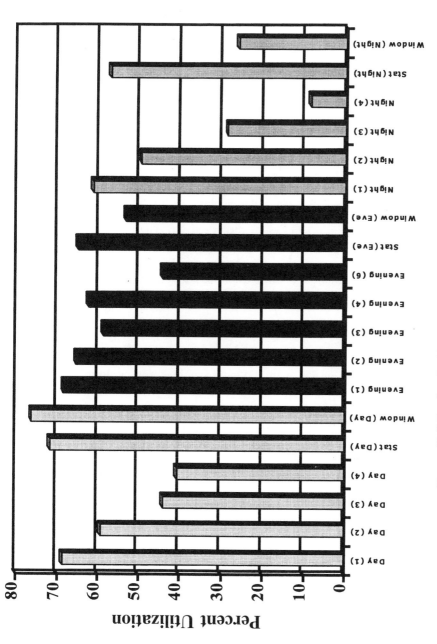

FIGURE 13-9. Predicted utilization of personnel according to shift.

that are batched before processing could be optimized. Simulation to optimize the two criteria of time and number of samples found that batching routine samples to a maximum of 24 arriving within a 10-minute time period would give the minimum TAT and the optimum utilization of centrifuges and order entry stations.

The conclusions and recommendations that resulted from the use of simulation to study receiving and processing follow:

- The existing process is capable of providing the stipulated TAT if there are no "call-ins."
- There is no buffer capacity in terms of labor during day and evening shifts. Hence, if more than one person calls in sick during either of these shifts, a delay in TAT of ~ 20% of stat samples will result.
- There are adequate numbers of centrifuges and order entry terminals.
- The layout of different stations in the laboratory is optimal and only 3% of time is spent walking from one station to another.
- Implementation of front-end automation without the prior implementation of physician order entry will cause a delay in TAT of stat samples.
- Implementation of physician order entry and front-end automation will provide a labor savings of four and three FTEs, respectively.
- Processing hematology samples on FE 500 will not result in a significant delay in TAT of other samples for this laboratory.

## Conclusion

Computer simulation has many potential applications in clinical laboratory management, including simulating clinical analyzers to predict optimum throughput, evaluating the impact of digital imaging technology on the overall efficiency of a hematology laboratory, estimating the excess capacity in existing instrumentation, optimizing work flow in anatomic pathology and histology laboratories, scheduling phlebotomy in outpatient clinics, optimizing work flow in microbiology and other labor-intensive areas such cytopathology and cytogenetics, and development of the best courier routes to allow efficient pickup of samples from outreach clinics. Simulation by itself should seen not as a solution but as a way to evaluate the processes within a laboratory. To make the best use of simulation, it should be performed as a part of a larger process improvement project.

In summary, simulation can be extremely useful: it fosters creative problem solving and exploration of alternatives at little added cost. It can also help predict outcomes and account for system variances. It is very effective for deriving solutions that will minimize the impact of variances, if not eliminating them entirely, it promotes a total solution that can be cost-effective, and finally and perhaps most important, it forces attention to the details in a process.

# Chapter Glossary

**continuous event:** In simulation studies, an action that continues without stopping and involves a change in a physical or chemical property over time.

**discrete event:** In simulation studies, an action that occurs at a unique point in time.

**simulation:** Use of a computer to construct a model designed to imitate and capture the dynamic behavior of a system in order to evaluate the different ways of improving its efficiency.

# *References*

1. Harrell CR, Bateman RE, Gogg TJ, Mott JRA. System Improvement Using Simulation, p. 1. Promodel Corporation, Salt Lake City, Utah, 4th ed.

# 14
# Artificial Intelligence and Expert Systems

DANIEL F. COWAN

Computer scientists and engineers, perhaps to make their activities more intelligible and more appealing to lay people, tend to use biological metaphors for the products of their activities. Prominent among these are artificial intelligence, neural networks, and genetic algorithms. All these are more or less expressions for categories of programs and the way they work. The intent (at least of some practitioners) is recreate the intelligence of a human in a machine. Whether this is possible or even desirable depends on how one looks at the processes of a machine and the processes of the human mind. History, folklore, and literature are full of accounts of attempts to create man or the intelligence of man in a robot or automaton: the Golem in Jewish folklore, the creature in Mary Shelley's *Frankenstein*, and HAL, the computer in Arthur Clarke's *2001: A Space Odyssey*. It is interesting to reflect on how many of these efforts failed or went out of control because of the lack of a human moral sense in the creation. One of the very best and most scholarly and thoughtful works on the subject of "computer intelligence" is Jaki's *Brain, Mind and Computers.*[1]

Part of the discussion about artificial intelligence centers on the meaning of the word "intelligence." According to the Oxford dictionary, intelligence is "the intellect; the understanding; quickness of understanding, wisdom," and artificial intelligence is "the application of computers to areas normally regarded as requiring human intelligence."

If the term "intelligence" refers to processing capability, then every computer is intelligent. But artificial intelligence implies *humanlike* intelligence, which includes considerably more than processing capacity; for example, intuition provides insights that cannot be accounted for by sequential processing. The notion that a biological system can be emulated by an engineering process may strike some as an example of reductionism carried to an absurd extreme—at least an egregious example of hubris.

## Artifical Intelligence

Apparently the phrase "artificial intelligence" was coined in 1950 at a conference at Dartmouth College. Artificial intelligence may be defined as devices and applications that exhibit human intelligence and behavior. Devices include expert systems, robots, voice recognition, and natural and foreign language processing. The term also implies the ability to learn or adapt through experience.

Those interested in artificial intelligence, or AI, tend to divide into three philosophical schools. One includes those who use AI as a model to study the nature of human intelligence and how to reproduce it. Some are simply interested in enlarging their understanding of intelligence, while others believe human intelligence is essentially computational and therefore accurately reproducible in a machine. Another group includes those who use AI as an engineering technique to solve problems, without caring whether the system mimics human intelligence or is even intelligent at all, as long as it works. The third group includes those who want their machines to behave intelligently and to learn and adapt to the environment in a way similar to humans.[2]

It is still a controversial subject, but the test of when a machine has AI was defined by the English scientist Alan Turing, who said, "A machine has artificial intelligence when there is no discernible difference between the conversation generated by the machine and that of an intelligent person." No such machine has yet been achieved.

In essence, AI is the attempt to learn how people think when they are making decisions or solving problems, identify the steps that make up the thought process, and then design a computer program that solves problems in the same stepwise fashion. The intention is to provide a relatively simple structured approach to designing complex decision-making programs. These steps can be simplified and summarized as setting a goal which sets the thinking process in motion; calling upon known facts and rules; pruning, or disregarding those facts or rules that do not relate to the problem, and drawing an inference from the relevant rules and facts.

- **Setting a goal.** This is one of the most important tasks in developing an AI system. Lacking intuition, the computer must be instructed in exactly what the problem to be solved is. It does not require that the problem be simple, but it must be well defined. The task may be as simple as producing a set of directions or as complex as selecting the colors to use in decorating a room in a particular period style or in transforming spoken words into text on a page. Further, the goals may be sequential; having arrived at a solution to one part of a problem, the result is used in addressing the second part of the problem, and so on.
- **Facts and rules.** A collection of facts and rules governing the application of the facts may be large or small, but all should relate in some way to the problem to be solved or the goal achieved. The facts and rules are conditionally related; that is, related in if-then sequences. *If* I cannot swim, *and* I fall into deep water, *then* I will drown.
- **Pruning.** Pruning is the process of selecting and disregarding alternatives in a logical sequence. Not all facts and rules are pertinent to a problem or to a subproblem in a sequence. The pruning process uses rules to select alternatives that diverge down different paths. If the result is *A,* then go to

*C.* If the result is *B*, then go to *D*. If the result is *A*, then alternative *D* and sequential alternatives derived from *D* are excluded from further consideration. Anyone who has used a taxonomic key is familiar with this process.

- **Inference.** The program completes the process by drawing inferences from the facts and rules sorted by the pruning process. The resulting bit of new knowledge (the solution to the problem originally set) is added to the collection of facts and rules for use in solving the next problem. In this way the program can be said to learn.

We can illustrate this process by setting up a simple problem: One of John's parents is a doctor. Which of John's parents is the doctor? (This problem statement makes facts about aunts, uncles, cousins, and friends irrelevant.) John's father is not a doctor (add a new fact or find it in the database). Therefore John's mother is a doctor (an inference based on general knowledge and the rule that a person has two parents, a mother and a father). The fact that John's mother is a doctor is added to the database.

An ordinary computer program tends to be highly task specific and can provide answers to problems for which it is specifically programmed. If a new problem requires new information, the program must be modified, with consequences that might be hard to predict. In contrast, AI programs are so constructed that they can accept new information without changing the underlying program. They incorporate modularized instructions and rules that work against an easily modified database.

# Expert Systems

Specific areas of interest for which AI systems can be developed are called **domains**. An AI system created to solve problems in a particular domain is called an **expert system**, which may be defined as a knowledge-intensive computer program that is intended to capture human expertise in a limited domain of knowledge. An expert system is also defined as a system of software or combined software and hardware capable of competently executing a specific task usually performed by a human expert.[3] The common characteristics of an expert system include the ability to do some of the problem work of humans; to represent knowledge as rules or frames; to interact with humans; and to consider multiple hypotheses simultaneously. A **frame** in AI parlance is a data structure that holds a general description of an object, which is derived from basic concepts and experience. (An **object** in object-oriented programming is a self-contained module of data and its associated processing).

All the knowledge in an expert system is provided by human experts in the domain. The rules and capacities built into an expert system (for example, the ability to perform particular calculations) are appropriate to the focus of the system and the problem or problems to be solved. Highly specific rules, generally known to the expert through study and experience but not to the public at large, are termed **heuristic rules**. A pruning mechanism that uses heuristic rules is called a **heuristic search mechanism.**

An expert system is defined in terms of its function, not its underlying programming and representational structures. The essential components of an expert system are the **domain-independent knowledge module** and the **domain-specific knowledge module**. This division between domain-dependent and domain-independent knowledge permits easy updating of the knowledge base. Domain-independent knowledge includes general problem-solving strategies that apply to any set of domain-specific knowledge held in the system. Problem-solving ability resides in an **inference engine** that deduces results based on input facts and rules extant in the database. The inference engine includes a **rule interpreter** and a **scheduler**, which controls the sequence of actions taken by the inference engine.

Occasionally a problem requires the knowledge of more than one expert. For example, my problem is that my car will not start. An expert system, through a series of diagnostic interactions involving symptoms and rules, may identify a bad solenoid. However, the diagnostic expert does not know how to replace a solenoid in my particular model of automobile. A second expert system is needed to take me through the steps of replacing the solenoid. The second expert system does not know how to identify the need for a new solenoid; it knows only how to replace it when the first expert system identifies the solenoid as the basis of the problem. The two expert systems need not run completely independent of each other. As a user, it does me little good to know that a bad solenoid is my problem if I do not know how to replace it, and further, it does me little good to be instructed in the replacement of a part if I don't know which one to replace. In the full expert system, the first program posts its solution, "bad solenoid" to a **blackboard**, a common reference point, where it is found by the second program, which now tells me which one to buy for my car, and displays the correct replacement sequence from among its repertoire of replacement procedures.

## *Chaining*

Let's assume that before my car went on the fritz it was slow in starting and delivered a series of clicks before finally starting. What can happen as a result of this? Am I liable for a worse problem in the future? I can set up a sequence:

**Rule 1:** *If* my car clicks before starting, and starting is slow, then the car is not working normally.
**Rule 2:** *If* this problem gets worse, then my car may not start at all.
**Rule 3:** *If* my car won't start when I am in the garage at work, then it will cost me a lot of money to have it towed and I will be late for supper and my wife will be annoyed.

Notice that the conditional events occur in a sequence, or **chain** of events. Because the chain is sequential, that is, the condition comes before the conclusion and results in events in the future, it is a **forward chain**. An expert system in the domain of automobile starting problems will require me to provide the symptom, clicking and slow starting, then using its database of facts and rules, will apply forward chaining techniques according to its algorithm to arrive at the conclusion that the solenoid is going bad, and that if it goes out when I am away from home I will have to spend money to have the care towed and figure out how to mollify my wife.

Suppose my car will not start, and I want to know why. My expert system begins with the conclusion then the car will not start and must explore a series of *if* statements that precede the conclusion: *if* the gas tank is empty; *if* the battery is dead; *if* a wire is loose; *if* the solenoid is bad, and so forth, to find which best explains the symptoms I provide when queried by the system. The condition preceded the consequence now being experienced, and the expert system must go back to find the appropriate condition using a **backward chain** technique.

## Commercial Expert System Software

Expert systems are often built using the expertise of two persons. The **domain expert** is the person who is expert in the specific knowledge to be incorporated into the expert system. The **knowledge engineer** is the person who is adept at using the software tool and the procedures and methods for incorporating the domain expert's knowledge into the system.

An expert system can be built using a conventional programming language such as FORTRAN or COBOL, but these languages are limited in their ability for symbolic representation, which makes programming unreasonably complex. For that reason, other languages, notably LISP and PROLOG, were developed, but they are now being superseded by yet other languages, especially C and its elaborations.

Several vendors sell the software on which an expert system is based as a completed package: the shell. A shell is the outer layer of a program that provides the user interface, or way of commanding the computer. Shells are typically add-on programs created for command-driven operating systems, such as UNIX and DOS. A shell provides a menu-driven or graphical icon-oriented interface to the system to make it easier to use. It captures knowledge and manages strategies for searching databases (the inference engine), and is capable of functions such as chaining.

## Reasoning with Uncertainty

Many of the limitations of traditional AI relate to its being based on first-order logic and symbol manipulation. This has allowed the development of interesting applications, but it fails to come to terms with the realities of the world. Either/or logic has its limitations, readily seen in the assertion "I always lie." If in fact I always lie, then the statement itself is true, but by being true, it falsifies itself; meaning "I don't always lie." If the statement is false, being one of the lies I always tell, it means "I don't always lie." When confronted with a logical paradox of this sort, we can simply say to hell with it, but what is a poor stupid logical machine to do? This problem precedes attempts to build intelligence into machines and has been dealt with by accepting that true/false is not binary but rather ends of a spectrum, with an indeterminate middle ground. While this may not be acceptable to some logicians and may be denigrated as fuzzy thinking, it does reflect the way life is lived and decisions are made. The brain recognizes patterns that cannot be defined. Explain in an objective way exactly how you can recognize your mother unerringly in a crowd of 100 women of the same age, dressed alike. This property is called **recognition without definition**. Most concepts are learned by pointing out examples. A child may learn colors by having diverse objects of the same color pointed out or may learn different varieties of rose by looking at many roses while being told their names, not by use of a taxonomic key. The higher cognitive functions of the brain include reasoning, decision making, planning, and control. "The asynchronous, nonlinear neurons and synapses in our brain perform these functions under uncertainty. We reason with scant evidence, vague concepts, heuristic syllogisms, tentative facts, rules of thumb, principles shot through with exceptions, and an inarticulable pantheon of inexact intuitions, hunches, suspicions, beliefs, estimates, guesses, and the like."[4] Yet it all seems to work, with this biological endowment refined by cultural conditioning.

Before getting much further into how computer systems are being used to imitate the cognitive functions of the brain, it is worthwhile to mention sets and set theory, since they are such an important aspect of logical systems. A **set** in mathematics and logic is a collection of distinct entities that are individually specified or that satisfy specified conditions that together form a unit. We can think of all fruit as forming a set and all oranges being a set within the larger set of fruit. Potatoes need not apply; they are excluded from this set. **Set theory** is a branch of mathematics or logic that is concerned with sets of objects and rules for their manipulation. Its three primary operations are UNION, INTERSECT, and COMPLEMENT, which are used as follows: Given a file of trees and a file of yellow flowers, UNION creates a file of all trees and all yellow flowers. INTERSECT creates a file of trees with yellow flowers, and COMPLEMENT creates a file of yellow flowers not occurring on trees and a file of trees without yellow flowers. In traditional logic, objects fall into sets or they do not. A set of oranges contains all oranges but no apples. This logical approach fails when dealing with concepts that are not either/or, given "fuzzy names" such as long, short, hot, cold, big, little. How big is big? Is warm hot or cold?

So far the logical sequences presented here have been treated in a binary fashion; that is, either it is this or it is that, clear-cut and black or white. This is very unrealistic in many situations, especially in medicine, when many decisions are made on the basis of informed opinion, or the "best guess" of an educated person. Events or observations may not fall into discrete sets. Expert systems that attempt to offer the informed judgments of human experts (heuristic rules) must work on the basis of probabilities. Given a group of signs and symptoms, the likelihood that a patient has condition X is so much, with a lesser probability that it is some other condition or perhaps no condition at all but merely physiological variation. This is not easy for a digital computer to deal with, since its circuits are binary and capable ultimately of only yes or no answers.

Typical logical systems assume that available knowledge is complete (or can be inferred), and accurate and consistent and can be accumulated. Such a system is designated **monotonic**. While it is useful, a monotonic system does not deal well with information that is incomplete, uncertain, or changing. Several other approaches are used (for a full discussion of this topic, see Finlay and Dix[2]). These are non-monotonic reasoning, reasoning with uncertainty factors, probabilistic reasoning, and fuzzy reasoning.

> **Nonmonotonic reasoning:** In nonmonotonic systems, new information may result in the modification or deletion of existing knowledge. Old knowledge may have been inferred from evidence that seemed good at the time but has now been shown to be false.
>
> **Certainty factors:** Heuristic rules are learned from experience and involve judgments and informed estimates. Our certainty about the correctness of a rule is specified by assigning a **certainty factor** or CF to the rule. The CF approximates the degree to which we think our rule is correct. Certainty factors range from -1 to +1, with -1 indicating that we are absolutely sure the rule is wrong and +1 indicating that we are absolutely sure the rule is right. CF reflect the expert's judgment about the facts and rules applying to the problem and are worked into calculations.
>
> **Probabilistic systems:** Probabilistic reasoning is used to deal with incomplete data. It depends on knowledge of relationships between evidence and hypotheses, assumed in applications of Bayes' theorem. The basic statement of probability (P) of an event occurring relates the number of ways a specific event may occur to the number of ways any event can occur.

$$P = \frac{\text{Total number of ways a specific event may occur}}{\text{Total number of ways any event can occur}}$$

Thus, if a coin is flipped twice, the specific event "heads" may occur both times or once (three events), but the total possibility is four events: heads/heads, heads/tails, tails/heads, tails/tails. Thus, in two tosses, the probability of heads is

$$P = \frac{3}{4} = 0.75$$

**Fuzzy reasoning:** Fuzzy reasoning, or *fuzzy logic*, is a mathematical tool for dealing with imprecise data and problems that have many possible solutions.[5] Fuzzy theory holds that all things are a matter of degree. Fuzzy logic works with a range of values solving problems in a way that is closer to human logic than simple yes or no approaches. "Fuzziness" means multivaluedness or multivalence. Three-valued fuzziness corresponds to truth, falsehood, and indeterminacy or to presence, absence, and ambiguity. Multivalued fuzziness corresponds to degrees of indeterminacy or ambiguity, partial occurrence of events or relations,[4] decidedly "non-set."

Much of the basis for fuzzy systems depends on theories of conditional probability. Conditional probability, that is, probability based on evidence, sets the problem of the coin flip a little differently. What is the probability that the specific sequential events, first toss heads, second toss tails, will occur? From the list of total possibilities given above, the probability is 1/4, or 0.25. However, if the first toss produces heads, then the conditional probability of achieving the sequence heads/tails on the next toss is ½ or 0.50.

A **fuzzy computer** is a computer specially designed with architectural components such as analog circuits and parallel processing for use in AI applications employing fuzzy logic. A **fuzzy search** is a special search for data that comes close to the desired data. It is used, for example, when exact spelling of a name is unknown or to help find information loosely related to the primary subject. Fuzzy searching is the basis for identifying particular persons in the University of Texas Medical Branch database of patients. The historical database contains (for example) about 1750 women named Maria Garcia. To find the right one, ancillary information such as date of birth, age, place of birth, and so on is entered to produce a ranking of all Maria Garcias in descending order of likelihood, based on this added information. Within this ranking, it is not guaranteed that the top-ranked one is the Maria Garcia of interest; the top-ranked one is merely the one most likely to be that person.

# Neural Networks

The human visual system behaves as an adaptive system. For example:

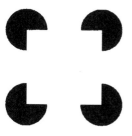

This pattern (the Kanizsa square) is readily seen by most people as a square with a bright interior and boundaries. Actually, we do not *see* a square at all, since it is not objectively there. We *recognize* or *perceive* a square, when in reality there are only four circles with missing quadrants (actually, only ink in patterns on paper). The square exists only because we perceive it. This perception, or **preattentive processing** is typical of sensory inputs, which are processed at great speed and largely at a subconscious level. Once the stimuli have been perceived at this level, we may then pay attention to them, analyze them, and make decisions about them. **Neural network theory** studies both preattentive and attentive processing of stimuli; does not address the higher cognitive functions of reasoning, decision making, planning, and control.[4]

Rather than modeling the cognitive architecture of the brain (how it works), neural networks focus on the brain's physical architecture (how it is built). A neural network is a modeling technique based on aspects of the observed behavior of biological neurons, and it is used to mimic the performance of a neural system. It consists of a set of elements that start out connected in a random pattern and, based upon operational feedback, are molded into the pattern required to generate the required results. It is used in applications such as robotics, diagnosing, forecasting, image processing, and pattern recognition. The neural network approach visualizes the brain as consisting of billions of basic processing units, the neurons, each of which is connected to many others to form a network. The neuron collects inputs, and when the reach a threshold level, the unit reacts. Successfully reacting connections are reinforced; those that do not react appropriately are degraded. The complexity and adaptability of the brain is therefore explained not by the complexity of its processors, which are in fact simple, but rather on its adaptable connectedness and the parallel operation of its billions of processing units.

It has been estimated that the human brain contains 100 billion neurons, about as many as there are stars in the Milky Way, with about $10^4$ synaptic junctions per neuron. This implies about 1 quadrillion synapses in the brain, an observation that inspired Kosko[4] to describe the brain as "an asynchronous, nonlinear, massively parallel, feedback dynamical system of cosmological proportions." Neural networks attempt to model this architecture, although the most complex systems incorporate hundreds, not billions, of processing units.

Parallel computing is the practice of solving a single problem with multiple computers or computers made up of multiple processors. A **neural network computer** is an interconnected set of parallel switches or processors that can be controlled by intervention; resistance can be raised on some circuits, forcing other units or "neurons" to fire. The computer may be specialized hardware or neural network software that runs on a traditional computer. The network is trained by controlling the flow of messages to adjust the resistors in the circuit. Eventually the network will be able to find a pattern of connections that allows it to carry out the desired computation. The neural network computer is said to simulate a brain in that it is influenced by experience and can change its responses according to experience. It learns without specific programming for the task, and it can recognize patterns that could not be presented to a traditional computer.[4]

# Genetic Algorithms

The essential purpose of synthetic intelligence research is to develop systems that show the ability to use prior instructions or semantic rules in pattern recognition, organization, and association. The goal is to replicate in machines the self-organization and adaptation to environmental pressures that characterize biological organisms. According to Darwinian theory, successful adaptive characteristics are selected for and inferior characteristics are selected against by the impersonal forces of nature—"natural selection." Natural selection results in structural and functional specializations, internal knowledge representations, and organization of information, passed along in the genes to later generations. Cumulative selection transforms random processes into nonrandom ones. Each incremental improvement becomes the basis for improvement in the next generation. The internal problem space has no knowledge of good or bad performance; there is no internal standard or internal "awareness" of which innovation is to be good or adaptive. This relies on an external environmental performance measure.

While Darwinian evolutionary theory has known weaknesses and cannot adequately explain the observed facts, it has inspired algorithms that have been successful when incorporated into the principles of functional optimization and machine "learning" and that have been used to model a wide range of phenomena.[5,6] These so-called "genetic algorithms" or "adaptive computation" are an important area of current research and applications development. They are conceptually based on the process of adaptation—"evolution"—shown by biological organisms as they resolve problems. Genetic algorithms control their own adaptive variations, selection and elimination of possible progressive solutions based on fitness, crossover of "genes," and mutation or random change of "genes." As solutions develop, inferior solutions are discarded and better ones are preserved.

**Genetic algorithm** has been defined as "an iterative procedure maintaining a population of structures that are candidate solutions to specific domain challenges. During each temporal increment (called a generation), the structures in the current population are rated for their efficiency as domain solutions, and on the basis of these evaluations, a new population of candidate solutions is formed using specific "genetic operators" such as reproduction, crossover and mutation."[5]

## *Modeling Assumptions*

Genetic algorithms are specified within a fairly general framework. The basic assumption is that the environment and its inputs and outputs can be represented as strings of symbols of a fixed length using a specified alphabet. This alphabet is usually binary, but other, arbitrary alphabets are under investigation. Each point in the problem space can be represented individually and uniquely within the system by a code string developed from the alphabet. Analogy to genetic material regards this string as the chromosome, with specific positions (loci) on the string containing unique symbols or tokens (genes) taking on values (alleles). At any moment the system maintains a population $P(t)$ of strings representing the current set of solutions to the problem. The process begins by random generation or specific design of a starting population of code strings. The only feedback available to an adaptive strategy is fitness; in this case, progress toward solution of the problem. The least information required for adaption is some indication of how well the adaption process is performing. Time is measured in discrete intervals (generations).

The "gene pool" of algorithms consists of strings of 1 and 0 (or some other arbitrary alphabet). Each string is evaluated for fitness, and the best strings "mate" and produce new strings (offspring) by means of crossover. Strings of intermediate fitness simply survive to the next generation, and the least fit perish. If particular patterns of bits improve the fitness of strings that carry them, repeated cycles of evaluating and mating will cause the proportion of these high-quality "building blocks" to increase. Holland,[5] regarded as the founder of genetic or adaptive computing, devised a "genetic code" of binary digits that could be used to represent any type of action in the computer program. With a long enough string of digits, a combination will be found to be "right" in relation to the problem; that is, to constitute a program that performs the combination of actions needed to progress toward or arrive at a desired solution.[6]

## Genetic Operators

There are three primary genetic operators: reproduction, crossover, and mutation. The primary population is chosen either heuristically or at random. The next generation is chosen (reproduced) by probabilistic selection, based on performance against the problem. In crossover, segments of two reproduced strings are swapped by choosing a random point in the strings (the crossover point) and exchanging segments to either the left or the right of the point. The new strings are tested against the problem, and the cycle is repeated by selecting the more successful strings among the new combinations for reproduction and crossover. Mutation modifies one or more segments (genes) of a string, which is then introduced into the cycle.

## Execution Cycle

From a set of existing solutions, some are selected according to performance ("fitness"). Those with the highest fitness rating are most likely to contribute "offspring." After reproduction, pairs are selected for crossover (exchange of genetic material). A mutation may be applied. Performance of the new population is evaluated and the weakest performers eliminated. The cycle is repeated.

Genetic algorithms provide a set of efficient, domain-independent search heuristics for use in a broad array of engineering applications.

# Data Warehouse

The "data warehouse" is a term applied most often to a system for storing and delivering large masses of accumulated data held in some kind of framework. The implication is that the data in a warehouse, like physical goods in a warehouse, are organized and accessible; that they are held in consistent cells or other units of storage. Often the data comes from a variety of sources, with a variety of formats and precision. Data are values collected through record keeping, observing, measuring, or polling (facts, figures, transactions), organized for analysis and decision making. To be storable in a data warehouse, the data must be classifiable and clean, that is, not encumbered with errors, gaps, or extraneous elements that might interfere with classification and retrieval. Small limited data warehouses may be relatively easy to develop, while large warehouses, populated with data of varied cleanness from diverse sources, may be costly in time and expertise to develop.

Two opinions exist regarding the data to be included in a warehouse. The inventor of the relational database (Dr. Codd) promoted an important principle of database design; that all data be "normalized." The normalization principle mandates that no data point is ever duplicated and that a database table should never contain a field that is not a unique attribute of the key of that table. Databases designed in this way are optimized for transactional systems and are relatively easy to maintain and update. As an example of this principle, we could not list a doctor in our database using both doctor name and doctor number. We would have to use one or the other but not both. Database architects and database administrators are commonly devotees of the principle of "normalization" of data (see Chapter 12).

A data warehouse based on rigorously normalized data can be a disaster for the user. In a user-friendly database, data is normalized as described in Chapter 12; however, a happy medium is struck so that the data is clean but also will allow flexible approaches to data searches. A user-friendly data warehouse contains different ways of getting at the data of interest; we would want both the doctor name and doctor number to work with and lots more replication besides. The data is to a degree selectively "denormalized." This approach permits greater flexibility and ease of use for query and analysis, which is after all the purpose of the warehouse in the first place. For example, an aggregation of tests done per day would also include columns for week, month, quarter, and year to permit easy migration up the hierarchy.

The issue comes down to who will do the work. Hackney, writing in *DM Review,* uses the analogy of a sandwich. You can go to the supermarket where all ingredients are laid out according to a plan that may or may not be known to the customer, who has to figure out where the bread, mayonnaise, meat, pickles, and mustard are shelved, gather them, take them to the checkout and pay for them, take them home and make the sandwich. Or you can go to a convenience store, where the sandwiches are ready made, and pick the one you want. The normalized database is like the supermarket, laid out for the convenience of the stockers, who know where everything is supposed to be and restock at a convenient hour; the denormalized database is like the convenience store, which exists to please the customer. The work of gathering the ingredients and making the sandwich is the same; the difference is whether it is done by the store people or the consumer.

However, the difference in the two approaches must not be pursued too hard. A too rigidly normalized data warehouse will not find many customers; an experienced and demanding user will find the convenience store approach ultimately unsatisfactory. The effective warehouse will be so structured as to satisfy a wide range of clients.

What is the point of a data warehouse at all? Consider the situation in a company in which data is stored in large files. An executive needing information discusses his or her needs with a programmer, an information intermediary, to develop queries. The programmer than writes programs to extract the information from the existing databases. A report is prepared for the requester, for whom it may not be entirely satisfactory. The format of the report may be awkward and less than clearly communicative, or the query might have been off just a bit, not giving exactly the information needed. To get it just right, another trip to the programmer is needed. With a well-developed data warehouse, there is no human information intermediary. The human intermediary is replaced by a software intermediary providing a set of tools that allow the user rapid and flexible approach to the database. The user, employing selected software, develops queries independently to address the data system. An interactive or iterative search can be done as often as necessary to get the needed information. As the data warehouse is sited on a different piece of hardware (a server, for instance), performance of the operational system is not impeded. Integration of data files in the warehouse enhances analytical ability and improved reporting.

## *Development of the Data Warehouse*

There are four conceptual steps or stages in the development of a data warehouse.

1. Define and plot a strategic direction. Determine organizational need. Does the enterprise need an organizationwide general data warehouse or one or more subject-specific data marts or both?
2. Select an appropriate database software product and the hardware plat-

form on which it will run. The issues are functionality (Will the tools do what needs doing?), reliability, scalability (Will function be essentially the same if the data store becomes very large?), compatibility with other software and hardware in the enterprise, and value for the organization. Will it contribute value in excess of its cost?

3. Devise a data acquisition/transformation strategy. Identify data sources and how to capture data and transform and replicate it in a manner consistent with decision support applications.

4. Through selection of appropriate tools, enable the user to be effective and productive. Select robust and user-friendly query, analytical processing, reporting, and presentation tools.

There may be advantages to developing a string of data marts rather than a single massive data warehouse. Among the advantages are the lower cost of multiple data marts in terms of data selection and preparation, focused function, adaptability, and speed with which the systems may be brought to a functional state.

## Making Data Accessible and Usable

The functional task is not so much to accumulate data in a warehouse as to convert data into usable information and make it accessible. Without appropriate tools to access and organize it, data is of little or no use. Two approaches to exploiting the potential information in the data warehouse are on-line analytical processing (OLAP) and data mining.

### OLAP

OLAP is a higher-level decision and support tool. OLAP enables users to view and analyze data across several dimensions, hence the designation **multidimensional analysis** (MDA). As a rough generalization, lower-level analytical tools describe what is in the data, while OLAP is used to test hypotheses about the data. It refers to database applications that allow the user to view, traverse, manipulate, and analyze multidimensional databases. For example, we might want to identify the factors that lead to liver failure. Our initial hypothesis is based on an idea that people who drink alcohol are likely to experience liver failure. If a query based on that hypothesis does not lead to a satisfactory (confirming) result, we might then query on a different hypothesis: that hepatitis leads to liver failure. If this new query still does not lead to a satisfactory result, we might try a new hypothesis that asks if alcohol use plus hepatitis lead to liver failure. This might give a better result and lead us to add to the query certain drugs: alcohol plus hepatitis plus drug $x$, $y$, or $z$. The result may be better yet. The OLAP analyst develops a series of hypothetical patterns and relationships and uses queries against the database to validate or repudiate them. This very powerful analytic tool suffers certain limitations. First, the analyst has to think of a testable hypothesis. If he or she does not think of a query, it cannot be run. Second, the more variables under consideration, the more difficult and time consuming it becomes to develop and test the hypothesis. Always unanswered are the questions "Is the hypothesis that has been set the best one? Is there something I haven't thought of?"

There have been two approaches to OLAP based on differing opinions about the best technology for supporting OLAP; multidimensional or relational. Using a multidimensional OLAP tool, data can be studied in a combination of dimensions, such as analyte, date, time, method, associated data. Special indexing schemes are used to access data. (An index is a directory listing maintained by the OS or the application in which an entry is created for each file name and location. An index has an entry for each key field and the location of the record.) This approach to OLAP gives good performance for summarized data with fewer than eight dimensions. The weakness of this approach is the lack of standardization from vendor to vendor, hence ease of data acquisition from diverse sources and difficulties with scalability; that is, the ability to handle large and increasing volumes of data. Relational OLAP (ROLAP) approaches data in a relational database that typically contains data in detail and as summaries. Typically, ROLAP is more flexible, but it is slower than the multidimensional approach. While the trend is toward ROLAP, since the slowness of that approach is compensated by ever-increasing hardware power, each has its virtues. ROLAP is best suited to dynamic processing of summarized and detailed data, a definite advantage for people dealing with large volumes of data, while multidimensional OLAP lends itself to predefined processing of derived and summarized data, essentially a spreadsheet approach, which is effective for study of financial data.

## Data Mining

Data mining is the attempt to find patterns and relationships in large volumes of data by building models. It is more formally defined as an information extraction activity whose goal is to discover hidden facts in databases. It is also referred to as knowledge discovery, or KD. Using a combination of statistical analysis, database technology, modeling techniques and machine learning, it aims to find subtle relationships and patterns in data and to infer rules that permit prediction of future events. Data mining has become possible through the development of tools and processes of AI and especially through the development of more powerful computers and cheaper and cheaper disk storage. The volumes of data involved made data mining prohibitively expensive for most potential users under the old technology.

Data mining uses two kinds of models, descriptive and predictive. **Descriptive models** find or describe patterns in existing data. They may give definition or precision to patterns or relationships already known or suspected to be there, or they may find new, subtle or indirect relationships. Descriptive models are used to make implicit predictions when they form the basis for decisions and to make predictive models. Since there are no previously known results to provide a frame of reference for algorithms, the three descriptive models, clustering, association, and sequence discovery are sometimes called *unsupervised learning models.*

**Clustering** divides the database into groups, looking for similarities in apparently dissimilar groupings. Since the search is for unspecified similarities, the number or characteristics of the groups is not known. The resulting clusters must be evaluated by someone familiar with the subject area or business to eliminate irrelevancies incorporated into the clusters. Once the clusters are evaluated and found to segment the database in a reasonable way, they can be used to classify new data.

**Associations** are events or data items that occur together in a record. Association tools discover the rules of the association. For example, if hepatitis is the event, then serological positivity for C virus is associated some percent of the time. The percent association is the confidence level of the association. If I have hepatitis, I can be 65% sure that it is hepatitis C. The sequence of the events might be reversed; if Hepatitis C seropositivity is the primary event, then hepatitis is associated some percent of the time. The order may change the confidence level of the association. If I am seropositive for Hepatitis C antibody, I can be 20% sure that I have hepatitis. Each association rule has a left-hand side (the antecedent) and a right-hand side (the consequent). Depending on the power of the software tool used, the antecedent and the consequent may both have multiple items. Remember that the rules merely describe associations that are not necessarily cause and event; we might find an association between the consumption of bananas and industrial accidents, not because bananas cause accidents or accidents cause consumption of bananas, but because both could relate to a third element, increased industrialization, higher wages, and the prosperity that permits the consumption of imported fruit.

**Sequence discovery** is a form of association analysis that incorporates time and the ability of the mining software to associate items spread over a period of considerable duration. Sequence discovery may discover associations between (for example) use of a drug and a later manifestation of liver injury, with a certain degree of confidence.

**Predictive models** of data mining use data of known value to construct models to predict values for different data. Thus the data that are associated with a high frequency of liver failure can be used to predict who will not go into failure. Three predictive models, sometimes referred to as **supervised learning models,** are classification, regression, and time series models. They all use data that is already classified to some degree.

**Classification models** are based on characteristics of cases that indicate to which group each case belongs. For example, one might specify examination of cases already classified as hepatitis. The classification mode finds predictive patterns by finding antecedent factors associated with later development of hepatitis, such as drugs, chemicals, travel to exotic locations, and so forth.

Having identified antecedents with high confidence levels, the antecedents can be used to predict who will develop (but does not currently have) hepatitis. The same sort of approach can be used to predict who is likely to respond to an appeal to donate blood by looking at characteristics of those people who have already done so.

**Regression models** are an elaboration of standard statistical techniques such as linear regression. The advantage of the regression model is its ability to incorporate several or many complex variables that themselves respond to other variables. Regression models use existing data values to predict what other values will be. When these models take into account special properties of time, (e.g., five-day work week vs. seven-day calendar week, calendar vs. lunar month, seasonality, holidays, and so on), they are called **time series models.**

# Knowledge Discovery Process

The knowledge discovery (KD) process is not simply a matter of approaching the data warehouse with a question or request such as "Show me the correlations." That kind of free-form, unguided approach will surely bring up such astounding information as the close association of age and date of birth, specious information such as the association of bananas and industrial accidents, and other information that may be equally false but less obviously so. An enormous amount of irrelevancy will defy comprehension.

The *sine qua non* for successful knowledge discovery is to understand the business operation and the data that will be used in the process. There will be no help for leaders who do not understand their business. The first step in KD is to be sure that the corporate data warehouse (all the databases of the organization, whether from internal or external sources) is properly and understandably organized, the constituent data is clean and relevant, and the business model is defined. The business model defines the kind of things relevant to the business organization and the relationships among them. Having done that, a model is built and used and the results monitored and validated. This process can be detailed as follows.

1. Definition of the business problem to be addressed
2. Collection and preparation of the data
   Collect the data.
   Evaluate the data.
   Organize and consolidate the data.
   Clean the data and standardize formats.
   Select the data, develop a data mart.
   Transform the data.
3. Development of the model
   Evaluate the model.

Interpret the model.
Validate the model.
4. Use of the model
5. Monitoring the performance of the model

## *Definition of the Business Problem to Be Addressed*

Formulate the definition as a discrete objective that can be used as the benchmark of success. It must be relevant to the needs or aspirations of the operation. If you don't know where you are going, you don't need a road map.

## *Collection and Preparation of the Data*

Data may come from internal or external sources. Internal sources may be consistent and structured, such as results from automated instruments, while data from external sources may be inconsistent and structured in a different way. It might include demographic information from a hospital or other client system or separate databases entirely. Similar information for a data item may come from different sources and need to be consolidated. Data about a particular element may disagree, for example, a patient's birthday may be reported as different days by the hospital system and by an insurance company. Birth dates must agree with stated age. A woman's parity may be recorded differently in different records. These discrepancies must all be reconciled. Laboratory results for the same parameter might have different reference ranges in different reporting laboratories. A particular analyte, e.g., glucose, may have been assayed under widely differing conditions: fasting or random, or after glucose loading challenge. All results must be cleaned and assigned to an appropriate data address. The data must be assessed for reliability and consistency. A data search cannot produce good results without good foundation data. This step in the process is usually the most protracted, demanding, and expensive. Many thousands or even millions of dollars in salary may have to be expended to prepare a large, multisource database.

Within the larger data warehouse, data must be organized into appropriate groupings. Not all data is needed to address a single question or a group of questions related to a single issue. Search and query can be simplified and speeded up and demand on computer resources moderated by creating issue-specific subdatabases. Subdatabases are often referred to as **data marts**, an extension of the analogy of the warehouse to the retail store. Software and representational tools may be very useful at this point.

Data must be selected for each model to be built. It will be used to train the model, and for a predictive model, will include dependent and independent variables and cases. This is an interactive process, as in building the model some data will be found to be useful, some not useful, and some, by introducing irrelevant variables, may impede the model. This is the point where the domain expert makes a major contribution. When the database is very large, a sample may provide as valid a result as a run of the entire database, at a fraction of the cost. The sample must be selected and validated using conventional sampling and statistical methods. At some point, it may be advisable to transform the data, reexpressing it by changing units of measurement, normalizing it, or aggregating it.

## Development of the Model

Models are either descriptive or predictive. Descriptive models help one to understand processes, while predictive models provide a set of rules that enable prediction of unknown or unmeasured values. Models are built around an algorithm. This may be logistic regression, a decision tree, or an AI tool such as a neural net. Various vendors offer products for algorithm construction. Whichever approach is chosen, it is necessary to regard it as an iterative, interactive process. The model requires shaping and working the data and the model together toward the objective. It is not unusual to realize that more and different data are needed or confusing data excluded. This iterative process of successive estimations is called **training the model.** At some point in this process a working version is arrived at, and it is tested on a sample of the database that has not been used in developing the model. During the course of development of the model, a set of data is used to build the model and a second set used to test it. A third set of data from the same database is often used to test the completed model. This test provides a further hedge against over-estimating the accuracy of the model, which strictly applies only to the data with which it was developed. If it provides satisfactory results, then it is applied to the data in the data mart.

When the model is done, it produces results that must be evaluated and interpreted. Evaluation involves comparisons of results predicted with the actual occurrences. The cost to the enterprise of deviations from the predicted outcomes is assessed. Interpretation of the results of the model may be simple or very complex or somewhere in between, and it is convenient to use a variety of methods, such as rules systems and decision trees, to explain the logic in the system and use graphical representations of outcomes in operations, which may be relatively small and incremental.

Every model is based on certain assumptions, which may not be valid. Therefore, a model may seem sound and consistent and give good-looking but wrong predictions. The hedge is to validate the model against some external standard, such as a sample trial. If a sample trial goes the way it has been predicted to go, then the model is probably valid. If the sample is not successful, then some integral assumptions have to be revisited.

## Use of the Model

The finished, validated model may be used in several ways. It can be used to estimate probabilities of success of a business initiative, to predict treatment outcomes, to predict the stock market, to monitor transactions in, for example, a security system, to identify deviant patterns of behavior, such as a laboratory technician browsing patient records for which there is no logical job connection. A model system may detect abrupt changes in the pattern of use of a credit card, suggesting that it has been stolen. The list of uses is endless.

## *Monitoring Performance of the Model*

The model is not done when it is done. Since so much is invested in the model and its use may be critical to the business success of the organization, it must be more or less continuously validated. After all, it is only a model; it can always be refined. More important is the recognition that the model was built on assumptions, data, and other factors that were good at the time but may have changed. The model may be an excellent representation of things as they no longer are. New data, new associations, and other changes must be incorporated into the model to keep it valid.

## Chapter Glossary

**artificial intelligence** (AI): Application of computers to areas normally regarded as requiring human intelligence. Also, devices and applications that exhibit human intelligence and behavior.

**backward chaining:** In expert systems, linking items or records to form a chain, with each link in the chain pointing to a previous item.

**certainty factor** (CF): Estimate about the correctness of a heuristic rule. The CF approximates the degree to which we think our rule is correct.

**chaining:** In expert systems, linking items or records to form a chain. Each link in the chain points to the next item.

**domain expert:** In expert systems, the person who is expert in the specific knowledge to be incorporated into the expert system.

**domain-independent knowledge:** In expert systems, general problem-solving strategies that apply to any set of domain-specific knowledge held in the system.

**expert system:** AI system created to solve problems in a particular domain; a knowledge-intensive computer program that is intended to capture human expertise in a limited domain of knowledge. Also, a system of software or combined software and hardware capable of competently executing a specific task usually performed by a human expert.

**forward chaining:** In expert systems, linking items or records to form a chain, with each link in the chain pointing to a subsequent item.

**frame:** In AI parlance, a data structure that holds a general description of an object, which is derived from basic concepts and experience.

**fuzzy computer:** Computer specially designed with architectural components such as analog circuits and parallel processing for use in AI applications employing fuzzy logic.

**fuzzy reasoning** (fuzzy logic): A mathematical tool for dealing with imprecise data and problems that have many possible solutions. Fuzzy theory holds that all things are a matter of degree.

**fuzzy search:** Special search for data that comes close to the desired data.

**genetic algorithm:** Iterative procedure maintaining a population of structures that are candidate solutions to specific domain challenges.

**heuristic rules:** Highly specific rules, generally known to the expert through study and experience but not to the public at large.

**heuristic search mechanism:** Pruning mechanism that uses heuristic rules.

**inference:** Formation of a conclusion from premises.

**inference engine:** Processing program in an expert system. It derives a conclusion from the facts and rules contained in the knowledge base using various AI techniques.

**knowledge engineer:** In expert systems, the person who is adept at using the software tool and the procedures and methods for incorporating the domain expert's knowledge into the system.

**neural network:** Modeling technique based on aspects of the observed behavior of biological neurons and used to mimic the performance of a neural system.

**neural network computer:** Interconnected set of parallel switches or processors that can be controlled by intervention; resistance can be raised on some circuits forcing other units or "neurons" to fire. The computer may be specialized hardware or neural network software that runs on a traditional computer.

**object:** In object-oriented programming, a self-contained module of data and its associated processing.

**pruning:** In an expert system, the process of selecting and disregarding alternatives in a logical sequence.

**scheduler:** In an expert system, a function that controls the sequence of actions taken by the inference engine.

**set:** In mathematics and logic, a collection of distinct entities that are individually specified or that satisfy specified conditions that together form a unit.

**set theory:** Branch of mathematics or logic concerned with sets of objects and rules for their manipulation.

# References

1. Jaki SL. Brain, Mind and Computers. Gateway Editions, South Bend, Indiana, 1978
2. Finlay J, Dix A. An Introduction to Artificial Intelligence. UCL Press, London. 1996
3. Bowerman RG, Glover DE. Putting Expert Systems into Practice. Van Nostrand Reinhold, New York, 1988
4. Kosko B. Neural Networks and Fuzzy Systems: A Dynamical Approach to Machine Intelligence. Prentice-Hall, Englewood Cliffs, New Jersey 1992
5. Holland JH. Genetic algorithms. Scientific American, July 1992
6. Grefenstette, JJ. Optimization of control parameters for genetic algorithms. IEEE Transactions on Systems, Man and Cybernetics SMC-16 1986; 1:122–128

# 15
# Imaging, Image Analysis and Computer-Assisted Quantitation
## Applications for Electronic Imaging in Pathology

GERALD A. CAMPBELL

The use of microscopic images in pathology dates back to the first users of the microscope. As early as the seventeenth century, Antoni van Leeuwenhoek measured the sizes of microscopic objects, including human erythrocytes, using reference objects such as hairs and grains of sand.[1] Drawings from observation and later from the camera lucida were the earliest means of recording microscopic images. With the development of photography in the nineteenth century, photomicrography came into use for the communication and archiving of microscopic images, and it has been the standard for well over a century.[2] The development of electronic imaging in the twentieth century had diverse roots in the fields of astronomy and medical radiology, the television and motion picture industries, the development of electronic copying, publishing, and printing technology, and of course the ascendance of the microcomputer. Only in the last decade has the technology for electronic acquisition, display, and storage of images become generally available, cost-effective and capable of sufficient resolution for effective routine use in pathology.

The uses of electronic imaging in modern pathology include documentation, communication, and preservation of microscopic and macroscopic observations supporting diagnoses and research results, analysis of images for primary data acquisition for research and diagnostic purposes, educational aids in the demonstration of pathologic changes, and clinical and experimental research publication.

# Mechanics of Imaging

The application of the technology of electronic imaging to the tasks of pathology requires consideration of a number of factors that depend on the intended use of the images and the availability of equipment and software. These considerations include, at a minimum, (1) image acquisition, (2) display of images, (3) storage and retrieval of images, and (4) transmission of images. Other requirements relevant to specialized applications of electronic imaging in pathology may include image processing, image analysis and computer-assisted morphometry.

## *Image Acquisition*

Devices for acquiring images range from electronic still and video cameras, which can obtain electronic images directly in real time, to various types of scanners, which convert photographs, projection slides, or other hard copy images to digital data sets suitable for display, processing, and storage by a computer. Still and video cameras use a lens to focus an optical image onto a photosensitive electronic chip, such as a CCD (charge-coupled device), to produce an electrical signal. Depending on the specific design, the output signal may be analog (video cameras) or digital (most still cameras and some video cameras) in character. Analog signals, which have continuously varying voltages, require an extra device such as a "frame grabber" card in the computer to convert the analog signal to digital image data that the computer can process. In this case the digital signal is input directly into the computer's bus through the card's mainboard connectors. Devices such as scanners and still cameras contain internal circuitry to interpret the CCD output and directly supply a digital signal, usually through a high-speed port or bus such as SCSI, USB, firewire, parallel or serial port, that the computer can input directly without additional specialized image capture circuitry.

The spectrum of electronic cameras available in terms of cost, resolution, and function is very broad and constantly changing. Thus, the choice of an instrument for a particular application depends heavily on the current state (and cost) of technology. Spatial resolution, defined for photographic film as the number of lines distinguishable per millimeter, is defined for electronic images as the "pixel" size. A pixel is an elemental image component that possesses position, intensity, and color when translated by a display device. Images are characterized by pixel size (e.g., $640 \times 480$ pixels for a standard VGA display), pixel or bit depth (the number of bits in computer memory required to hold the data for a pixel, usually 8, 16, 24, or 32) and file format (how the data is stored). File formats are discussed at the end of this chapter. File size for the digital representation of an image depends on all these characteristics. For example, a high-resolution image of 1536 × 1024 pixels would have a file size of 1.5 Mb at 8-bit depth (256 colors) and 4.5 Mb at 24-bit depth (16.7 million colors).[3] Various types of file compression can significantly reduce the size of these files, although the calculations required for compression and decompression increase processing time, and image quality and other characteristics may be changed by some processes.

Still cameras, which range in price from hundreds to tens of thousands of dollars (~$30,000 at the top of the scale), range in resolution from 320 × 240 (76,800) pixels to 2036 × 3060 (6.2 million) pixels. Although digital images and film images are not directly comparable because of the large number of variables influencing resolution (e.g., grain size, lens factors, development conditions, and so on), a rough figure for the equivalent number of "pixels" in a 35-mm frame for an average resolution film is 3.5 million.[3] Still cameras usually provide internal memory for storage of a number of images comparable to a roll of film. Cameras at the low end of the resolution scale (320 × 240 and 640 × 480) provide a serial interface for communication with a computer. High-end cameras may use any of a variety of interfaces, depending on the manufacturer. SCSI is currently most common, but newer, more user-friendly technologies (USB and firewire) are beginning to supplant SCSI interfaces. Some cameras also come with TWAIN drivers, allowing direct acquisition of images into certain image-processing applications.

Still cameras in the medium-to-high resolution range are probably the best choice for microscopic and gross imaging where single frames are acceptable and real-time capture of motion is not required. Very few "consumer" electronic cameras are easily adapted to the microscope, since the lenses are not removable, unlike the photographic SLR cameras for which microscope adapters are usually readily available from microscope manufacturers. The result of this situation is that special versions of electronic cameras with microscope adapters or cameras specifically designed for microscopes must be purchased at premium prices. In addition, the standard photoeyepiece used to interface the microscope to the camera does not possess sufficient flexibility to adjust for the wide variety of sizes and shapes of detectors to adequately sample the microscope field, even for dedicated microscope cameras. Engineering solutions to adapt off-the-shelf cameras to microscopes would make this technology available to many more pathologists at a reasonable cost. Such cameras with over 2 million pixels are currently (mid-2001) available for under $1000. For imaging gross specimens, on the other hand, such cameras are ideal; they adapt readily to handheld use in the autopsy room or for use on gross photographic stands. Several articles have appeared in the literature describing uses of consumer-type digital cameras.[4,5]

Video cameras also use CCD chips to acquire images, but they convert the image data to a continuous analog, television-type signal for output (known according to the standard: NTSC for the USA, SECAM for France, and PAL for the rest of Europe). Video cameras can also capture images in a frame-by-frame mode similar to still cameras, but the output signal is analog. The output signal is reconstructed on a television monitor by interlaced scanning from the top to the bottom of the screen. First the even lines and then the "interlaced" odd lines are scanned, resulting in two alternating partial images per frame. (Most modern computer monitors use a noninterlaced scan method to reduce "flicker.") Cameras with resolution in the range of 2.5 to $4 \times 10^5$ pixels ($512 \times 512$, $640 \times 480$, $768 \times 512$) are suitable for standard television display (525 to 625 scan lines). HDTV (high definition television) display will use ~1000 scan lines and require images with resolution on the order of 1.5 million pixels ($1536 \times 1024$). Because of the somewhat lower inherent resolution of video cameras and the losses in image quality associated with conversion of the image first to analog and then to digital signal, video images are somewhat poorer than still camera images of the same pixel size for computer display. Another issue is the interlacing of even and odd scan lines required by the television standards, which can produce flicker in some settings where video images are viewed on computer monitors. Thus video cameras are most useful for applications where continuous display of rapidly changing images is required or where analog signals are needed for compatibility with equipment and software for image capture and display. For example, in telepathology applications where the ability to scan a microscopic slide robotically from a remote location is needed, a video camera would be an appropriate choice. Clearly, real-time digitization of video images generates massive amounts of data (about 10 Mb per second for a $640 \times 480$ pixel image at 30 frames per second and 8-bit color depth and 30 Mb per second for 24-bit true color, equivalent to the television standard). Image file compression can here again significantly reduce file size, but the amount of digital data to be transmitted is still enormous and requires sophisticated engineering solutions and compromises to transmit such images over telephone lines or computer networks.

Specialized cameras with image-intensifier tubes and cooling devices for the CCD chips to reduce electrical (thermal) noise have been designed for very low-light-level images, such as those obtained from fluorescent dyes used in immunocytochemistry and other biological labeling techniques. Confocal microscopy, due to its restricted depth of focus and scanning method, usually requires such low-light cameras. These cameras also often have special circuitry to electronically build up, or integrate, the image from multiple exposures or a prolonged exposure time, in comparison to standard video cameras, which have a fixed exposure time. This is another way to reduce the effects of electronic noise in a low-signal setting. As a result, these cameras are very expensive ($10,000 and up) and are consequently used primarily for specialized applications, such as confocal microscopy, that are still predominantly in the research arena.

Scanners range from very expensive, highly precise spinning mirrored drum designs to inexpensive hand scanners that are manually moved across a document. Desktop scanners that economically provide high-quality graphics include the flatbed type scanners and 35-mm film or slide scanners. Both types use a lens and a linear array of detectors, usually a CCD, which is scanned across the document, either by moving the document past the detector (in film scanners) or by moving the detector, lens, and light source (in flatbed scanners). Color is produced either by three sequential passes with a single (monochrome) line of detectors and, alternately, red, green, and blue (RGB) filters, or by a single pass with a tricolor scanning array composed of three lines of RGB filtered pixel detectors. The three-pass designs are more expensive to produce, but currently they provide higher image quality in the same price range than single-pass scanners.

Resolution for scanners is measured in dots per inch (dpi). Detector (optical) resolutions are in multiples of 300 dpi (300, 600, and 1200 are the standard values), although some scanners provide interpolation technology to achieve the equivalent of 4800 or 9600 dpi. The current color output standard for scanners is 24-bit pixel depth ("true color" or 16,777,216 colors). Some higher-quality (and higher-priced) scanners use 32- or 36-bit pixel depth for internal scanning and processing to produce more reliable color reproduction.

Some, but not all, scanners have software drivers that support the TWAIN interface standard, allowing software applications such as Adobe Photoshop and Optimas to directly access the device, obviating the need to transfer the image from proprietary image acquisition software to the image processing application.[6] For some film scanners, a special attachment is available (PathScan Enabler, Meyer Instruments, Inc., Houston, TX) that allows glass microscopic slides to be inserted in place of film, allowing images of the entire slide to be obtained without the need to use a digital camera attached to a dissecting microscope or macro camera lens to produce a global image of a tissue section.

Relatively inexpensive photo/slide scanners (such as the Artec SCANROM 4E), which use a moving plastic tray to hold photos or slides, can also accomplish the same purpose. In fact, the image quality and resolution of the better flatbed scanners can, with some image manipulation, reproduce stained tissue sections with quality sufficient for applications in which imaging the entire section at low magnification is required. Examples of such applications are three-dimensional reconstruction of serially sectioned structures and area measurements of whole-mount tissue sections.

## Image Display

Display of images is usually targeted for computer display monitors, RGB monitors, or printers. Image resolution on display monitors depends on the dot pitch (distance between active screen elements of the same color), screen size, and pixel resolution of the video output card. Two basic methods are utilized by CRT (cathode ray tube) monitors to interrupt the electron beam to create a pixilated image: a shadow mask consisting of a metal plate with punched holes, preferred for precision graphics and text, and an aperture grill or stripe mask that uses vertical rectangular openings to create brighter, more saturated colors preferred for desktop publishing and graphic arts. Dot pitch for currently available monitors varies from 0.25 mm to 0.31 mm, the smaller distances giving higher resolution, all other factors being equal. For aperture grill monitors, the measure of resolution is stripe pitch, which is not directly comparable to dot pitch due to the difference in the way pixels are represented. However, using a rough conversion, a stripe pitch of 0.25 mm is comparable to a dot pitch of 0.27 mm.[7] The highest pixel resolution routinely achieved on computer monitors is currently $1280 \times 1024$ for 17-inch monitors and $1600 \times 1200$ for 19-inch monitors, although for special applications, higher resolutions may be obtainable with larger monitors and special processing. Of course, achieving these resolutions also depends on the use of graphics adapter cards that support them. In dpi, for comparison with scanners and printers, computer monitors achieve resolutions of less then 100.

RGB or television monitors are used for the display of analog signals such as those directly output by video cameras or the output of frame grabbers. Thus, for imaging systems using video cameras and frame grabbers, two monitors are usually required, one for the computer display and another for the working image. A rapidly developing technology is flat panel (as opposed to CRT) displays, most of which use liquid crystal technology analogous to the displays used in laptop computers. Due to the differences in display technology and the way image size is measured, the image quality of a 15-inch flat panel display is roughly equivalent to that of a 17-inch CRT monitor. Advantages of flat panel displays include lower power consumption, weight, and size ("footprint") on the desktop. Prices for these displays currently begin in the $500–$1000 range, however.

Printer resolution is expressed, as with scanners, in multiples of 300 dpi, and ranges up to 1200 dpi for commonly available laser and ink jet printers. The quality and sharpness of color images depends not only on resolution but also on the type of color rendition, ink or substrate. Ink jet printers, laser printers, and color copiers can, at their highest resolution, produce "near-photographic" quality images on plain paper, transparencies, and coated papers. Dye sublimation printers, given digitized images of sufficient resolution, can produce photographic-quality images on photographic-type paper or transparencies.

All these printers use a CMYK (cyan, magenta, yellow, black) printing model, based on the inks used; therefore software must be used to convert colors digitized using a RGB color system to the CMYK system. Most image processing applications, such as Adobe Photoshop, are able to make this conversion to communicate with drivers supplied by the printer manufacturers. For these and other reasons, printed images are not necessarily exactly the same as when viewed on a monitor.

Yet another type of printer is the film recorder, which scans a laser beam through RGB filters across a 35-mm film frame, producing a positive photographic image on film. With this type of printer, images can be transferred from a computer to 35-mm photographic slides. Typical resolution for these instruments is $4096 \times 2731$ (>10 million pixels) and 36-bit depth (>68 billion colors), capable of producing true photographic image quality from suitable image files.

## Image Transfer, Storage and Archiving

Image files, as noted, tend to be large, making floppy disks unsuitable for transfer or storage of more than a few files. Most image files suitable for high-resolution printing will not fit on a 1.44-Mb diskette. Image files can be stored on the computer's hard disk while actively using them, but hard disk storage over the long term is subject to loss due to disk crashes and congestion of the disk because of the large space requirements. Solutions utilizing magnetic media include removable hard drives, magnetic tape, and removable high-capacity diskettes, such as the Iomega Zip drive. These media have the advantage of relative economy and availability, but they have limited storage life for archiving (5–10 years). A higher-capacity storage solution is magnetooptical media. This medium has the advantages of being erasable and rewritable, longer storage life, and very high capacity (several Gb), but the drives are expensive (thousands of dollars) and relatively few computers have them, limiting the utility of the drive for file transfer.

Finally, an optical medium (CD-ROM), has recently become economical and easy to produce. CDs hold on the order of 650 Mb of data and practically all new computers now have CD-ROM drives for reading the medium. Drives capable of writing CDs (CD-R) are now available for a few hundred dollars. In addition, optical discs have very long data storage life, especially if not used regularly and protected from scratches and physical deterioration. Thus, CDs are highly suited for archiving large image files, combined text and images and video. Other recent developments in this area include rewritable CD medium (CD-RW) and higher capacity DVD (digital video disc) technology.

Transmission of image files from one computer to another, either locally or over long distances, is another issue that is increasingly important. The ability to move images over local networks may be essential, since all the devices and software needed to acquire, analyze, and print images for a variety of purposes are usually not available on a single computer. It is frequently the case that images must be acquired using a specialized device, such as a microscope-camera system, moved to an office computer or workstation for convenience in editing and analysis, and finally moved to a third device for printing. Local area networks and intranets are the usual means of communication in such cases.

Where links such as Ethernet are used for these networks, transmission speeds of 10–100 Mbps (million bits per second) are achieved, and transmission of large files is feasible. Where files must be transmitted long distances—as for publication, telepathology, diagnostic consultation, and so on—the options currently available are direct links by telephone and indirect communication through the Internet via e-mail or downloads using FTP (file transfer protocol) or on World Wide Web (WWW) pages. Analog telephone lines that are readily accessible through modem without special setup can support transmission speeds up to 56 Kbps (thousand bits per second), although it is frequently the case that lower speeds in the 28–38 Kbps range are routinely achievable. At these speeds, transmission of a single 10-MB file requires about 30 minutes. Faster connections include dedicated digital telephone lines (DSL, ISDN) and dedicated multichannel connections (T1, T3), which range from up to 128 Kbps for ISDN to 43 Mbps for T3) but require special installation and interface equipment and are progressively expensive to lease.

The Internet provides an alternative solution where real-time transmission is not an issue. In this setting, information is sent in discrete packets and reassembled at the destination into a complete file (image, text, binary file, Web page, and so on). Because the Internet is a highly shared system, transmission speeds are very variable and can be much slower than even analog telephone lines. This may be an issue for images used on WWW pages, where it is desirable to have image files as small as possible for rapid display. Technical issues related to WWW display of images also include the image file type, file compression algorithm, resolution, and bit depth and variability in appearance of images when displayed by a variety of computers and viewing software (browsers). In addition, patient confidentiality concerns require that proven safeguards of the security of transmissions be in place prior to using the Internet for diagnostic consultation.

# Image Analysis

Image analysis involves two separate activities: image processing and quantitation, or morphometry. Image processing may be hardware-based, i.e., incorporated into cameras, scanners, or frame grabbers, software-based, or (usually) both. Although extensive image processing abilities are generally incorporated into quantitation software packages, specialized software, such as Adobe Photoshop or Jasc Paint Shop Pro, is available for that purpose only. Such software is an economical solution where image acquisition and editing or enhancement are the only goals, but it also offers flexibility in producing finished images for publication as an adjunct to the more expensive morphometry systems.

Image processing software, in addition to supporting some forms of image acquisition and the ability to open, convert, and save many types of image files, provides facilities for editing, enhancing, and modifying the image in a variety of ways. Editing capabilities include sizing and cropping, rotation, horizontal and vertical reflection, cutting and pasting parts of the image, and adding text, arrows, and other labels. Enhancement tools allow adjusting the density, contrast, and color balance of the image. The color system used to represent the image (RGB or CMYK) can also be chosen at this point in the more sophisticated programs. Another feature that is usually available is the ability to apply "filters" that modify the image based on mathematical algorithms applied to contiguous groups of pixels to achieve blurring, sharpening, convolution, and so on. These filters may be useful for special effects or for bringing out features that are to be measured later. Examples of special algorithms that morphometry systems usually provide are detection, enhancement, and outlining of edges, skeletonization (reduction of areas to lines), separation of touching or overlapping areas, and background correction. These capabilities may be useful for some purposes, but success in their use depends highly on the nature of the original image (contrast, complexity, and so on) and on the experience and judgment of the operator in applying them. In most cases, the operator must also use manual editing capabilities such as drawing and painting tools to retouch the image so that appropriate objects are selected for measurement.

Morphometry software generally provides two modes for making measurements from images. A manual mode provides for directly marking and counting objects, drawing lines for length and orientation measurements, and outlining areas for geometric measures such as area, boundary, shape, and orientation parameters. In addition, intensity or optical density measures can be made in a pointwise mode (individual pixels), as distributions along lines, or averaged across areas. Some software packages also provide a choice of grids to be used as overlays over the image so that traditional stereologic methods for determining object densities and areas can be used. The automatic mode of measurement requires the software to choose the objects to be measured, either by a process such as the outlining of edges or by using a density or intensity threshold to set the criteria that determine which pixels are included in the object selection and which are excluded. It is usually also possible to include size and shape criteria in these selection processes. For automatic selection, the operator is required to outline one or more specific areas of the image (range of interest, or ROI) in which measurements are to be made. Where many adjacent fields are to be measured sequentially, it is also necessary to provide instruction whether to include or exclude objects touching or overlapping the ROI boundary. It is imperative that the operator check each step of the automatic selection and measurement process to ensure that objects are being chosen appropriately and that the measurements are reasonable. A useful, although expensive, adjunct that can greatly facilitate such repetitive measurements in microscopic images is a step-motor-controlled stage.

The choice of image analysis software may depend on the pathologist's previous experience and preferences, whether it is for general-purpose use or for a specific task, whether it is to be used with existing equipment or purchased as an integrated system, and, obviously, on the budget available. Adobe Photoshop or equivalent software is almost a requirement for any multiuse installation for image preparation, file conversion, and production of a finished product for reporting or publication. Morphometry programs are produced by a limited number of companies and range from $1000 to $10,000 in initial purchase price. Specific considerations are (1) equipment compatibility, especially with regard to frame grabbers, and (2) general-purpose utility and programmability versus dedicated use and/or "turnkey" characteristics, depending on the task(s) to be accomplished and the operator's anticipated level of skill.

Image analysis software companies such as Optimas and Media Cybernetics (Image Pro) usually provide only software, but some (BioQuant) also offer systems including microscope, camera, computer, and printers or other accessories. Independent imaging specialty firms, such as Meyer Instruments of Houston, TX, can serve as system integrators, providing functional packages of equipment and software to meet specific requirements. Such firms are also a source for programs, or macros, written to accomplish specific tasks using the general software packages. Examples of such specific software include routines for DNA ploidy measurements, object size classification for cytology, analysis of *in situ* hybridization, fluorescent or stained specimens, and measurement of cross-sectional, or Martin's, radii of objects such as nerve or muscle fibers.[8] Some microscope manufacturers (Zeiss, Olympus) also offer image analysis packages integrated with their microscopes, both general purpose and specific. Most of these companies also provide, for additional fees, training in the use of the software and/or equipment. Finally, a sophisticated morphometry package for the Macintosh computer has been extensively developed at the National Institutes of Health (NIH *Image*) and is available free of charge for downloading. It also has programming capability for adaptation to various tasks and applications, and versions for the PC have also recently become available (see the NIH web site).

A separate issue in image analysis is the process of three-dimensional reconstruction using collated sequences of images, which may be derived from ultrastructural, microscopic, or macroscopic imaging. Software to produce such reconstructions may be provided with certain types of systems (scanning electron microscopes, confocal microscopes) or it may be a separate item. Different types of reconstructions are also offered, including stereo pairs, depth-shaded renderings, projections, and volume or surface representations with variable shading and transparency. Examples of specific system-independent programs performing these functions are T3D (Fortner, Inc.) and Voxblaster (Media Cybernetics).

## Typical Imaging Systems

Clearly, imaging systems vary widely depending on function and available resources. However, most such systems contain many of the elements described in this discussion. A typical system is depicted in Figure 15-1, consisting of a computer system, digital cameras for image acquisition from a microscope and a gross specimen stand, a flatbed scanner, and a scanner for 35-mm (and possibly glass

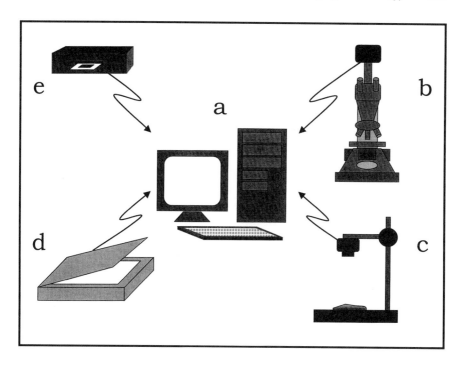

e

a

b

d

c

FIGURE 15-1. Typical configuration of a computer imaging system for pathology. (a) Computer system of either PC or Macintosh type. (b) Light (and possibly fluorescence) microscope with digital camera suitable for the images to be acquired. (c) Gross photographic stand with digital camera. (d) Flatbed scanner. (e) 35-mm slide scanner (possibly with adapter for scanning glass microscope slides).

microscopic) slides. Such a configuration is suitable for both "digital darkroom" use as well as computer-assisted morphometry. The principal difference in these two functions is the type of software provided. In the former, a "photoshop"-type application may be sufficient, although other software to facilitate organizing and archiving images would also be desirable. In the latter case, the more expensive general- or special-use image processing and analysis applications would also be needed. The computer systems appropriate for both uses are those manufactured since 1998, with processor speeds starting at 300 MHz, hard drives with a minimum capacity of 10 GB, and high-capacity removable storage media of both magnetic and optical types.

# Image Files

Image files exist in two broad categories, vector and raster types. **Vector-type files** contain instructions for drawing objects from segments, or vectors, on a display monitor or a plotter. Such files are used in drawing and design software because they allow multiple objects to be represented and moved or altered as units, independent of the background. They also support multiple layers that can be manipulated independently. **Raster-type** files consist of arrays of data that represent pixels in images, mapped on a one-to-one basis to an output device, and are used to represent continuous-tone images such as photographic images. Raster-type images are the natural output format of scanners and digital cameras. Mixed file formats also exist, and most formats have a header that may store titles and other text information, file size, data needed for decompression, and other information. Files may also be compressed using a variety of algorithms. Compression methods may be lossy, or not totally faithful to the original image, or lossless. The most commonly used algorithms are Huffman coding, which is a two-pass statistical method, and LZW (Lempel-Ziv-Welch), which uses pointers to a dictionary of repeating bit phrases. File types frequently used in imaging are described in the following list.[9,10] Table 15-1 presents a listing of vendors of imaging software and hardware.

**bitmap.** With respect to image files, a set of bits holding image data in which each pixel corresponds to a group of bits holding its data in a raster-type format. The Microsoft Windows file of this type has the extension BMP.

**Windows metafile.** A mixed file type, holding vector graphics as well as bitmaps and text, that is used primarily for image transfer between Microsoft Windows applications. The file extension is WMF.

**TIFF** (Tagged Image File Format). A raster-type format developed by Aldus and Microsoft for use with a wide variety of images, including monochrome, gray scale, and 8-bit and 24-bit color. LZW and other forms of lossless compression are used and there are at least six different versions, so not all TIFF files are readable by all software supporting TIFF. This file type is extensively used for transfer of images between different applications because image integrity is preserved. The file extension is TIF.

**Targa.** A raster-type file format developed by Truevision, Inc., for high-resolution (16- bit, 24-bit and 32-bit) color images. The file extension is TGA.

**PICT** (Picture). A vector-type file format developed for Macintosh computers and transported to PC's with the file extension PCT.

**GIF** (Graphics Interchange Format). A raster-type file developed by CompuServe for network transmission of images. It uses lossless compression but is limited to 8-bit depth (256 colors). It is one of the most popular formats for transmission of pictures over the Internet. The file extension is GIF.

**JPEG** (Joint Photographic Experts Group). A 24-bit depth file, developed for the representation of color photographic images, that is capable of high (but lossy) compression to ratios of 100:1 and higher. It is also a popular format for transmission of images over the Internet because of the small file size and high color depth. Display time may not be reduced compared to GIF, however, because of the extra time required for decompression. It

**TABLE 15-1.** Imaging Company Web Site Addresses (December 15, 1999)

| Company | Web site | Product |
|---|---|---|
| ACD Systems | http://www.acdsystems.com | Image viewing and management software |
| Adobe | http://www.adobe.com | Photoshop image-processing software |
| Artec | http://www.artec.com.tw | Scanners |
| Canon | http://www.usa.canon.com | Digital cameras, scanners, projectors, printers |
| Eastman Kodak | http://www.kodak.com | Digital cameras |
| Epson | http://www.epson.com | Digital cameras, scanners, projectors, printers |
| Fortner | http://www.fortner.com | Data analysis and visualization software, T3D |
| Hewlett-Packard | http://www.hp.com | Printers and digital imaging equipment (scanners, cameras) |
| Jasc Software | http://www.jasc.com | Paint Shop Pro image-processing software |
| Leeds Precision Instruments, Inc. | http://www.leedsmicro.com | Custom imaging systems integrators, equipment, and software |
| Leica | http://www.leicamicrosystems.com | Digital camera systems and equipment for microscopes |
| Media Cybernetics | http://www.mediacy.com | Image Pro image analysis software |
| Meyer Instruments | http://www.meyerinst.com | Custom imaging systems integrators, equipment, and software |
| NIH Image | http://rsb.info.nih.gov/nihimage/ | Free image analysis software |
| Nikon | http://www.nikonusa.com | Digital cameras, film scanners, and microscopes |
| Olympus | http://www.olympusamerica. com | Digital cameras, microscopes, imaging systems, and software |
| Optimas | http://www.optimas.com | Image analysis software; now owned and supported by Media Cybernetics |
| R&M Biometrics | http://www.bioquant.com | Bioquant image analysis software and systems |
| Research Systems | http://www.rsinc.com | Data analysis and visualization software |
| SPSS | http://www.spssscience.com | SigmaScan image analysis software |
| Zeiss | http://www.zeiss.com | Microscopes, imaging systems, and software |

may not be suitable for some types of quantitation because the final (de-compressed) image is not faithful to the original (before compression). The file extension is JPG.

**EPS** (encapsulated PostScript). A file containing PostScript (printer) code as well as (optionally) preview images in several raster formats. The file extension is EPS.

# Chapter Glossary

**bitmap:** As applied to image files, a set of bits holding image data in which each pixel corresponds to a group of bits holding its data in a raster-type format.

**BMP:** See **Windows bitmap file.**

**CCD** (charge-coupled device): Silicon chip that integrates an array or matrix of photosensitive elements that acquire an electronic charge corresponding to the intensity of the incident light with associated circuitry to scan these elements and produce a digital output signal that can be reconstructed into an image by appropriate devices and software.

**CD** (compact disk): Plastic disk medium that can store large amounts of digital data by means of microscopic pits in one or more metallic layers.

**CD-R** (CD-recordable): CD drive technology that permits data to be recorded on a blank CD to produce a CD-ROM or audio CD. Data can be written to an area of the CD only once, but "multisession" technology permits the data to be added to the CD in multiple sessions.

**CD-ROM** (CD-read-only memory): CD format that stores digital data, usually around 650 MB/disk, in a file form that can be read by a computer.

**CD-RW** (CD-rewritable): CD medium and drive technology that permits data to be written and overwritten many times. Standard CD-ROM drives cannot read CD-RW disks, but CD drives with "multiread" technology can read both types.

**CMYK** (cyan-magenta-yellow-black): A color system used for printing, based on the primary colors of the inks that are combined to generate colors.

**DIB:** See **Windows bitmap file.**

**DS1, DS3** (Digital signals 1 and 3): See **T1, T3.**

**DSL** (digital subscriber line): Digital transmission technology that uses modulation techniques to transmit data at high speeds (up to 32 Mbps upstream and 1 Mbps downstream) over dedicated standard telephone wires for short distances (less than 20,000 feet) from telephone switching offices to users.

**EPS** (encapsulated PostScript): File containing PostScript (printer) code as well as (optionally) preview images in several raster formats. The file extension is EPS.

**firewire:** Hardware computer interface that allows serial transfer of digital signals between a computer and up to 63 peripheral devices at transfer speeds of 100 to 400 Mbps, compared to 20 Kbps for ordinary serial ports and 150 Kbps for parallel ports. Developed by Apple Computer and Texas Instruments.

**frame grabber:** Electronic device or computer accessory that accepts analog video signals as input and produces a digitized representation of the current video frame, which is then stored in a memory array and used to construct a digital signal that can be interpreted by a computer and, in some cases, an analog signal representing the "frozen" frame for display or recording by analog devices.

**GIF** (Graphics Interchange Format): Raster-type file developed by CompuServe for network transmission of images. It uses lossless LZW compression but is limited to 8-bit depth (256 colors). It is one of the most popular formats for transmission of pictures over the Internet. The file extension is GIF.

**ISDN** (integrated services digital network): Telephone communication standard that uses two dedicated 64-Kbps digital telephone lines to transfer data at rates up to 128 Kbps from a telephone switching office to a user (baseband ISDN). Broadband ISDN is much faster but requires fiberoptic cables.

**JPEG** (Joint Photographic Experts Group): 24-bit depth file developed for the representation of color photographic images that is capable of high (but lossy) compression to ratios of 100:1 and higher. It is also a popular format for transmission of images over the Internet because of the small file size and high color depth. Display time may not be reduced compared to GIF, however, because of the extra time required for decompression. It may not be suitable for some types of quantitation because the final (decompressed) image is not faithful to the original (before compression). The file extension is JPG.

**JPG:** See **JPEG.**

**Kbps** (kilobits [thousand bits] per second): Data transmission-rate unit.

**LZW** (Lempel-Ziv-Welch): Patented lossless file compression algorithm, used in GIF image files, which uses pointers to a dictionary of repeating bit phrases.

**Mbps** (million bits per second): Data transmission-rate unit.

**NTSC** (National TV Standards Committee): U.S. standard for television signals, allowing for 525 lines/frame at a frequency of 30 frames/second (60 half-frames interlaced).

**PAL** (phase alternating line): Dominant European standard for television video that uses 625 lines/frame at 50 half-frames/second, differing from the U.S. standard in both resolution and frequency. See **NTSC.**

**pixel** (picture element): Smallest element making up a digital image, represented by a dot of light on a display monitor or a dot of ink on a printed image; contains coded information defining location, intensity, and color.

**PCT:** See **PICT.**

**PICT** (Picture): Vector-type file format developed for Macintosh computers and transported to PCs with the file extension PCT.

**PNG** (portable network graphics, pronounced "ping"): New raster-type (bit-mapped) graphics format similar to GIF but free of patent restrictions imposed on GIF by use of the patented LZW compression algorithm. The file extension is PNG.

**RGB** (red-green-blue): Color system used primarily for display monitors, scanning, and film printing, based on the primary colors represented by monitor pixels and scanning or printing filters.

**ROI** (range of interest): Area of an image, usually selected by the operator, on which image analysis procedures are to be performed.

**SCSI** (small computer system interface, pronounced "scuzzy"): Hardware computer interface that allows communication between a computer and up to seven peripheral devices by simultaneous (parallel) transfer of 8- to 64-bit signals at speeds of 5 to 80 Mbps, using a single computer expansion slot and set of resources (interrupt, and so on). Different versions with increasing speed and bit width are SCSI-1, SCSI-2, fast wide SCSI-2, and ultra, ultra wide, ultra2, and ultra2 wide SCSI.

**SECAM** (Système Electronique Couleur avec Mémoire): Television video standard used primarily in France and eastern Europe. Compare **NTSC.**

**T1, T3 (DS1, DS3):** Multiplexed high-speed digital transmission technology ("T-carrier") providing 24 or 672 channels, respectively, with speeds of 64 Kbps each. T1 at full width (using all channels) supports transmission speeds of 1.544 Mbps and is used mainly for connecting larger users to the Internet and internet service providers (ISPs) to Internet nodes (or "backbone"). T3 supports maximal rates of around 43 Mbps and is used to connect larger ISPs to the Internet and for the Internet backbone connecting nodes.

**Targa:** Raster-type file format developed by Truevision, Inc., for high-resolution (16-bit, 24-bit, and 32-bit) color images. The file extension is TGA.

**TGA:** See **Targa.**

**TIF:** See **TIFF.**

**TIFF** (tagged image file format): Raster-type format developed by Aldus and Microsoft for use with a wide variety of images, including monochrome, gray scale, and 8-bit and 24-bit color. LZW and other forms of lossless compression are used, and there are at least six different versions, so not all TIFF files are readable by all software supporting TIFF. This file type is extensively used for transfer of images between different applications because image integrity is preserved. The file extension is TIF.

**TWAIN** (ostensibly from "Ne'er the twain shall meet"): A software interface (data source manager) that allows an imaging application program to activate and receive images from image acquisition devices (cameras, scanners, and so on).

**USB** (universal serial bus): Hardware computer interface that allows serial transfer of digital signals between a computer and up to 127 peripheral devices at transfer speeds of up to 12 Mbps, compared to 20 Kbps for ordinary serial ports and 150 Kbps for parallel ports.

**Windows bitmap file:** Bitmap image file format developed for Microsoft Windows; may be device dependent or device independent (DIB). The file extension is BMP.

**Windows metafile:** Mixed file type, holding vector graphics as well as bitmaps and text, that is used primarily for image transfer between Microsoft Windows applications. The file extension is WMF.

**WMF:** See **Windows metafile.**

# Cited References

1. Meijer GA, Belien JAM, van Diest PJ, Baak JPA. Origins of . . . image analysis in clinical pathology. J Clin Pathol 1997; 50:365–370
2. Delly JG. Photography Through the Microscope. Eastman Kodak, Rochester, New York, 9th ed 1988:2.
3. Langford LA. Electronic imaging: a guide for anatomic pathologists. Advances in Anatomic Pathology 1995; 2:141–152
4. Tse CC. Anatomic pathology image capture using a consumer-type digital camera. Am J Surg Pathol 1999; 23:1555–1558
5. Leong AS, Visinoni F, Visinoni C, Milios J. An advanced digital image-capture system for gross specimens: A substitute for gross deception. Pathology 2000; 32:131–135
6. Scanning Essentials. Nikon, Melville, New York, 1994.
7. ViewSonic Corp. The Monitor Buyer's Guide [Online]. Available: http://www.monitorbuyersguide.com/ [1999, December 15].
8. Catalog of Custom Macros for Optimas and Optimate. Meyer Instruments, Houston, 1994.
9. Weinman L. <preparing web graphics>. New Riders, Indianapolis, 1997.
10. Freedman A. The Computer Glossary. 7th ed. AMACOM, New York, 1995.

## *Additional References*

Aller RD. The pathologist's workstation. Clin Lab Med 1997; 17:201–228

Andrew SM, Benbow EW. Conversion of a traditional image archive into an image resource on compact disc. J Clin Pathol 1997; 50:544–547

Cheong S-K, Micklem K, Mason DY. Computerised image handling in pathology. J Clin Pathol 1995; 48:796–802

Cohen C. Image cytometric analysis in pathology. Hum Pathol 1996; 27:482–493

Furness PN. The use of digital images in pathology. J Pathol 1997; 183:253–263

Internet.com. Webopedia [Online]. Available: http://webopedia.internet.com/ [1999, December 15].

Nazaran H, Rice F, Moran W, Skinner J. Biomedical image processing in pathology: a review. Australasian Physical & Engineering Sciences in Medicine. 1995; 18:26–38

Oberholzer M et al. Telepathology: frozen section diagnosis at a distance. Virchows Archiv 1995; 426:3–9

O'Brien MJ, Sotnikov AV. Digital imaging in anatomic pathology. Am J Clin Pathol 1996; 106(Suppl. 1):s25–s32

Oliver WR. Image processing in forensic pathology. Clin Lab Med 1998; 18:151–180

Weinberg DS, Doolittle M. Image management in pathology. Am J Clin Pathol 1996; 105 (Suppl. 1):s54–s59

Weinberg DS. Digital imaging as a teaching tool for pathologists. Clin Lab Med 1997; 17:229–244

# 16
# Introduction to Telepathology

MICHAEL B. SMITH

The practice of medicine has been subject to economic, social, scientific, and technological forces that have altered the practice of the profession over the last several decades. In many cases, pressures have been applied by forces that have seemingly contradictory goals. Economic forces applied by the evolution of managed care have led to a reorganization of the medical infrastructure in the United States, which have resulted in increasing numbers of patients for individual providers to care for and the unavailability of medical care to larger and larger segments of the population. Concurrently, medicine has been under constant pressure, from both inside and outside the profession to find a way to care for the medically underserved, not only those created by the economic restructuring, but those who were underserved in the past, such as the geographically remote. While the appeasement of contradictory forces and pressures on priorities in medicine at a national level are a laborious, complicated process involving many social, economic, and philosophical issues, medical practitioners are having to deal with the problem of providing care to more and more patients dispersed over a greater and greater geographic area on a daily basis. Pathology by its nature has been particularly prone to the pressures and problems of centralized care. Fortunately, advancements in the technology of telecommunications and computer science have offered practitioners an effective option in dealing with this problem.

Telemedicine, or the use of telecommunications technology to send data, graphics, audio, or images between practitioners physically separated by a distance for the purposes of clinical care has been proffered as one aid in providing increased access in the face of centralized medical care.[1] As a subset of telemedicine, telepathology is the transmission of histopathological images between different sites for diagnostic, consultative, educational, or quality assurance purposes. Great interest has been generated in the use of telepathology to increase the efficiency of histopathology laboratories in serving larger populations with either the same or decreasing resources.

Although isolated incidences of the transmission of microscopic images for diagnosis occurred in the United States during the late 1960s and early 1970s, the first functioning long-distance telepathology network used on a routine basis was implemented in Europe at the University of Tromsø, Tromsø, Norway, in 1989.[2-4] The university constructed a telepathology system utilizing telephone lines to allow the evaluation of frozen sections performed at a remote hospital 400 km away above the Arctic Circle. Also in 1989, a telepathology network was established in France (Resintel) that evolved to link 32 sites throughout France and the islands of Martinique and Guadeloupe.[5] Although the French network was not a commercial success, it was important because it proved that the technology available was capable of linking a complex network of stations, including some very remote sites, into a functioning telepathology system. Extensive networks of telepathology stations have not been developed in the United States, but many centers have carried out evaluations of telepathology systems that involve either a small number of submitting sites in this country or submissions from other countries. An example of a viable and functioning system is the telepathology link between the Iron Mountain, Michigan, and Milwaukee, Wisconsin, Veteran's Medical Centers.[6] Pathologists at the medical center in Milwaukee, Wisconsin, are able to offer surgical pathology services to a remote facility that has an active surgical service without local pathology support. The U.S. military has been using telepathology to provide services to remote facilities on the Pacific rim, and in 1994 the Armed Forces Institute of Pathology instituted a telepathology service that reaches worldwide.[7-8] Other telepathology services began going on line in recent years, with most originating from university systems such as the University of Arizona.[9]

## Telepathology Systems

Although there are number of options to choose from when constructing a telepathology system, the basic framework includes an image acquisition method, a method to compress and store the image, a way to transmit the image to a remote receiving station, and a way to display the image at the receiving station. When considering whether or not to institute telepathology, other issues such as format, reimbursement, and legal issues must also be taken into account.

## *Acquiring the Image*

The most common use of telepathology to date has been as a method to perform histopathologic assessment from a site remote to the tissue section and microscope. The first step in this process is acquiring the image with a camera mounted to a light microscope. Of two options, the cheapest is to capture the image with a video camera, a method used in many large pathology practices for local microscopic video conferencing. It must be remembered, however, that most inexpensive video cameras on the market have not been configured for medical uses and as a consequence may not be adequate for telepathology in terms of resolution or color representation. Resolution is expressed in terms of pixels (picture elements) in columns and rows. The video camera uses a silicon grid of light-sensitive wells arranged in columns and rows termed a **charge-coupled device** (CCD). Each well in the CCD detects photons that are converted to an electrical charge, whose intensity depends on the amount of light striking the well, and then to a voltage signal, which is used to generate an image (analog signal). In general, the number of wells in the CCD reflects the clarity or resolution of the image produced. Many video cameras have 640 rectangular wells in the horizontal plane and 480 in the vertical plane (640H × 480V). As a point of reference, this is the standard established by the National Television Standards Committee (NTSC) and is the resolution seen on the home television set. The degree of resolution for telepathology has not been standardized, and the literature reports a wide range of degrees of spatial resolution, although 800H × 600V and 1024H × 1024V are reported with frequency.[10]

In contrast to radiology, whose use of teleradiology is much further advanced than pathology's use of telepathology, color information in the image is of importance with both routine and special histologic stains. Since the CCD is a monochromatic device, it is necessary to manipulate the image to obtain three images in the primary colors, red, green, and blue (RGB). The most commonly utilized method is to place color filters over the CCD, devoting one third of the wells to each one of the primary colors. This method has the disadvantage of reducing resolution; hence, these types of cameras may not be optimal for telepathology. The image produced by the second method, having the light split by a prism to three separate CCDs, each with a separate color filter, is superior in both resolution and color. These types of cameras are, however, more expensive. The third method, using pulsed light of each of the primary colors to capture three separate images on a single CCD and then integrating the three images by computer, is a strategy used with great frequency in endoscopy cameras.

To allow for storage, manipulation, and eventual transmission of an image, the analog video signal must be converted to the binary language of the computer. Conversion is accomplished with the use of the image capture board, usually in a desktop computer. The **image capture board** contains a device that samples the continuous voltage signal from the video camera and converts it to a numeric value, "digitizing" the image. The location and digital value of each pixel is stored in a second part of the image capture board, the **image frame buffer,** from which the computer can extract the data. Monochromatic video signal is encoded as 8 bits of data, with the value corresponding to the level of brightness or intensity of light. For "true color" imaging, imaging that approximates the range of the human eye, this means that $2^8$ or 256 different shades of each primary color are encoded on each of three different channels. The total number of colors will be $2^{24}$ ($2^8$ for each of the three primary colors), or $16.7 \times 10^6$ colors, with obvious implications for the size of the file necessary for the resultant image.

An alternative to video cameras for capturing still images are digital cameras. Digital cameras convert light from the image into binary code within the camera, and as, no image capture board is required, the image can be downloaded to the desktop computer via serial cable or PC card. Until recently, digital cameras were prohibitively expensive, but prices are now competitive with quality video cameras. The image sensor in many digital cameras is the CCD. However, some cameras have made use of a new sensor technology, **complementary metal oxide conductor sensors** (CMOS), which can be produced cheaper than CCDs. Additionally, other functions such as image stabilization and compression can be built into the CMOS chip, making the camera smaller, lighter, and more efficient. Like video cameras, digital cameras have built-in image delay times, which vary with the make and model of the camera. The delay time in digital cameras is a reflection of the refresh rate, the time delay between pressing the shutter button and capturing the image (the camera first clears the image sensor, sets the white balance to correct for color, sets the exposure, and focuses, if using autofocus), and the recycle time (the time it takes to capture the image, process it, and store it).

The time delay inherent in digital cameras may be negligible or of no importance depending on the make and model of camera or the system it is being used in, or it may cause a constant irritation for the users of the system. While it is possible to obtain some information about different cameras from specifications provided by the manufacturer and from the literature, there is no substitute for an on-site trial performing the function for which it is intended.

## Image Storage and Compression

After the image has been acquired by the camera and converted to binary code, the image is stored in a desktop computer that is part of the workstation until it can be transmitted to the receiving station. Image files are large files, with consequencies for both storage and transmission. To determine the file size, you need to know the resolution of the image in pixels and the color depth in bits.[7] For example, if the camera you are using produces an image with a resolution of $1024 \times 1024$ and 24-bit color, the formula would be

file size = $1024 \times 1024 \times 3$ (number of bytes per pixel; 24/8 bits = 3 bytes)
file size = 3,145,728 bytes, or about 3.2 megabytes for each image

Since image files are kept for documentation, quality assurance, teaching, and possibly medical-legal reasons,[10] you can see that storage space will be utilized at a steady clip if cases are imaged with frequency. For example, if a site using the example camera images 5000 cases per year with an average of 5 images,

storage space/year required = 5000 cases $\times$ 5 images/case average $\times$ 3.2 megabytes/image
storage space/year required = 80,000 megabytes = 80 gigabytes

To reduce storage space required (and to make transmission of the image practical), **compression algorithm software** is utilized. This software uses numeric algorithms to represent an image with a reduced amount of information that can be re-added at a later time. There are two classes of algorithms, lossless and lossy. In **lossless compression,** the algorithm is reversible to the point that the decompressed image is numerically identical to the original. The compression ratio for lossless compression is generally no greater than 6:1. With **lossy compression,** much greater degrees of compression can be accomplished, up to 1000:1 depending on the algorithm. The disadvantage of lossy algorithms is that with decompression, the image is numerically similar but not identical to the original. The implications for telepathology, from both a diagnostic standpoint and a medical-legal standpoint, have not been addressed in the literature.

Of the lossless compression formats available, Graphics Interchange Format (GIF) and variants of Joint Photographic Experts Group (JPEG) are two of the most common. GIF is limited in the amount of color that can be represented and therefore may not be optimal for imaging in pathology. Both lossless JPEG and lossy JPEG algorithms exist. JPEG, however, is dependent on redundancy in the image to function efficiently, and with high-quality images (and less redundancy), JPEG is not as efficient and can result in loss of image quality.[11] Very high compression ratios (reportedly up to 1000:1) can be achieved with the lossy algorithms (wavelet transforms) associated with Digital Imaging and Communications in Medicine (DICOM) standards.[12] DICOM is being used by radiologists to facilitate uniformity in teleradiology, and the College of American Pathologists has initiated efforts to develop revisions that allow use of the standards in pathology imaging.[10]

As mentioned, some of the compression algorithms have color limitations. As is the case with many of the variables associated with imaging in pathology, the color range necessary for adequate histopathological assessment of images in telepathology has not been extensively evaluated; however, preliminary studies have suggested that true color ($16.7 \times 10^6$ colors) may not be necessary or even preferred. Doolittle and colleagues[13] showed that pathologists in their study actually preferred images with 256 colors (8 bits) to those with $16.7 \times 10^6$ colors (24 bits), indicating that the 8-bit images were of "better quality". Reducing a 24-bit color image to 8 bits could reduce the size of an image file by approximately 66%. If this preference is borne out in subsequent studies, it could provide way to reduce image file size to facilitate storage and transmission.

Storage of the images can be accomplished by a number of drives with removable magnetic, magneto-optical, or optical disks or cartridges. These platforms are characterized by large capacity (megabytes to gigabytes), easy accessibility and quick access, and durability. An example of magnetic disk technology is the Iomega Zip Drive (Iomega Corp., Roy, UT) with 100 or 250 megabyte disks. Improvements in optical technology have occurred in the last several years, with such systems as Panasonic's PD/CTM optical drive with cartridges that hold 650 megabytes coming on the market. Older technologies arranged in novel architectures, such as CD-ROMs in jukebox library configurations, are capable of storing tremendous amounts of image data (terabytes, or trillions of bytes). WORM (write once, read many times) optical disks allowing storage of data that cannot be edited can be utilized, enabling one to secure archived data from inadvertent or intentional change. RAID (redundant array of independent disks) architecture also allows storage of tremendous amounts of data. Pathology systems that are connected to networks can use the large data storage capacity associated with the server, and in some cases, it may be possible to store an uncompressed image in a large image server for medical-legal purposes and a compressed image locally for easy access for such purposes as teaching. Image security in telepathology is another issue that has been little addressed in the literature but will become increasingly important as telepathology practices become more prevalent.

Currently, there is no universally accepted software standard for archiving and transmitting images in pathology as there is in radiology. The DICOM standard has enabled standardization of file format and compression algorithms, facilitating labeling of images with patient information, coding, archiving, retrieval of images, and development of new hardware. Such an image file format standard not only facilitates transmission and receiving of images for consultation, but makes it easier to include the image in an electronic medical record (EMR) that could be transmitted between medical care facilities. Anyone who has had to contend with the problems associated with a patient referred for care from another hospital without records, radiographs, or diagnostic histology can understand how an EMR transmitted from the referring facility directly could enhance care for the patient.

As previously mentioned, the College of American Pathologists has been cooperating with the American College of Radiology and the National Electrical Manufacturer's Association, the authors of the DICOM standards, in producing an extension of DICOM to include pathology and laboratory medicine.[11] The extension to the most recent version of DICOM, version 3.0, will provide standards for accessioning cases, gross and microscopic image descriptions, and SNOMED international coding of cases.[11] The creation of standards for image file folders has been a high priority in Europe for a number of years. The Association pour le Developpement de l'Informatique en Cytologie et en Anatomie Pathologique (ADICAP) has since 1980 been using an image file folder standard to facilitate archiving pathology computer images, and in 1994 it extended the standard to image transmission applications both within networks in France and to the Internet.[14] One of the stated goals of this project has been to develop an internationally accepted standard for histological image exchange.

## *Transmitting the Image*

Whether the image is transmitted in a compressed form or as a large noncompressed file, a number of different transmission options are available

TABLE 16-1. Digital Transmission Modes and Maximum Transmission Speeds

| Electronic Transmission Mode | Maximum Transmission Speed |
|---|---|
| Dialup modem and POTS[a] | 56 Kbps[d] |
| ISDN[b] | 128 Kbps |
| T-1 | 1.5 Mbps[e] |
| LAN[c] token ring | 4–16 Mbps |
| LAN Ethernet | 10 Mbps |
| Cable | 30 Mbps |
| T-3 | 45 Mbps |
| LAN Fast Ethernet | 100 Mbps |

[a] POTS = plain old telephone service
[b] ISDN = integrated services digital networkL
[c] LAN = local area network
[d] Kbps = kilobits per second
[e] Mbps = megabits per second

depending on the technology available in the area and whether the sending station is part of a communications network. The data capacity of an electronic line is expressed as bandwidth, which can be expressed in different ways but for digital transmission is expressed most commonly as bits per second (bps). Some of the more commonly available lines available with the maximum transmission rates are listed in Table 16-1.

The table is not all-inclusive, as other types of transmission modes exist, albeit at higher cost and limited availability at the present time. Other modalities with much greater speed, such as asynchronous transfer mode (ATM), are expected to become widely available in the near future. ATM is capable of speeds of up to 2488 Mbps.

It should be noted that the actual transmission rate for a line is not the maximum rate because of various overhead factors. For example, a local area network (LAN) with a token ring topology can transmit anywhere from 4 to 16 Mbps. To determine an approximation of the actual rate of transmission, assuming the LAN transmits 4 Mbps, one first divides bps by 8 to get the number of bytes per second. In this case, our lines can transmit about 500,000 bytes per second. To account for the technical overhead, the convention is to halve this value. Our LAN will be capable of transmitting about 250,000 bytes per second. A 3-megabyte file would require 12 seconds to transmit over the network.

An additional consideration is cost. Although using a 56.6-Kbps modem and POTS (plain old telephone line) will incur only the cost of local telephone service, the slow and sometimes capricious nature of this type of connection could cause a submitting telepathology station to obtain a dedicated line such as an ISDN or T1 line. Cost to the facility to obtain these lines would be approximately several hundred and several thousand dollars per month, respectively, depending on the local market.

## Display of the Received Image

Once the transmitted image has been received at the receiving telepathology site, the image must be displayed on a color monitor. Most color monitors in use today in pathology are of the cathode ray tube (CRT) type, although with recent improvements in liquid crystal display (LCD) technology, LCDs may become more popular in the future. There are two types of CRT technologies, the trio-dot system and the Trinitron system (Sony, Japan). In the trio-dot system, the red, green, and blue phosphorus are arranged on the display screen as three dot groupings in a hexagonal pattern with a hexagonal filter between the electron beam and the display screen, allowing each beam to excite only the appropriate color phosphorus. The advantage of this type of CRT system is that because there are three axes of symmetry (from the hexagonal trio-dot arrangement), vertical and horizontal resolution characteristics are similar.[12] In contrast, the disadvantage is that the system is susceptible to beam misalignment with resultant color smearing.[12] The Trinitron system differs in that the three colors of phosphorus are arranged as alternating columns with a slit filter between the display and the electron source. This system is less susceptible to beam misalignment, however, because there is only one axis of symmetry; the horizontal resolution is only one third that of the vertical.[12] With a Trinitron monitor, the horizontal resolution of an image displayed cannot exceed the horizontal resolution of the display monitor.[12]

Resolution capability in CRT monitors is indicated by dot pitch, or the size in millimeters of a group of three phosphor elements (red, green, and blue) on the display surface. Current monitors have a dot pitch of .31, .28, or .25 mm.[12] To determine the pixel display capability (resolution) of a given monitor, dot pitch is divided into the length of the displayable image surface. For a 21-inch monitor with a dot pitch of .25 mm, the horizontal displayable length is approximately 16 inches or 400 mm, resulting in a maximal horizontal resolution of 1600.[12] Monitors are now capable of changing displayed resolution to either a lower or higher (up to the maximum) resolution under software control, allowing images taken at differing resolutions to be displayed on the same monitor. It is important to keep in mind that one cannot improve the resolution of an image beyond the resolution it was photographed at by displaying it on a monitor with a higher resolution.

Another factor that must considered in displaying images on computer monitors is the aspect ratio, or the ratio of the number of pixels on the horizontal axis to the number of pixels on the vertical axis.[12] Most monitors have been calibrated such that a circle will appear to be a circle at an aspect ratio of 4:3. If an image of a circle with an aspect ratio of 5:4 is displayed on a monitor calibrated to an aspect ratio of 4:3, it will appear as an ellipse. Image distortion can occur unless the aspect ratio of the image photographed by the submitting telepathology station corresponds to the aspect ratio of the receiving stations monitor.[12]

Finally, as higher-resolution monitors display more pixels, more memory is required in the video card to allow the RAMDAC (random access memory digital-to-analog converter) to produce a sufficient refresh rate to prevent flickering. Flickering results in fatigue and eyestrain for the viewer. The RAMDAC in the video card is the device that converts the digital image to analog signal and sends it to the monitor. The number of times per second the RAMDAC converts the image and sends it to the monitor is the refresh rate, expressed in Hertz (Hz). It is generally accepted that refresh rates below 60 Hz commonly produce flicker and rates above 72 Hz rarely do, although these thresholds vary with the individual. The prevention of flickering depends both on the ability of the RAMDAC to process the necessary number of images per second and on the ability of the monitor to handle that number of images per second.

# Telepathology System Formats

Telepathology system formats are of three basic types: static, dynamic, and hybrid. In the **static format,** representative images are selected at the sending station and sent to the receiving station where the pathologist views the preselected images. With a **dynamic system,** the pathologist views the original slide on a microscopic stage that is controlled from the receiving station by remote control. The stage is moved and areas to be viewed at a higher power are selected by the viewing pathologists, then the images are viewed, all in real time. **Hybrid systems** combine elements of both static and dynamic systems. Each type has strengths and weaknesses.

Purely dynamic telepathology, where "live" viewing of the tissue section is completely controlled by the viewing pathologist at a site remote from the location of the microscope, was a strategy used early in trials of telepathology. This format was associated with a number of difficulties, as available video teleconferencing equipment did not provide sufficient resolution necessary for histopathologic detail. Additionally, this approach was associated with certain technical considerations. To avoid distracting and disorienting start-and-stop motion, the video had to been sent at a rate of 30 frames per second, requiring transmission of a very large amount of data, either compressed or uncompressed.[15] This application required high-resolution video cameras, broadband telecommunications, and robotic microscopes, all of which proved too expensive to be practical.[7] A commercially constructed dynamic telepathology system (Corabi International Telemetrics, Inc.) using a dedicated microwave telecommunications system went into operation between Emory University Hospital and Grady Memorial Hospital as far back as 1990, but few such systems can be found in the more recent literature.[2]

In contrast, telepathology systems using the static format have become increasingly popular and are currently the dominant system format in use. In a recent review,[16] 19 of 22 systems were of this format.[16] This type of system can also be termed the "store and forward" format, a label that explains the popularity of this type of system. Images are selected, stored, and transmitted to the receiving station where they can be either viewed on reception or stored and viewed at the convenience of the pathologist. The advantages of this format are that the pathologist is not tied up waiting for the image, and since time of transmission is not crucial, it can be transmitted over low bandwidth lines during off hours. Cost is reduced through the use of low bandwidths, the absence of need for robotics, and more efficient use of the pathologist's time.

Examples of static telepathology systems using a wide variety of hardware and telecommunication modes are present in the literature. Vazir, Loane, and Wooten[17] constructed a system using a single-chip video camera, a codec ($352 \times 288$ pixels), a commercial television set, and commercial television lines. Off-the-shelf components were used by these authors to test the feasibility of constructing a functional yet inexpensive system that could be used in undeveloped areas. The introduction of the MIME (Multimedia Internet Mail Extension) message format, allowing inclusion of static images, video, and voice components in a message, unlike SMTP (Simple Mail Transfer Protocol) or POP (Post Office Protocol), has led to the use of e-mail for static telepathology. Access to the Internet has been via various modes such commercial telephone lines, T1 lines, or ISDN lines.[18–19] High-end-systems, such as that described by Weinstein and Epstein[20] using a commercial imaging system (Roche Image Analysis System, Elon College, NC), a digital video camera, and a 17-inch color monitor (resolution not specified for either the camera or the monitor), have also been described.

The wide variety of system architectures is but one of the difficulties in assessing the accuracy of telepathology in providing diagnoses. While the literature is replete with studies assessing the "accuracy" of static pathology systems, it is important to remember that many of these studies involve having pathologists make diagnoses on preselected archival cases under conditions that do not necessarily reflect actual practice.[3,18–24] These studies, termed feasibility (performed prior to implementation of a system) and validation (performed after the system is in operation) studies by Weinstein, Bhattacharyya, and colleagues,[5] are useful in assessing the performance of specific pathologists, examining interobserver variability, and detecting reasons for errors. A better assessment of the performance of static telepathology systems is achieved by looking at studies that correlate prospectively the diagnosis rendered using a functioning system, with glass slides of the case after the telepathology case has been signed out. This type of study, termed a clinical study, assesses the performance under conditions of actual practice and as such can give an assessment of how often static image telepathology is unable to lead to a diagnosis, that is, how often the pathologist is forced to defer a diagnosis until glass slides can be examined.[5] Diagnostic accuracy in clinical studies has been demonstrated to range from 88% to 100%, with a deferral rate of 2% to 23%.[4,25–27]

Incorrect diagnoses in telepathology result from one of three etiologies: the quality of the image, the fields selected for viewing, and interpretive error. Errors in interpretation are a function of experience and not limited to telepathology, while errors due to poor image quality do occur but are cited by most authors as an infrequent cause of misdiagnosis.[23] The pathologist has the option of deferring the diagnosis if there is uncertainty. Misinterpretation of small cells due to insufficient resolution has been cited as a potential problem in the use of telepathology for the assessment of Pap smears.[21] The major cause of diagnostic error in static telepathology studies has been due to selection of nonrepresentative fields by the sending station. In the study by Halliday and colleagues,[25] 9 of the 17 misdiagnoses (out of 127 total diagnoses rendered) were due to nonrepresentative field selection by the referring pathologist. All serious errors (5) that would have resulted in improper therapy were due to improper field selection. The remaining incorrect diagnoses were due to interpretive errors; none were due to poor image quality. In a study in which 200 archived cases were reviewed by four pathologists in a simulated static telepathology system, there were 27 misdiagnoses among the four pathologists: 10 were due to nonrepresentative field selection, 15 to interpretation errors, and 2 to image quality.[23] Image quality was felt to have contributed to four of the interpretive errors.

Nonrepresentative field selection resulting in misdiagnosis is a problem that is associated with static telepathology systems alone. In the dynamic system, the pathologist at the receiving station controls viewing of the slide via a remote-controlled robotic stage and can select the areas to be closely inspected. While no studies assessing the accuracy of purely dynamic systems or comparing static and dynamic systems are in the literature, it is generally accepted that dynamic systems afford the opportunity for greater accuracy. Dynamic-robotic systems are felt to more accurately mimic the routine intellectual processes that pathologists use during light microscopy. The tissue section can be viewed in its entirety, contributing to confidence and accuracy.[5] The viewing pathologist selects the fields to be closely viewed, greatly reducing improper field selection as a source of error. As previously discussed, however, dynamic systems have not gained popularity due to technical and cost considerations. In an effort to allow the pathologist to retain control of the viewing process inherent in the dynamic system, yet have the technical and cost flexibility associated with the static system, hybrid systems have been developed.

Because of the expense associated with developing the robotic microscope and controlling software, initial hybrid systems were developed by or in cooperation with commercial companies. These dynamic-static hybrid systems allow various combinations of low-power dynamic viewing of the entire slide with static imaging of areas chosen by the viewing pathologists on high power. To obviate the need to send data at 30 frames per second, necessary to avoid lag motion of the image, the Telepath System (TeleMedicine Solutions,

Birmingham, AL) uses discrete commands rather than continuous remote control to form a lower-power image of the tissue section out of multiple small image tiles, and the image is then transmitted to the receiving station.[15] By moving a cursor to an area of interest and clicking on the spot, the objective on the microscope is changed, autofocus is performed, and a high-power image is captured and transmitted. No image compression is used and all images are stored with coordinates relative to the low-power image in a remote server. Dunn and colleagues[6] describe a similar system (Apollo Systems, Alexandria, VA) that has been in use between two hospitals in the VA medical system for a number of years. A similar type of system has been adapted by Nagata and Mizushima[28] to serve multiple clients who need only a PC with an Internet connection. The "World Wide Microscope" is essentially a robotic microscope with a digital camera and a URL, a WWW server with a special CGI, and a Java applet for clients. In feasibility studies, accuracy rates for the Telepath and Apollo systems have been 97% and 98%, respectively.[6,15]

Along similar lines, Petersen and colleagues[29] have constructed software that runs as Java applets from a Web browser and allows remote control of a robotic microscope and transforms a personal computer into a Web server with an image grabber that can be used to display static microscopic images in real time for multiple receiving clients. Additionally, the software incorporates a chat function that allows real-time communication between sending and receiving stations. The authors have made this software available without cost to interested parties in order to foster use of the Internet for telepathology.

Recently, e-MedSoft.com Illumea Product Group (Newport Beach, CA) has begun marketing a purely dynamic telepathology system, which uses a proprietary streaming technology to produce real-time images in true color (24 bits) without lag. The system, FiberPix, can use 56.6-Kb modems and POTS for transmission, rather than expensive dedicated lines, and will accept input from either analog or digital cameras. According to the company, high-power images from the low-power view are obtainable instantly. To accommodate the large image files for storage, Illumea offers storage space on a remote server.

## Legal Issues

In many cases, transmission of telepathology images and patient data will be across state lines. Since the practice of medicine is regulated at the state level, licensing issues come into play when a telepathologist views and gives an opinion on a case that originates in another state. Ten states have enacted legislation that requires a physician practicing telemedicine to be licensed in their state even if the physician is not physically present in the state.[30] Regulations are not uniform from state to state, however, and in an effort to establish consistency, the American Medical Association (AMA) has issued a policy statement (H-480.969) calling for states to require "full and unrestricted license" for physicians involved in situations where there is "telemedical transmission of individual patient data from the patient's state."[31] In contrast, the Federation of State Medical Boards[32] issued in 1996 a model statute that calls for a special license limited to the practice of medicine across state lines rather than the full and unrestricted license as recommended by the AMA. For the foreseeable future, licensing issues for telepathology with respect to interstate consultations will vary from state to state, and the respective state medical boards involved in a given situation should be consulted.

Finally, the issue of liability in telepathology must be considered. Similar to the situation with licensing, liability issues are unresolved. As Bargnesi and Naegely[33] point out in an on-line article from the law firm of Damon and Morey, LLP, as of late 1998 when their article was published there were no published medical malpractice cases involving telemedicine. While some claims had been filed involving telemedicine prior to their review, all had been settled out of court. Many questions will need to be resolved with respect to medical liability in telemedicine:[34]

- Has a patient-physician relationship been established by telecommunications?
- For interstate practice, which state's law will apply, the one the patient is in, the one the doctor is in, or both?
- Who is liable for the failures of technology, the doctor, the manufacturer, or both?
- As malpractice policies exclude coverage for unlicensed activities, will the insurer deny coverage on a telemedicine claim unless the physician is licensed in the state in which the suit is filed and judgment rendered?

Most of these questions generalize to all specialties of medicine that could potentially have involvement in telemedicine, and for some, telepathology could potentially pose unique variations on these questions. For example, if a misdiagnosis that results in improper treatment is made because of compression–decompression-induced artifact in a telepathology image, is the pathologist totally liable for damages or does the software manufacturer also bear partial (or complete) liability?

## Economic Issues

Determining the cost-benefit ratio of installing and operating a telepathology system is of prime importance in deciding whether or not to institute telepathology in a healthcare facility. Depending on the system, cameras, personal computers, software, monitors, and transmission lines can result in a significant initial investment. In the current environment of cost containment in medicine, labor savings and generated revenue must offset any incurred costs. In the previously described Veteran's Administration telepathology system initiated between Iron Mountain, MI, and Milwaukee, WI, the ability of pathologists in Milwaukee to sign out cases in Iron Mountain enabled the VA to not replace a retiring pathologist at the Iron Mountain facility, saving the system the cost of a pathologist.[35]

While reimbursement for telemedicine has been an ongoing difficulty for the discipline, services that do not require personal contact between patient and provider, such as telepathology and teleradiology, have been covered by Medicare for some time using traditional procedural codes.[36] Additionally, private insurance companies have paid for such noncontact services, primarily teleradiology. One issue that has been a cause of contention between teleradiology providers and payors, which in all probability will also involve telepathology in the future, is whether or not transmission costs can be factored into the reimbursement rates.[34]

# Future of Telepathology

While telepathology has been the subject of numerous studies since the 1970s, approximately the time period studies on teleradiology have been in the literature, it has yet to achieve the same status and popularity enjoyed by teleradiology. There are probably several reasons. One is that despite the attention given to telepathology by researchers and the implementation a number of functioning programs, standards (*de facto* or agreed on by the profession or regulatory entities) for the different aspects of telepathology, unlike teleradiology, are not currently available. The efforts on the part of the College of American Pathologists to foster the development of extensions to the DICOM standards for data management and transmission and HIPAA-mandated standards for security and confidentiality as applied to telepathology will aid in promoting uniformity in these areas. Additionally, in an effort to define clinical practice guidelines for telepathology, the American Telemedicine Association Special Interest Group for Telepathology[37] has published on-line proposed standards for the practice of telepathology. The proposal, for which the ATA is soliciting public comment, addresses the practice of primary diagnosis telepathology and second opinion telepathology with respect to responsibilities of the pathologists, training of support personnel, quality control, documentation and archiving, and data integrity and security.

Probably of much greater significance than the need for standards, however, is what Mairinger and colleagues[38] found in their survey on telepathology of the Austrian Society of Pathology. The authors describe a "deep but unfocused skepticism expressed in questions dealing with transferring telepathology techniques into routine work". Of the major concerns expressed by respondents ($n =118$), 67% were concerned about liability issues, 53% about data security, 49% about cost, and 43% about image quality. One of the central issues with telepathology is the adequacy of static telepathology in making diagnoses, and of the respondents in this survey, only 19% felt that high-resolution still images would be sufficient to render a diagnosis on a case. Despite the fact that a number of studies have claimed that static imaging pathology has an accuracy rate close to that of conventional light microscopy, this inexpensive and relatively easy-to-implement format has not been embraced by pathologists, seemingly because it is foreign to how pathologists normally work. It is the contention of several authors that until it is feasible for telepathology to more closely approximate the routine intellectual processes a pathologist goes through when reviewing a microscopic slide, it will not be readily accepted as a diagnostic modality.[5,39] With the advent of the commercial dynamic hybrid and dynamic systems described, it may now be possible to accomplish this.

The potential uses of telepathology include primary diagnosis, either frozen section or permanent section, consultation, education, quality assurance, and image archiving for research purposes. Progress in the establishment of electronic and clinical practice standards along with technological advancements now make the practice of telepathology a more viable option for pathology departments and healthcare facilities. Whether telepathology becomes an integral part of medical practice in the United States similar to teleradiology remains to be seen.

# Chapter Glossary

**ATM** (asynchronous transfer mode): Network technology based on transferring data in packets of a uniform size with a fixed channel or route between two points. This is different than **TCP/IP** (transmission control protocol/internet protocol), the *de facto* data transmission protocol of the Internet, where packets of data can take a different route from source to end point.

**CRT** (cathode ray tube): Technology used in television and computer display screens, based on the movement of an electron beam back and forth across a screen, lighting up phosphor dots on the inside of the glass screen.

**CCD** (charge-coupled device): Instrument used in digital and video cameras where semiconductors are connected so that the output of one serves as the input of the next.

**CD-ROM** (compact disc read-only memory): Optical disk capable of storing about the equivalent of 700 floppy disks (650MB–1GB)—about 300,000 pages of text.

**CGI** (common gateway interface): Specification that allows dynamic interaction between a World Wide Web server and a user. The user must be running a CGI-compatible program that is designed to accept and return information conforming to the CGI specification.

**codec** (coder/decoder): General term for a device that encodes and decodes a signal, such as converting an analog signal to a binary (digital) signal.

**CMOS** (complementary metal oxide semiconductor): Type of semiconductor chip that uses both negative and positive polarity circuits (although only one at a time), requiring less power than chips that use just one type of transistor.

**dot pitch:** Measurement that indicates in millimeters the diagonal distance between phosphor dots of the same color. The smaller the distance, the sharper the image.

**Ethernet:** LAN protocol developed by Xerox, DEC, and Intel that uses a bus or star topology and allows data transfer at up to 10 Mbps. One of the most common LAN standards used.

**fast Ethernet** (100Base-T): LAN protocol based on the older Ethernet standard but allowing 10 times the speed of data transfer (up to 100 Mbps).

**GIF** (graphics interchange format): Lossless image compression format, based on a substitution algorithm that has limitations with respect to pathology images in that the color palette is limited to 256 or fewer colors.

**ISDN** (integrated services digital network): International communication standard for transmission of voice, data, and images over telephone lines at 64 Kbps (kilobits per second). Most commercial ISDN lines are B channels, providing two lines, allowing transmission rates of 128 Kbps if the same data type is transmitted over both lines.

**Java:** High-level programming language with features that make it particularly suitable for use on the World Wide Web.

**JPEG** (Joint Photographic Experts Group): Compression algorithm, based on the discrete cosine transformation, which is useful for color images, allowing a greater variety of color. JPEG until relatively recently was available only as a lossy algorithm,

**LAN** (local area network): Computer network that encompasses a relatively small area, such as one building or a group of buildings such as a university campus. Each node (individual workstation) is usually a PC that can run its own programs but can access data and hardware anywhere on the LAN. LANs differ in topology (geometric arrangement of nodes, i.e., straight line, star, and so on), data protocols, and type of transmission lines (coaxial cables, fiber-optic cables, etc.).

**LCD** (liquid crystal display): Display that uses two layers of polarizable material separated by a liquid crystal solution, through which is passed an electric current that causes the crystals to align so that light cannot pass through. LCD technology is used extensively in laptop computers.

**lossless compression:** Data or image compression algorithm in which no data is lost during the compression and decompression process.

**lossy compression:** Data or image compression algorithm in which data is lost during compression and decompression. An image, for example, will be very similar but not absolutely identical after compression/decompression with a lossy algorithm.

**MIME** (multipurpose Internet mail extensions): Format specifications allowing messages that include images, video, and audio via the Internet e-mail system.

**POP** (post office protocol): Protocol used to retrieve e-mail from a mail server; the most common protocol used for this purpose.

**POTS** (plain old telephone service): Standard telephone lines, which are limited to a data transmission rate of 52 Kbps.

**RAMDAC** (random access memory digital-to-analog converter): Chip in video adapter cards that converts digitally encoded images into analog signals that allow display on a monitor.

**RAID** (redundant array of independent [or inexpensive] disks): Storage strategy that uses two or more disk drives in combination to improve performance and error correction. There are four levels, 0, 1, 3, and 5; 5 provides the highest level of performance and fault tolerance.

**SMTP** (simple mail transfer protocol): Protocol most commonly used to send e-mail between servers. Note that when an e-mail application is configured, both the POP and SMTP server must be specified.

**T1 line** (T-1 carrier or DS1 lines): Dedicated phone-line connections that consist of 24 channels, each allowing a data transmission rate of 64 Kbps, for a total transmission rate of 1.544 Mbps. These are used by businesses and Internet service providers to connect to the Internet "backbone" (see **T3**).

**T3 line** (T-3 carrier or DS3 lines): Dedicated phone-line connections that consist of 672 channels, each allowing a data transmission rate of 64 Kbps, for a total transmission rate of 43 Mbps. T3 lines are used as the "backbone" of the Internet and by some Internet service providers to connect to the Internet.

**token ring network:** LAN protocol in which the individual nodes are arranged in a geometric circle. A special bit pattern, the token, travels continuously around the circle, carrying messages from one node to another.

**true color:** Software or imaging device that uses 24 bits to represent each pixel, resulting in $16 \times 10^6$ colors.

**wavelet transforms:** Lossy image compression algorithm that transforms its component parts as a frequency representation. It is similar to JPEG but with a different mathematical basis function. There is less compression/decompression artifact, but transmission speed is up to three times slower.

**WORM** (write once, read many times): An optical disk technology, also known as CD-R, that allows one to write data to a disk only once, after which it cannot be altered but can be read many times. A limitation is that there is no standard for WORM disks, and most can be read only on the same type of drive that created them.

**Zip drive:** Floppy disk system developed by Iomega Corporation that can hold 100 MB of data. Zip drives are often used to back up PC hard drives.

# *References*

1. Brecht RM, Barrett JE. Telemedicine in the United States. In: Dunn K, Viegas, SF, editors. Telemedicine: Practicing in the Information Age. Philadelphia, Lippincott-Raven, 1998
2. Weinstein RS. Telepathology comes of age in Norway. Hum Pathol 1991; 22:511–513
3. Weinstein LJ, Epstein JI, Edlow D, et al. Static image analysis of skin specimens: The application of telepathology to frozen section evaluation. Hum Pathol 1997; 28:30–35
4. Nordrum I, Engum B, Rinde E, et al. Remote frozen section service: At telepathology project in northern Norway. Hum Pathol 1991; 22:514–518
5. Weinstein RS, Bhattacharyya AK, Graham AR, et al. Telepathology: A ten-year progress report. Hum Pathol 1997; 28:1–7
6. Dunn BE, Almagro UA, Choi H, et al. Dynamic-robotic telepathology: Department of Veterans Affairs feasibility study. Hum Pathol 1997; 28:8–12
7. Weinberg DS. How is telepathology being used to improve patient care? Clin Chem 1996; 42:831–835.
8. Mun SK, Elasayed AM, Tohme WG, et al. Teleradiology/telepathology requirements and implementation. J Med Sys 1995; 19:153–164
9. Winokur S, McCleelan S, Siegal GP, et al. A prospective trial of telepathology for intraoperative consultation (frozen sections). Hum Pathol 2000; 31:781–785
10. Weinberg DS, Doolittle M. Image management in pathology. Am J Clin Pathol 1996; 105(Suppl 1):S54–S59
11. O'Brien MJ, Takahashi M, Brugal G, et al. Digital imagery/telecytology: IAC task force summary. Acta Cytologica 1998; 42:148–164
12. Balis U. Image output technology. Clin Lab Med 1997; 17:175–188

13. Doolittle MH, Doolittle KW, Winkelman Z, et al. Color images in telepathology: How many colors do we need? Hum Pathol 1997; 28:36–41
14. Klossa J, Cordier JC, Flandrin G, et al. A European de facto standard for image folders applied to telepathology and teaching. Int J Med Informatics 1998; 48:207–216
15. Winokur TS, McClellan S, Siegal GP, et al. An initial trial of a prototype telepathology system featuring static imaging with discrete control of the remote microscope. Am J Clin Pathol 1998; 110:43–49
16. Zhou J, Hogarth MA, Walters RF, et al. Hybrid system for telepathology. Hum Pathol 2000; 31:826–833
17. Vazir MH, Loane MA, Wooton R. A pilot study of low-cost dynamic telepathology using the public telephone network. J Telemed Telecare 1998; 4:168–171
18. Singson PC, Natarajan S, Greenson JK, et al. Virtual microscopy and the internet as telepathology consultation tools. Am J Pathol 1999; 111:792–795
19. Della Mea V, Cataldi P, Boi S, et al. Image selection in static telepathology through the Internet. J Telemed Telecare 1998; 4(Suppl. 1):20–22
20. Weinstein MH, Epstein JI. Telepathology diagnosis of prostate needle biopsies. Hum Pathol 1997; 28:22–29
21. Ziol M, Vacher-Lavenu M, Heudes D. Expert consultation for cervical carcinoma smears: Reliability of selected-field videomicroscopy. Analyt Quant Cytol Histol 1999; 21:35–41
22. Della Mea V, Beltram CA. Telepathology applications of the Internet multimedia electronic mail. Med Informatics 1998; 23:237–244
23. Weinberg DS, Allaert FA, Dusserre P, et al. Telepathology diagnosis by means of digital still images: An international validation study. Hum Pathol 1996; 27:111–118
24. Raab SS, Zaleski MS, Thomas PA, et al. Telecytology. Am J Clin Pathol 1996; 105:599–603
25. Halliday B, Bhattacharyya AK, Graham AR, et al. Diagnostic accuracy of an international static-imaging telepathology consultation service. Hum Pathol 1997; 28:17–21
26. Eusebi V, Foschini L, Erde S, et al. Transcontinental consults in surgical pathology via the Internet. Hum Pathol 1997; 28:13–16
27. Dawson PJ, Johnson JG, Edgemon LJ, et al. Outpatient frozen sections by telepathology in a Veteran's Administration Medical Center. Hum Pathol 2000; 31:786–788.
28. Nagata H, Mizushima H. World wide microscope: New concept of Internet telepathology microscope and implementation of the prototype. In: Cesnik, B, et al., editors. MEDINFO 98. Amsterdam: IOS Press, 1998:286–289
29. Petersen I, Wolf G, Roth K. Telepathology by the Internet. J Pathol 2000; 191:8–14
30. Frishmann R. Telemedicine healers in cyberspace. Harvard Health Letter 1997:9–12
31. American Medical Association. H-480.969: The promotion of quality telemedicine [Online]. 1999. Available: http://www.ama-assn.org/cmeselec/cmeres/cme-7-1.htm
32. Federation of State Medical Boards. A model act to regulate the practice of medicine across state lines [Online]. 1996. Available: http://www.fsmb.org/telemed.htm
33. Bargnesi JM, Naegely EC. Telemedicine: Will technology expand medical liability? [Online] 1998. Available: http://www.damonmorey.com.pubs/autumn98_1c.html
34. Miller NW. Telemedicine legalities for physicians in PA [Online]. Physician's News Digest 1999. Available: http://www.physiciansnews.com/law/699miller.html
35. Titus, K. Labs making leap to telepathology. CAP Today 1997; 11:1
36. Office for the Advancement of Telehealth. Telemedicine reimbursement. [Online] 1998. Available: http://telehealth.hrsa.gov/reimb.htm

37. American Telemedicine Association Special Interest Group for Telepathology. Clinical guidelines for telepathology: A draft version 2.4 [Online]. Available: http://telepathology.upmc.edu/ata/guideline.html

38. Mairinger T, Netzer TT, Schoner W, et al. Pathologists' attitudes to implementing telepathology. J Telemed Telecare 1998; 4:41–46

39. Dervan PA, Wooton R. Diagnostic telepathology. Histopathol 1998; 32:195–198

# Glossary

**acceptance validation** (acceptance testing): Initial approval process for live use of a system by the user.

**AIM:** Automatic Identification Manufacturers Inc., a trade association.

**alphanumeric:** Character set that contains the letters A–Z and numerals 0–9.

**application software:** Programs written to fulfill a specific purpose, e.g., text editor, spreadsheet.

**ASCII** (American Standard Code for Information Interchange): Standard code for representing characters as binary numbers, used on most microcomputers, terminals, and printers. Each character represents 7 bits for a total of 128 possible symbols.

**ASCII character set:** 128 characters, including both control and printing characters.

**ASCII file:** Text file on a machine using the ASCII character set.

**ASP:** (application service provider): Third party whose main business is providing a software-based service to multiple customers over a wide-area network in return for payment.

**aspect ratio:** Expressed as $X:Y$. When referring to two-dimensional bar codes, either the ratio of module height to module width, or the height to the width of the entire symbol.

**assembly language:** "Language" in which each statement corresponds to a machine language statement, the statements themselves are written in a symbolic code that is easier for people to read.

**authentication:** Generally automated and formalized methods of establishing the authorized nature of a communications partner over the Internet communications channel itself (an "in-band" process); may include formal certificate authority, based on use of digital certificates; locally managed digital certificates; self-authentication by the use of symmetric private keys; and tokens or "smart cards."

**background:** In bar coding, the spaces, quiet zones, and area surrounding a printed symbol.

**band:** Range of frequencies used for transmitting a signal. A band is identified by its lower and upper limits; for example, a 10-MHz band in the 110–110-MHz range.

**bandwidth:** Transmission capacity of a computer channel, communications line, or bus. It is expressed in cycles per second (Hertz), the bandwidth being the difference

Sources: Hershon P. Electronic Computer Glossary. Computer Language Co., 1993. Downing D, Covington M. Dictionary of Computer Terms. Barron's Business Guides, New York. 2nd ed, 1989. Whatis.com. Webopedia.com.

between the lowest and highest frequencies transmitted. The frequency is equal to or greater than the bits per second. Bandwidth is also often stated in bits or bytes or kilobytes per second.

**bank:** Arrangement of identical hardware components.

**bar:** Darker element of a printed bar code symbol

**bar code:** Automatic identification technology that encodes information into an array of adjacent varying, width parallel rectangular bars and spaces.

**bar code character:** Single group of bars and spaces that represents a specific number (often one) of numbers, letters, punctuation marks, or other symbols. Smallest subset of a bar code symbol that contains data.

**baseband:** Communications technique in which digital signals are placed onto the transmission line without change in modulation. It is usually limited to a few miles and does not require the complex modems used in broadband transmission. Common baseband LAN techniques are token passing ring (token ring) and CSMA/CD (Ethernet). In baseband, the full bandwidth of the channel is used, and simultaneous transmission of multiple sets of data is accomplished by interleaving pulses using TDM (time-division multiplexing). Contrast with **broadband** transmission, which transmits data, voice, and video simultaneously by modulating each signal onto a different frequency using FDM (frequency division multiplexing).

**baud:** Modem transmission rate. A transmission range of 120 characters per second is 1200 baud. Modern systems available for PCs run up to 56,000 baud and include facsimile (fax) transmission capabilities (FaxModem).

**biometrics:** Method of identification based on a physical characteristic, such as a fingerprint, iris pattern, or palm print.

**BIPS:** billions of instructions per second.

**bit:** Contraction of "binary digit," represented in a computer by a two-stage (on/off) device. Microcomputers are rated by the number of bits each register can contain. The early Apples and IBM PCs are 8-bit machines. The 80286 processor is a 16-bit device. The 80486 is a 32-bit device. In general, the more bits, the faster the processor runs.

**bitmap:** As applied to image files, a set of bits holding image data in which each pixel corresponds to a group of bits holding its data in a raster-type format.

**BMP:** See **Windows bitmap file.**

**boot sector:** Area on a disk, usually the first sectors in the first disk partition, used to store the operating system. When the computer is started up, it searches the boot sectors for the operating system, which must be loaded into memory before any program can be run.

**boot-sector virus:** Virus that overwrites the boot sector with bad information, preventing the computer from booting.

**bridge:** Computer system that connects two similar LANs.

**broadband:** Technique for transmitting large amounts of data, voice, and video over long distances. Using high-frequency transmission over coaxial cable or optical fibers, broadband transmission requires modems for connecting terminals and computers to the network. Using the same FDM technique as cable TV, several streams of data can be transmitted simultaneously.

**browser** (Web browser): Interface to the Web that permits the display of Web pages and other Web services, such as e-mail, discussion groups, and so on.

**bus topology:** Network topology built around a common cable (bus) that connects all devices in the network.

**byte:** Number of bits that represent a character, usually 8. A kilobyte (KB) is 1024 bytes. A megabyte (MB) is 1,048,576 bytes = 1024 KB. 20 MB is the equivalent of 10,000 typed pages.

**cache:** Reserved section of memory, either on disk or in a chip, used to improve performance.

**CAN** (campus area network): Network of two or more LANs that span several buildings.

**CCD** (charge-coupled device): Silicon chip that integrates an array or matrix of photosensitive elements that acquire an electronic charge corresponding to the intensity of the incident light with associated circuitry to scan these elements and produce a digital output signal that can be reconstructed into an image by appropriate devices and software.

**CD** (compact disk): Plastic disk medium that can store large amounts of digital data by means of microscopic pits in one or more metallic layers.

**CD-R** (CD-recordable): CD drive technology that permits data to be recorded on a blank CD to produce a CD-ROM or audio CD. Data can be written to an area of the CD only once, but multisession technology permits the data to be added to the CD in multiple sessions.

**CD-ROM** (CD read-only memory): CD format that stores digital data, usually around 650 MB/disk, in file form that can be read by a computer.

**CD-RW** (CD rewritable): CD media and drive technology that permits data to be written and overwritten many times. Standard CD-ROM drives cannot read CD-RW disks, but CD drives with "MultiRead" technology can read both types.

**certificate authority:** Third party providing digital certificates for the purpose of validating certificate holder's identity.

**change control:** Process of tracking all revisions, alterations, and fixes applied to a hardware or software component of a computerized system; all changes are formally authorized and documented.

**check character:** In bar coding, a character within a symbol whose value is used to perform a mathematical check to ensure that the symbol has been decoded correctly.

**chip:** Integrated circuit. Chips are squares or rectangles that measure approximately from 1/16 to 5/8 of an inch on a side. They are about 1/30 of an inch thick, although only the top 1/1000 of an inch holds the actual circuits. Chips contain from a few dozen to several million electronic components (transistors, resistors, etc.). The terms chip, integrated circuit, and microelectronic are synonymous.

**client/server network:** Communications network that uses dedicated servers for all clients in the network. A central database server or engine performs all database commands sent to it from client workstations, and application programs on each client concentrate on user interface functions.

**clock:** Circuit that generates a series of evenly spaced pulses. All switching activity occurs when the clock is sending out a pulse. The faster the clock rate, the more operations per second can be carried out. Clock speeds are expressed as megahertz (MHz), or millions of cycles per second.

**closed system:** Computer architecture that uses proprietary elements that cannot be adapted or joined with products from two or more vendors. Closed systems are vendor-dependent and designed not to interconnect and work smoothly with a variety of products. See **open system.**

**CMYK** (cyan-magenta-yellow-black): Color system used for printing, based on the primary colors of the inks that are combined to generate colors.

**code word:** In bar coding, a symbol character value.

**compatible:** Capable of running the same programs. A matter of degree, since some programs contain hardware-dependent features.

**compiler:** Program that translates a high-level language into machine-language. The generated machine-language program is called the object program. Compilers translate the entire source program into machine language once, before running it.

**computer system:** Component of an information system consisting of the central processing unit (CPU), which processes data; the peripheral devices, which store and retrieve data; the operating system, which manages the processes of the computer system; and the interfaces, which connect the system to analytical devices and to foreign computer systems.

**computer cracker:** Person who gains illegal entrance into a computer system.

**confidentiality:** Restriction of access to data and information to individuals who have a need, a reason, and permission for access.

**coprocessor:** Separate circuit inside a computer that adds features to the CPU or does a specific task while the CPU is doing something else.

**customization:** Generally taken to mean vendor modification of code or provision of new code specifically for a particular client.

**data:** Uninterpreted material facts or clinical observations collected during an assessment activity.

**data accuracy:** Absence of mistakes or error in data.

**database:** Collection of information related to a particular subject or purpose; an information storage/retrieval facility where data is collected for the purpose of generating information/ discovering patterns. It does not have to be stored on a computer. It may have a user interface or not; it may be relational or not.

**database application (database system):** Collection of forms, screens, tables, queries, and reports utilizing a database managed by a database engine. For example, an LIS can be a database application.

**database engine:** Internal, highly technical file management system into which a logical database design is physically implemented. Some database engines Microsoft Jet, Microsoft SQL Server, IBM DB2, and Oracle.

**database management system** (DBMS): Collection of utility and administrative functions supporting the database engine. Its level of sophistication directly affects the robustness of any database system. It provides additional security and file management practices beyond what is delivered with the computer/network on which it runs. This level varies from vendor to vendor. For example, Oracle is a complete database management system; DBase, FoxPro, and Access are not.

**database server:** Fast computer in a local area network used for database storage and retrieval.

**data capture:** Acquisition or recording of data or information.

**data definition:** Identification of data to be used in analysis.

**data dictionary:** In essence, a database about data and databases, which holds the name, type, range of values, source, and authorization for access for each data element in the organization's files and databases. It also indicates which applications use the data so that when a change in a data structure is made, a list of affected programs can be generated.

**data integrity:** Desirable condition of data frequently taken for granted by users. It means that there are no duplicate records contained within the database, that there are no "orphan" records within the database (a test result without a patient), and that steps have been taken to ensure that the database retains integrity remains over time and activity.

**data normalization:** Process of making data and tables match database design standards. The objective of these standards is to eliminate redundant information to make managing data and future changes in table structure easier. If the tables are normalized, each data element/table attribute will be a fact about the key, the whole key, and nothing but the key.

**data reliability:** Stability, repeatability, and precision of data.

**data transformation:** Process of changing the form of data representation, for example, changing data into information using decision analysis tools.

**data transmission:** Sending of data or information from one location to another.

**data validity:** Verification of correctness; reflects the true situation.

**decision support system (DSS):** Information system similar to MIS, but tends to be more analytical, and deal with semi-structured problems using data from both internal and external sources.

**denial-of-service attack:** E-mail system attack in which a mail server or Web server is deliberately overloaded with (usually computer-generated) phony communications to prevent it from responding to valid ones. A line of defense is to identify the IP address of the sender and refuse to accept any communication from that address.

**desktop management interface** (DMI): Management system for microcomputers that provides a bidirectional path to interrogate all the hardware and software components within a computer system.

**developmental validation:** Validation procedures integrated into the process of customizing, configuring, adapting, or inventing a new system or component; the responsibility of the vendor who offers the product for sale or license.

**DIB:** See **Windows bitmap file.**

**digital certificate:** Secret, tamperproof electronic file issued by a third party, the certificate authority, for the purpose of verifying the identity of the certificate holder. They may permit or restrict access to specific files or information.

**DIR** (diffuse infrared system): Communication system using infrared frequency bands ranging from 3 micrometers ($3 \times 10^{-6}$ meters) to 750 nanometers ($7.5 \times 10^{-7}$ meters), just beyond the visible light range.

**direct costs:** Recognized, budgeted costs of operating an information system. Different models are used. One uses five categories: hardware and software, including capital purchases and lease fees; management (network, system, and storage administration, labor and outsourcing fees, management tasks); support (help desk, training, purchasing, travel, maintenance contracts, overhead); development and customization; communications fees (lease lines, server access). Another model uses four categories: capital costs; administrative costs; technical support, and end-user operations.

**direct sequence coding:** Simultaneous broadcasting over many radio frequencies, using unique spread codes known only to the transmitter and the intended receiver.

**disaster plan:** Group of detailed instructions formulated as SOPs that define what is to be done in the event of a major malfunction; a catastrophic interruption of function.

**distributed denial-of-service attack:** E-mail system attack in which the attacker recruits a large number of machines, often using Trojan horses, to send false messages, requiring the target to block a very large number of IP addresses.

**DS1, DS3** (digital signal 1 & 3): See **T1, T3.**

**DSL** (digital subscriber line): Digital transmission technology that uses modulation techniques to transmit data at high speeds (up to 32 Mbps upstream and 1 Mbps downstream) over dedicated standard telephone wires for short distances (less than 20,000 feet) from telephone switching offices to users.

**element:** In bar coding, a single bar or space.

**element width:** In bar coding, the thickness of an element measured from the edge closest to the symbol start character to the trailing edge of the same element.

**encryption:** Using an algorithm, conversion of original plain text into a coded equivalent ("ciphertext") to provide security for transmission over a public network.

**end node:** In a network, the object terminal device—a hand-held unit, a computer, or a stationary instrument.

**EPS** (encapsulated PostScript): File containing PostScript (printer) code as well as (optionally) preview images in several raster formats. The file extension is EPS.

**error correction** (*also referred to as* data redundancy): In bar coding, symbol characters reserved for error correction and/or error detection. These characters are calculated mathematically from the other symbol characters.

**error detection** (*also referred to as* **data security**): In bar coding, a system that prevents a symbol from being decoded as erroneous data. Error correction characters can be reserved for error detection. These characters then function as check characters.

**ESDI** (enhanced small device interface): Hard disk interface that transfers data in the 1–3 MByte/sec range. Originally, the high-speed interface for small computers but now being superseded by IDE and SCSI drives.

**Ethernet system:** Network topology consisting of up to 1024 nodes connected by electric wire or optical cable (bus topology). Ethernet broadcasts messages over its wires. All stations can "hear" all traffic and must sort out messages by specific address.

**executable virus:** Virus that attaches itself to a file header located at the end of an EXE file or the beginning of a COM file. The virus corrupts the header, either changing the command that initiates the program or simply preventing the program from working.

**executive support system (ESS):** Information system used at the strategic decision level of an organization, designed to address unstructured decision making using advanced graphics and communication representing vast amounts of structured and processed information.

**extract file:** Subfile or extract (sometimes called a superfile) of a larger database focused on a particular topic, series of issues, group of patients or type of data.

**fat client:** In client/server architecture, a client that performs the bulk of the data processing operations, while the data itself is stored on the server. It usually has substantial computing power.

**file server** (network server): Fast computer in a local area network used to store many kinds of programs and data files shared by users on the network. It is used as a remote disk drive.

**finder pattern (recognition pattern):** In bar coding, a pattern used to help find the symbol, determine the symbol version, and determine the symbol's tilt and orientation, as well as providing additional reference points to calculate the data square positions and to account for surface curvature.

**firewall:** Network node set up as a boundary to prevent traffic from one segment to cross over into another.

**firewire:** Hardware computer interface that allows serial transfer of digital signals between a computer and up to 63 peripheral devices at transfer speeds of 100–400

Mbps, compared to 20 Kbps for ordinary serial ports and 150 Kbps for parallel ports. Developed by Apple Computer and Texas Instruments.

**firmware chip:** Permanent memory chip that holds its content without power, e.g., ROM, PROM, EPROM, and EEPROM .

**foreign key:** In database design, a field or set of fields within a table that equal the primary key of another table. Foreign keys are how one table is related to another. For example, a patient table contains a field called location code, which is also the primary key of the location table. Used by the relational database system to be able to find the location name whenever it needs it while storing only the location code with the patient record. When the location changes its name, it needs to be changed only once in the location table to make the change appear in all subsequent uses of the location code.

**frame grabber:** Electronic device or computer accessory that accepts analog video signals as input and produces a digitized representation of the current video frame, which is then stored in a memory array and used to construct a digital signal that can be interpreted by a computer and, in some cases, an analog signal representing the "frozen" frame for display or recording by analog devices.

**frequency hopping spread spectrum** (FHSS): Transmission of radio signals over frequencies that shift every few milliseconds according to a defined sequence known only to the transmitter and the intended receiver.

**function:** Goal-directed, interrelated series of processes, such as patient assessment or patient care.

**GAN** (global area network): Many LANs around the world connected together.

**gateway:** Computer subsystem that performs protocol conversion between different types of networks or applications; e. g., a gateway can connect a personal computer LAN to a mainframe network. An electronic mail, or messaging, gateway converts messages between two different messaging protocols. See bridge.

**GIF** (graphics interchange format): Raster-type file developed by CompuServe for network transmission of images. It uses lossless LZW compression, but it is limited to 8-bit depth (256 colors). It is one of the most popular formats for transmission of pictures over the Internet. The file extension is GIF.

**hacker:** Person who writes programs in assembly language or in system-level languages, such as C; term implies very tedious "hacking away" at the bits and bytes. Increasingly, the term is used for people who try to gain illegal entrance into a computer system. Compare **cracker.**

**hand-held unit (walk-around unit):** Device designed to carry out certain functions without direct connection to a computer; typically contains an RF or DIR transceiver, its antenna, and a battery; may have a graphical user interface (GUI) screen for display and a keyboard or a touch-screen input system, or both.

**handshakes:** Signals transmitted back and forth over a communications network that establish a valid connection between two stations.

**handshaking:** Process used by two devices to define how they will send and receive data from each other. It defines the transfer speed, number of bits that make up a data packet, number of bits that will signal the beginning and end of a packet, and use of parity bit for error checking and mode of operation.

**hazard analysis:** Determination of the potential degree of human harm that might result from the failure of a device or system; i.e., specification of the penalty for failure.

**header:** First record in a file, used for identification. It includes the file name, date of last update, and other status data.

**high-level language:** Description of a computer programming language. The closer the program is to natural language, the higher it is said to be.

**HIPAA** (Health Insurance Portability and Accountability Act of 1996 (PL 104-191), the "Kennedy/Kassebaum Law"): Law that regulates patient privacy and electronic communication of medical-related information, including over the Internet or an intranet.

**HL7** (Health Level 7): Dominant interface protocol used in healthcare applications. Acceptance and support have increased to the point where many people consider HL7 the standard interface protocol in healthcare related applications.

**horizontal function:** Horizontal refers to a function that is similar in diverse industries, such as truck fleet management, tax preparation services, and so on.

**hot backup:** Alternative computing site to which operations are shifted in the event of catastrophic failure of the primary system.

**HTML** (hypertext markup language): Computer language used to create Web pages. HTML documents consist of text and embedded special instructions called tags. HTML documents are read using a Web browser, which interprets the tags and displays the document as a Web page.

**HTTP** (hypertext transfer protocol): Connection-oriented protocol used to carry World Wide Web traffic between a WWW browser and the WWW server being accessed.

**hub:** Central connecting device for communications lines in a star topology. "Passive hubs" merely pass data through; "active hubs" regenerate signals and may monitor traffic for network management.

**hyperlink:** Predefined linkage between one object and another.

**IDE** (integrated drive electronics): Hard disk that contains a built-in controller. IDE drives range in capacity from 40MB up to 1GB. Widely used in small computers.

**identification:** Method of establishing the authorized nature of a communications partner, which is usually manual, involves human interaction, and uses not the Internet data channel itself but another "out-of-band" path such as the telephone or postal service; may include telephone identification of users and/or password exchange by telephone, certified mail or bonded messenger, personal contact exchange of identities or passwords, and tokens or "smart cards."

**indirect costs:** Unbudgeted and therefore largely unaccountable costs associated with operation of an information system. They include costs incurred by users who do their own support or provide help or advice to peers, time spent learning applications, unauthorized time spent playing games, for example; and productivity lost to either scheduled or unscheduled downtime.

**informatics:** Information science; the science of processing data for storage and retrieval.

**information:** Interpreted sets of data that can assist in decision making.

**information structure:** Component of an information system consisting of the database, which defines the data structures and to a certain extent defines the organization; procedures, which define data flow; and the application programs, including data entry, queries, updating, and reporting.

**integrated circuit (chip):** Electronic device consisting of many miniature transistors and other circuit elements on a single silicon chip.

**integrated software suite:** Term used when all the components of the suite can exchange information with one another requiring minimal effort for the individual using the software.

**intelligent hub:** Computer that provides network management; may include bridging, routing, and gateway capabilities.

**interface:** Method by which two independent entities interact with a resultant interchange of data or information.

**Internet:** Global information system logically linked by unique addresses based on Internet protocol (IP); able to support communications using the transmission control protocol/Internet protocol (TCP/IP).

**interpreter:** Device that translates and runs the source program line by line each time it is run.

**intranet:** Internal information system with a single user interface, based on Internet technology, using TCP/IP and HTTP communication protocols.

**IP address:** Under Internet protocol, the specific address of a site or user.

**ISDN** (integrated services digital network): Telephone communication standard that uses two dedicated 64-Kbps digital telephone lines to transfer data in the 56–128-Kbps range from a telephone switching office to an user (baseband ISDN). Broadband ISDN is much faster but requires fiberoptic cables.

**ISP** (internet service provider): Company that offers Internet access on a fee-per-time-spent basis.

**JPG:** See **JPEG**.

**joystick:** Small vertical lever mounted on a base that steers the cursor on a computer display screen. The name derives from the control stick in an aircraft.

**JPEG** (Joint Photographic Experts Group): 24-bit depth file developed for the representation of color photographic images that is capable of high (but lossy) compression to ratios of 100:1 and higher. It is also a popular format for transmission of images over the Internet because of the small file size and high color depth. Display time may not be reduced compared to GIF, however, because of the extra time required for decompression. It may not be suitable for some types of quantitation because the final (decompressed) image is not faithful to the original (before compression). The extension is JPG.

**Kbps** (thousand bits per second): Data transmission-rate unit.

**kernel:** Fundamental part of a program, typically an operating system, that resides in memory at all times. It is also the most machine dependent part of the operating system and is usually written in the assembly language of its CPU family.

**key:** Numeric code used by an algorithm to create a code for encrypting data for security purposes.

**knowledge-based information:** Collection of stored facts, models, and information that can be used for designing and redesigning processes and for problem solving.

**knowledge work system (KWS):** Information system used by knowledge workers (scientists, engineers, and so on) to help create and distribute new knowledge.

**laboratory informatics:** Field that concerns itself with the theoretical and practical aspects of information processing and communication, based on knowledge and experience derived from processes in the laboratory and employing the methods and technology of computer systems.

**LAN** (local area network): Network that services a work group within an organization.

**light pen:** Penlike input device used by pressing against a special receptive computer display screen. Light pens are most suitable when the user has to interact with (e.g., select) a particular item on the screen.

**LINUX:** UNIX-like operating system meeting POSIX specification. It works like

UNIX but is built around a different kernel. The basic LINUX program is free, and the source code is public. The LINUX kernel is combined with different sets of utilities and applications to form complete operating systems, also called LINUX, available from various vendors.

**logic bomb:** Virus that is intended to destroy data immediately. In contrast to a virus, it may insert random bits of data into files, corrupting them, or it may initiate a reformatting of a hard drive.

**logic chip:** Single chip that can perform some or all of the functions of a processor. A microprocessor is an entire processor on a single chip.

**logical model:** In database design, a visual representation of how the database components relate one to another. There are multiple levels in the logical model; the highest is the topics within the database, the lowest is all the data elements about all the topics and all their relationships.

**LOINC** (Logical Observation Identifiers Names and Codes): Database providing a standard set of universal names and codes for identifying individual laboratory results and diagnostic study observations. Developed and copyrighted by The Regenstrief Institute.

**LZW** (Lempel-Ziv-Welch): Patented lossless file compression algorithm, used in GIF image files, which uses pointers to a dictionary of repeating bit phrases.

**machine language:** "Language" or set of instructions that a machine can execute directly. Machine languages are written in binary code, and each statement corresponds to one machine action.

**macro virus:** Virus that affects prewritten machine language subroutines that are called for throughout the program. At assembly, macro calls are substituted with the actual subroutine or instructions that branch to it. The high-level language equivalent is a function.

**MAN** (metropolitan area network): Network of two or more LANs connected within a few miles, usually without wires.

**management information system (MIS):** Information system used to provide current and historical performance data to middle managers who use it in planning, controlling and decision making.

**management system:** Component of an information system that sets the organization's goals and objectives, develops strategies and tactics, and plans, schedules, and controls the system.

**mainframe computer:** A large computer. Formerly, all computers were called mainframes, as the term referred to the main CPU cabinet. Today, it refers to a large computer system able to handle a variety of computing tasks. (See supercomputer)

**management information base** (MIB): Data structure that defines what can be obtained from a computer or peripheral device and which processes can be controlled, e.g., turned on or off.

**matrix code:** In bar coding, an arrangement of regular polygon-shaped cells where the center-to-center distance of adjacent elements is uniform. The arrangement of the elements represents data and/or symbology functions. Matrix symbols may include recognition patterns that do not follow the same rule as the other elements within the symbol.

**Mbps** (million bits per second): Data transmission-rate unit.

**medical informatics:** Field that concerns itself with the cognitive information processing and communications tasks of medical practice, education, and research, including the information science and technology to support the tasks.

**memory resident virus:** Virus that avoids detection by placing its code in different areas of memory; activated when an application program is launched.

**memory chip:** Chip that stores information in memory. Random access memory (RAM) chips, the computer's working storage, contain from a few hundred thousand to several million storage cells (bits). They require constant power to keep the bits charged.

**metadata:** Collection of data about data, a data dictionary that defines what the data is, where it originated, where it is stored, how frequently is it updated, and so on.

**microcomputer:** Computer in which all parts of the CPU are integrated on one chip.

**microprocessor:** Ultimate integrated circuit: a single chip containing the complete logic and arithmetic unit of a computer.

**minimum data sets:** Collections of related data items.

**MIPS** (millions of instructions per second): Measure of computational capacity.

**modem** (modulator-demodulator): Device that encodes data for transmission over a particular medium, such as telephone line and optical cable. The standard modem format is designated RS-232.

**module:** In bar coding, the narrowest nominal width unit of measure in a symbol. One or more modules are used to construct an element.

**module validation** (module testing): Testing of the function of a product as a whole.

**mouse:** Input device consisting of a palm-sized electromechanical mechanism in an oval or ergonomically suitable plastic housing; used as a pointing and drawing tool. As it is rolled across a surface, the screen cursor (pointer) moves correspondingly. Selections are made by pressing buttons on the mouse. So called because its low, smooth surface and trailing tail-like wire bear a fanciful resemblance to a mouse.

**multipath interference:** Form of radio interference caused by the broadcast frequency bouncing off surfaces such as walls and doors.

**NTSC** (National TV Standards Committee): U.S. standard for television signals, allowing for 525 lines/frame at a frequency of 30 frames/second (60 half-frames interlaced).

**numeric:** Character set including only numeral 1–9.

**office automation system (OAS):** Information system used to increase the productivity of data workers (secretaries, bookkeepers, and so on), but may also be used by knowledge workers.

**open architecture:** Computer system in which the specifications are made public in order to encourage or permit third-party vendors to develop add-on products.

**open system:** Computer architecture for which standards have been derived by a consensus of interested parties. Open systems are vendor-independent and designed to interconnect and work smoothly with a variety of products.

**operating system:** Program that controls a computer and makes it possible for users to operate the machine and run their own programs. Under control of the operating system, the computer recognizes and obeys commands entered by the user. It contains built-in routines that allow the application program to perform operations without having to specify detailed machine instructions. Examples: CP/M, MS/DOS, UNIX, OS2, Apple DOS.

**OSI** (open system interconnect): Standard for vendors to conform to specifics that enable most systems to work together.

**overhead:** In bar coding, the fixed number of characters required for start, stop, and checking in a given symbol. For example, a symbol requiring a start/stop and two check characters contains four characters of overhead. Thus, to encode three characters, seven characters are required to be printed.

**packet:** Frame or block of data used for transmission in packet switching and other communications methods.

**PAL** (phase alternating line): Dominant European standard for television video that uses 625 lines/frame at 50 half-frames/second, differing from the U.S. standard in both resolution and frequency. See **NTSC.**

**partition:** Part of a disk reserved for some special purpose.

**partition table virus:** Virus that either moves or destroys the computer's partition table information and loads the virus code in place of the partition table.

**PCMCIA** (Personal Computer Memory Card International Association): Nonprofit trade association founded to standardize the PC card or PCMCIA card.

**PC card (PCMCIA card):** Removable module that can hold memory, modems, fax/modems, radio transceivers, network adapters, solid-state disks or hard disks. All are 85.6 mm long by 54 mm wide (3.37 in. × 2.126 in.) and use a 68-pin connector. Thickness varies with the application.

**PCT:** See **PICT.**

**physical model:** In database design, a representation of how the database is physically stored in the computer's file system.

**PICT** (Picture): Vector-type file format developed for Macintosh computers and transported to PCs. The file extension is PCT.

**pixel** (picture element): The smallest element making up a digital image, represented by a dot of light on a display monitor or a dot of ink on a printed image; contains coded information defining location, intensity, and color.

**PNG** (portable network graphics, pronounced "ping"): New raster-type (bit-mapped) graphics format similar to GIF but free of patent restrictions imposed on GIF by use of the patented LZW compression algorithm. The file extension is PNG.

**polling:** Network communications technique that determines when a terminal is ready to send or receive data. The computer continually interrogates its connected terminals in sequence. If a terminal has data to send or is ready to receive, it sends back an acknowledgment and the transmission begins.

**portal:** Internet Web site or service that offers a broad array of resources and services, such as e-mail, discussion forums, search engines, and on-line shopping.

**presentation software:** Software that interacts with an individual developing, editing, and arranging slides for presentations.

**primary key:** In database design, a field or set of fields that uniquely identify each record stored in the table. The power of a relational database system comes from its ability to quickly find and bring together information stored in separate tables using queries. To do this, each table should include a primary key to ensure the uniqueness of each record. A primary key may be one or multiple fields within the record.

**process validation:** Establishment of documented evidence providing a high degree of assurance that a specific process will consistently produce a product meeting its predetermined specification and quality attributes.

**processing gain:** In broadcasting, an increase in signal-to-noise ratio; an improvement in the clarity of the signal.

**programming language:** Language in which a program is actually written by a programmer; it is designed so that people can write programs without having to understand the inner workings of the machine. Examples: BASIC, C, COBOL, ADA, PASCAL, FORTRAN.

**project management software:** Software that interacts with an individual planning or coordinating the effort needed to accomplish a change in the status quo. The individual identifies the tasks to be done, the time and resources needed for each, task dependencies, and available resources. The software calculates the critical path of the project and when effort expended and project completions are input calculates the status of the project.

**protocol:** Rules governing the transmitting and receiving of data.

**query:** In database design, a means of retrieving data from the database using criteria you specify and displaying it in the order you specify. Queries create a logical view of a subset of the data in the database and do not permanently occupy physical storage. Example: a query that pulls all patient test results received during a specific time period and includes the patient data with each test result.

**quiet zone:** In bar coding, spaces preceding the start character of a symbol and following a stop character. Sometimes called the "clear area."

**RAM** (random access memory): Memory usable for performing computer functions. Information is maintained in RAM during operations but is lost when the machine is turned off. For modern applications, 8 megabytes RAM is minimal; 12, 16, or 32 are much better.

**raster graphics:** In computer graphics, a technique for representing a picture image as a matrix of dots. It is the digital counterpart of the analog method used in television. However, unlike television, which uses one standard, there are many raster graphics standards.

**record:** In database design, the technical term for a row of data in a relational database. Table records contain facts or attributes or data elements or columns. For example, in a patient table we might expect to find a single record with facts about that patient, e.g., the patient's date of birth, sex, race, social security number. A record is similar to a row in a spreadsheet in appearance only.

**relationships:** In database design, definitions of how pieces of data relate to one another. A one-to-one relationship exists when one record in the primary table corresponds to one record in the related table. A one-to-many relationship exists when one record in the primary table corresponds to multiple records in the related table. Many-to-many relationships exist in the real world and are implemented in databases via two one-to-many relationships through a cross-reference table.

**referential integrity:** Something database engines have as a result of the relationships established in a database design. It ensures that data necessary for the relationship is not accidentally deleted, and it cascades updates and deletes through the relationship per the designer's specs. Referential integrity means that a patient record must exist in the patient table prior to adding a patient test result record to the test results table. If it is turned off, a test result can be added to the table without its corresponding patient. Referential integrity is a feature that comes with relational database engines and does not require any programming to be available.

**regressive validation:** Testing process that ensures that changes in a system have had no unexpected effect on existing functions.

**repeater:** Communications device that amplifies or regenerates a data signal to extend the transmission distance.

**retrospective validation (concurrent validation):** Determination of the reliability, accuracy, and completeness of a system in use.

**RF:** Radio frequency system broadcasting over a variety of wavelengths.

**RFI** (request for information): Document that invites a vendor to submit information about hardware, software, and/or services offered.

**RFP** (request for proposal): Document that invites a vendor to submit a bid to provide hardware, software, and/or services.

**RGB** (red-green-blue): Color system used primarily for display monitors, scanning, and film printing, based on the primary colors represented by monitor pixels and scanning or printing filters.

**ring topology (ring network):** Communications network architecture that connects terminals and computers in a continuous loop.

**risk analysis:** Systematic process for evaluating the vulnerability of a data-processing system and the information it contains to hazards in its environment.

**ROI:** 1. Range of interest. Area of an image, usually selected by the operator, on which image analysis procedures are to be performed. 2. Return on investment

**ROM** (read-only memory): Portion of the operating system built into a chip that allows the basic functions of the machine to be carried out, including accessing the remainder of the operating system either from a floppy disk or in internal disk memory. During the time the machine is on, the operating system may be held in RAM.

**router:** Computer subsystem in a network that routes messages between LANs and WANs. Routers deal with network addresses and all the possible paths between them; they read the network address in a transmitted message and send it based on the most expedient route.

**RS-232 serial interface** (recommended standard): Serial connection that consists of several independent circuits sharing the same cable and connectors. Nomenclature used by the Electronic Industry Association. (EIA)

**SCSI** (small computer system interface, pronounced "scuzzy"): Hardware computer interface that allows communication between a computer and up to seven peripheral devices by simultaneous (parallel) transfer of 8- to 64-bit signals at speeds of 5 to 80 Mbps, using a single computer expansion slot and set of resources (interrupt, and so on). Different versions with increasing speed and bit width are SCSI-1, SCSI-2, fast wide SCSI-2, and ultra, ultrawide, ultra2, and ultra2 wide SCSI.

**SECAM** (Système Electronique Couleur avec Mémoire): Television video standard used primarily in France and eastern Europe. Compare **NTSC.**

**security:** Protection of data against unauthorized access.

**security hole:** Point of deficiency in a security system.

**semantics:** Study of the meaning of words; in the case of computers, implies consistency of use. See **syntax.**

**server:** Computer in a network shared by multiple users.

**shareware:** Software distributed on a trial basis through BBSs, on-line services, mail-order vendors, and user groups. A fee is due the owner if the software is used beyond the trial period.

**sideband:** In communications, the upper or lower half of a wave. Since both sidebands are normally mirror images of each other, one of the halves can be used for a second channel to increase the data-carrying capacity of the line or for diagnostic or control purposes.

**SIMM** (single in-line memory module): Narrow, printed circuit boards about 3 inches long that hold eight or nine memory chips. Each memory chip is rated in terms of its megabit (Mb) capacity. SIMMs plug into sockets on the circuit board.

**smart card:** Device about the size of a credit card containing sufficient processing power to hold data and applications and do its own processing. Can be used as an identity verification device.

**SNOMED** (Systematized Nomenclature of Human and Veterinary Medicine): Encoding system developed and copyrighted by the College of American Pathologists. It is a coded vocabulary of names and descriptions used in computerized patient records.

**SOP** (standard operating procedures): Procedural instruction, written in a standard form, that specifies the steps required to perform tasks.

**source program (source code):** Original high-level program (before compiling or interpreting).

**spread spectrum transmission:** Radio frequency transmission that continuously changes carrier frequency across the spectrum according to a unique pattern recognized by both sending and receiving devices.

**spreadsheet software:** Program that interacts with an individual processing numbers, creating graphs and charts from the numbers, and financial, statistical, and other mathematical reports.

**SQL** (structured query language): Software tool or language used to interrogate and process data in a relational database. Term is used both generically to refer to such a tool and specifically to refer to the product developed by IBM for its mainframes and variants created for minicomputer and microcomputer database applications.

**stacked code:** In bar coding, a long multirow symbol broken into sections that are stacked one on another similar to sentences in a paragraph.

**star topology (star network):** Communications network in which all terminals are connected to a central computer or central hub.

**status change:** Action that affects a database, such as entry of an order, assignment of an accession number, and entry of a test result.

**stealth virus** (polymorphic virus): Virus that changes its binary pattern each time it infects a new file to keep it from being identified.

**stress test:** Form of testing in which a load approximating the maximum designed work capacity is placed on the system. The purpose is to determine whether a system operates with expected reliability at the limits of its capacity.

**string:** Continuous set of alphanumeric characters that does not contain numbers used in calculations.

**string testing:** Proving that a single function within a computer system works as intended.

**supercomputer:** Large, very fast computer, highly specialized by design to run a few complex computations quickly. It is typically used for simulations in fields such as petroleum exploration and production, structural analysis, computational fluid dynamics, physics and chemistry, electronic design, nuclear energy research, meteorology, and animated graphics.

**surge protector:** Device between a computer and a power source used to filter out power surges and spikes.

**symbol character:** In bar coding, a unique bar and/or space pattern that is defined for that symbology. Depending on the symbology, symbol characters may have a unique associated symbol value.

**syntax:** Rules governing the structure of a language statement; specifies how words and symbols are put together to form a phrase.

**system validation (system testing):** Testing of the performance of functions and modules working together as an integrated whole.

**T1, T3 (DS1, DS3):** Multiplexed high-speed digital transmission technology ("T-carrier") providing 24 or 672 channels, respectively, with speeds of 64 Kbps each. T1 at full width (using all channels) supports transmission speeds of 1.544 Mbps and is used mainly for connecting larger users to the Internet and internet service providers (ISPs) to Internet nodes (or "backbone"). T3 supports maximal rates of around 43 Mbps, and is used to connect larger (ISPs) to the Internet and for the Internet backbone connecting nodes.

**table:** In database design, the technical term for a file in a relational database, a collection of data about a single, specific topic such as a patient or a clinic or a test result. Tables contain records or rows of data, one record per patient or clinic or test result. Using a separate table for each topic means that you store that data only once, which increases your efficiency and reduces data entry errors. Tables organize data into columns (called fields) and rows (called records). Table records contain facts or attributes or data elements. For example, in a patient table we might expect to find a single record with facts about that patient, e.g., the patient's date of birth, sex, race, and social security number. A database table is similar to a spreadsheet in appearance only.

**Targa:** Raster-type file format developed by Truevision, Inc. for high resolution (16-bit, 24-bit and 32-bit) color images. The file extension is TGA.

**TCO** (total cost of ownership): Total of all costs, direct and hidden, associated with the information asset over its life cycle.

**test script:** Description of the exact procedures followed for testing and documenting a successful or unsuccessful test. Scripts are developed in conjunction with the test plan and must indicate the action taken when a test is not successful.

**TGA:** See **Targa.**

**thin client:** In client/server architecture, a low-cost, centrally managed client designed to be small and with deliberately limited, essential functions so that the bulk of data processing occurs on the server.

**TIF:** See **TIFF.**

**TIFF** (Tagged Image File Format): Raster-type format developed by Aldus and Microsoft for use with a wide variety of images, including monochrome, gray scale, and 8-bit and 24-bit color. LZW and other forms of lossless compression are used and there are at least six different versions, so not all TIFF files are readable by all software supporting TIFF. This file type is extensively used for transfer of images between different applications because image integrity is preserved. The file extension is TIF.

**token ring network:** Communications network that uses token-passing technology in a sequential manner. Each station in the network passes the token on to the station next to it. Messages are passed in the form of "tokens," repeating frames (packets of data transmitted as a single entity) that are transmitted along the network by the controlling computer.

**topology:** (1) Pattern of interconnection between nodes in a communications network. See **bus, ring, star topologies.** (2) Interconnection between processors in a parallel processing architecture; bus, grid, or hypercube configuration.

**touch screen:** Input mechanism whereby selections are made by touching a specially constructed computer screen.

**TP monitor** (transaction processing monitor or teleprocessing monitor): Communications control program that manages the transfer of data between multiple local and remote terminals and the application programs that serve them.

**trackball:** Input device consisting of a sphere rotating in a base (essentially, an inverted mouse) it steers the cursor on the screen. Used mainly when a desk does not have enough space to permit use of a mouse.

**transaction file:** Collection of transaction records. Data in transaction files is used to update master files, which contain the subjects of the organization. Transaction files can be used as audit trails.

**transaction log:** Running record of every event transpiring on a system, including at a minimum, who, what, where, and when.

**transaction processing system (TPS):** Basic business systems used at the operations level of an organization to keep track of daily transactions in the course of business; might include databases and spread sheets.

**Trojan horse:** An attack program designed to be attractive to a potential victim who voluntarily takes it into his system; designed to cause the system to respond and cede some level of control to the attacker.

**TWAIN** (ostensibly from "Ne'er the twain shall meet"): Software interface (data source manager) that allows an imaging application program to activate and receive images from image acquisition devices (cameras, scanners, and so on).

**unit validation (unit testing):** Testing of a functional module or unit of some complexity.

**UNIX:** Multiuser, multitasking, command line interface, open source operating system developed by AT&T. It is written in C, which can be compiled into many different machine languages, allowing UNIX to run in a wider variety of hardware than any other operating system. UNIX has three major components: the kernel, which governs fundamental tasks; the file system, which is a hierarchical directory for organizing the disk; and the shell, the interface that processes user commands.

**UPS** (uninterruptible power supply): Alternate power source automatically accessed when primary electrical power fails or drops to an unacceptable voltage level. A battery-based UPS provides power for a few minutes, allowing the computer to be powered down (shut off) in an orderly manner.

**URL** (uniform resource locator): Unique Web page address.

**USB** (universal serial bus): Hardware computer interface that allows serial transfer of digital signals between a computer and up to 127 peripheral devices at transfer speeds of up to 12 Mbps, compared to 20 Kbps for ordinary serial ports and 150 Kbps for parallel ports.

**user definable:** Software of a system allows for individuation or accommodation to the needs of a particular laboratory through the provision of built-in options—menus or tables from which the laboratory selects those that apply.

**user interface:** Methods and techniques used to interact with a computer and the software running on the computer at the behest of the user. There are two major types of interface: character and graphical. A character interface utilizes the keyboard as its input provider and happens character by character and line by line (command line interface). The individual is restricted to following a set course of actions every time an activity is worked through completion. A graphical interface is visual and utilizes the mouse and "images" and events as its input provider. Everyone's graphical interface may be different in appearance, whereas all character interfaces look pretty much the same.

**validation:** Continuing process of proving an information system fit for its intended use, initially and over time.

**verify:** 1. Insure that information has not been changed in transit or in storage. 2. Approve a result from a laboratory for release.

**version control:** Management of source code in a large software project in a database that keeps track of the revisions made to a program by all the programmers involved in it.

**vertical industry:** Industry in which all participants are in the same business, large or small, such as medical, legal, engineering, and architectural practices, funeral services, and the like.

**virus:** Program written to insert itself into an existing program and when activated by execution of the "infected" program, to replicate and attach copies of itself to other programs in the system. Infected programs copy the virus to other programs.

**virtual:** Simulated, conceptual, or extended.

**VUP** ( VAX unit of productivity): Roughly equivalent to one MIP. (VAX is a proprietary line of equipment made by Digital Equipment Corporation, DEC.)

**WAN** (wide area network): Two or more LANs connected across different areas, such as towns, states, or countries.

**Web page:** Document stored on the Web.

**Windows bitmap file:** Bitmap image file format developed for Microsoft Windows; may be device dependent or device independent (DIB). The file extension is BMP.

**Windows metafile:** Mixed file type holding vector graphics as well as bitmaps and text that is used primarily for image transfer between Microsoft Windows applications. The file extension is WMF.

**wireless LAN:** Network in which some part or all of the cable of the conventional system is replaced by broadcast energy, either radio waves or infrared light.

**WMF:** See **Windows metafile.**

**word:** Computer's internal storage unit. Refers to the amount of data it can hold in its registers and process at one time. A word is often 16 bits, in which case 32 bits is called a double word. Given the same clock rate, a 32-bit computer processes 4 bytes in the same time it takes a 16-bit machine to process 2.

**word processing software:** Software that interacts with an individual typing, changing, formatting, spellchecking, and printing textual documents.

**worm:** Destructive program that replicates itself throughout disk and memory, using up the computer's resources and eventually causing the system to fail.

**WORM drive** (write once, read many times CD device): Device that allows production of laser disks. Data is written to the disk once, and can only be read thereafter.

# Index

# Health Informatics Series
*(formerly Computers in Health Care)*

*(continued from page ii)*

Public Health Informatics and Information Systems
P.W. O'Carroll, W.A. Yasnoff, M.E. Ward, L.H. Ripp,
and E.L. Martin

Advancing Federal Sector Health Care
*A Model for Technology Transfer*
P. Ramsaroop, M.J. Ball, D. Beaulieu, and J.V. Douglas

Medical Informatics
*Computer Applications in Health Care and Biomedicine,* Second Edition
E.H. Shortliffe and L.E. Perreault

Filmless Radiology
E.L. Siegel and R.M. Kolodner

Cancer Informatics
*Essential Technologies for Clinical Trials*
J.S. Silva, M.J. Ball, C.G. Chute, J.V. Douglas, C.P. Langlotz, J.C. Niland,
and W.L. Scherlis

Clinical Information Systems
*A Component-Based Approach*
R. Van de Velde and P. Degoulet

Knowledge Coupling
*New Premises and New Tools for Medical Care and Education*
L.L. Weed

Healthcare Information Management Systems
*Cases, Strategies, and Solutions,* Third Edition
M.J. Ball, C.A. Weaver, and J.M. Kiel

Organizational Aspects of Health Informatics, Second Edition
*Managing Technological Change*
N.M. Lorenzi and R.T. Riley